Praise for *The Great Cholesterol Myth*

"This book reveals the true dietary villain when it comes to heart disease and it's not saturated fat! Backed by scientific research from peer reviewed journals, this is an excellent read with potentially life-saving information."

—NINA TEICHOLZ, *New York Times* best-selling author of *The Big Fat Surprise* and executive director of The Nutrition Coalition

"Jonny Bowden, Ph.D., and Stephen Sinatra, M.D., have brought the science of cholesterol into the 21st century. This book significantly moves the needle on our understanding of health and disease."

—SHAWN BAKER, M.D., author of *The Carnivore Diet*

"If you want to know the truth about cholesterol, and what you absolutely must do to improve your heart health, this is the book for you. Jonny Bowden and Dr. Stephen Sinatra reveal the facts in a compelling and insightful way. This invaluable book belongs on the bookshelf of anyone who cares about the truth in medicine and healing."

—DANIEL AMEN, M.D., CEO, Amen Clinics, Inc., author of *The Daniel Plan*, Change Your Brain Change Your Life, and *The End of Mental Illness*

"There's a persistent myth in our current culture: cholesterol and saturated fat are the enemy, leading to heart disease and a short life. Jonny Bowden and Steven Sinatra break that antiquated paradigm with a hammer of balanced truth! Highly recommended!"

—DR. WILL COLE, best-selling author of *The Inflammation Spectrum* and *Ketotarian*

"If you have any lingering fears about cholesterol and what it means for your health, read this book! When you're done with it, pass it on to your physician!"

—JENNIFER ISENHART, writer/director, *Fat Fiction*

"Thanks to the extensive scientific evidence provided by Bowden and Sinatra, the truth about cholesterol will hopefully end the utter madness that has plagued our society for far too long. Don't even think about taking another statin drug, cutting your fat and cholesterol intake, or other 'heart-healthy' measures until you read The Great Cholesterol Myth."

—JIMMY MOORE, host of *Livin' La Vida Low-Carb*, and co-author of *Keto Clarity*, *Cholesterol Clarity*, and *The Complete Guide to Fasting*

"*The Great Cholesterol Myth* shows that the primary cause of heart attacks is not cholesterol but insulin resistance. Timely and important—it will show you what steps to take to prevent and reverse heart disease"

—STEVEN MASLEY, M.D., FAHA, FACN, C.N.S., best-selling author of *The 30-Day Heart Tune-Up*

"A must-read for anyone interested in learning how deception and financial gain have dominated current diet and cholesterol treatment recommendations, with evidence-based advice on which foods and behavioral strategies can optimize your health."

—DAVID DIAMOND, PH.D., Professor, Departments of Psychology, Molecular Pharmacology and Physiology, University of South Florida

"Education is the key to health for both the patient and the health care provider. The updated 'Cholesterol Myth' is there for everyone's education. It is a sign of maturity for all to admit when you do not know something and here's a great introduction to your learning."

—GARY FETTKE, once sanctioned Australian orthopedic surgeon and real-food advocate

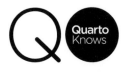

Brimming with creative inspiration, how-to projects, and useful information to enrich your everyday life, Quarto Knows is a favorite destination for those pursuing their interests and passions. Visit our site and dig deeper with our books into your area of interest: Quarto Creates, Quarto Cooks, Quarto Homes, Quarto Lives, Quarto Drives, Quarto Explores, Quarto Gifts, or Quarto Kids.

© 2020 Quarto Publishing Group USA Inc.
Text © 2012, 2020 Jonny Bowden and Stephen Sinatra
Second edition published in 2020
First Published in 2012 by Fair Winds Press, an imprint of The Quarto Group,
100 Cummings Center, Suite 265-D, Beverly, MA 01915, USA.
T (978) 282-9590 F (978) 283-2742 QuartoKnows.com

Fair Winds Press titles are also available at discount for retail, wholesale, promotional, and bulk purchase. For details, contact the Special Sales Manager by email at specialsales@quarto.com or by mail at The Quarto Group, Attn: Special Sales Manager, 100 Cummings Center, Suite 265-D, Beverly, MA 01915, USA.

24 23 22   6
ISBN: 978-1-59233-933-4
Digital edition published in 2020
Originally found under the following Library of Congress Cataloging-in-Publication Data
Bowden, Jonny.
The great cholesterol myth : why lowering your cholesterol won't prevent heart disease—and the statin-free plan that will / Jonny Bowden and Stephen Sinatra.
p . cm.
ISBN 978-1-59233-521-3
1. Heart--Diseases--Etiology--Popular works. 2. Heart--Diseases--Prevention--Popular works. 3. Cholesterol--Physiological aspects--Popular works. 4. Cholesterol--Health aspects--Popular works. I. Sinatra, Stephen T. II. Title.
RC682.B68 2012
616.1'2--dc23
2 012023479

Graphs shown on pages 120 and 122 are courtesy of David Diamond, Ph.D. Use with permission.

Page Layout: Claire MacMaster, barefoot art graphic design

Printed in China

The information in this book is for educational purposes only. It is not intended to replace the advice of a physician or medical practitioner. Please see your health-care provider before beginning any new health program.

THE

GREAT CHOLESTEROL

MYTH

Revised and Expanded

WHY LOWERING YOUR CHOLESTEROL
WON'T PREVENT HEART DISEASE—
AND THE STATIN-FREE PLAN THAT WILL

JONNY BOWDEN, PH.D. , C.N.S.
and STEPHEN SINATRA, M.D., F.A.C.C.

FAIR WINDS

DEDICATION

To anyone who ever fought against bullying by the medical establishment.
I celebrate your courage.
And to every doctor who had the courage to treat the *patient* instead of the symptom,
I celebrate your wisdom.

–Jonny

To my daughter, Marchann, who is the publisher of www.heartmdinstitute.com, my website. You have assisted me enormously in getting the truth out about integrative medicine. You are a dedicated patient advocate seeking out the truth in a sea of camouflage. I'm so blessed to have you in my life. Love, Dad

–SS

CONTENTS

"The mind is like a parachute—it only works if it's open."
—Anthony J. D'Angelo

FOREWORD

TWO HUNDRED YEARS AGO physicians routinely bled, purged, and plastered their patients. Bloodletting was the standard treatment for a host of diseases and had been so since the time of the philosopher-physician Galen almost 2,000 years before. The theory was that there were four humors: blood, phlegm, black bile, and yellow bile. Blood was dominant, requiring the most balancing for returning an ill patient to health.

Every doctor's kit was equipped with a variety of lancets, brutal-looking scarificators, and, starting in the early nineteenth century, leeches. In fact, the latter were used so often that physicians were themselves commonly referred to as leeches. Learned physicians conferred on the best veins to tap for given diseases and the optimal placement of leeches for the most therapeutic value, and countless protocols dictated the proper amount of blood to be let or number of leeches to be applied. Doctors wrote lengthy papers describing their own bleeding techniques and presented them at august medical conferences.

The whole idea was nonsense, of course, and has been shown to be so in the early 1600s by William Harvey, the discoverer of how the circulatory system actually works. But the fact that the "scientific" basis for bloodletting was nonexistent didn't give pause to physicians 200 years ago, some of whom applied as many as fifty leeches to a single patient and, in the case of George Washington, relieved him of almost two quarts of blood in an effort to treat the throat infection that, coupled with the physician-caused anemia, ultimately killed him.

We look back today and can only shake our heads. And be thankful we, ourselves, don't have to worry about getting bled by lancet or leech or that with today's modern, truly science-based medicine, we would ever be exposed to such nebulously grounded treatments. Surely with all the scientific studies performed in great institutions the world over, today's doctors would never ignore the actual evidence and pursue unnecessary and possibly even harmful treatments. Would they?

Sadly, many doctors today have the same herd mentality as those doctors of yore. By the tens of thousands, they treat a nonexistent disease with drugs that are far from benign. And they do so based not on any hard scientific data, but because they, like

> Cholesterol is an essential molecule without which there would be no life, so important that virtually every cell in the body is capable of synthesizing it.

their colleagues of 200 years ago, are firmly in the grip of group think. What is the nonexistent disease? Elevated cholesterol.

The vast majority of laypeople have been bombarded with so much misinformation about cholesterol that most take it as a given that cholesterol is a bad thing and that the less they have the better. The reality is that nothing could be further from the truth.

Cholesterol is an essential molecule without which there would be no life, so important that virtually every cell in the body is capable of synthesizing it. Among its other duties, cholesterol is a major structural molecule, a framework on which other critical substances are made. Were we able to somehow remove all its cholesterol, the body, would, in the words of Shakespeare, "melt, thaw and resolve itself into a dew." And that's not to mention that we wouldn't have bile acids, vitamin D, or steroid hormones (including sex hormones), all of which are cholesterol-based.

Despite the essential nature of cholesterol, doctors the world over administer billions of dollars' worth of drugs to try to prevent its natural synthesis. The fact that only a tiny minority of patients actually

extend their lives by taking these drugs is lost on the multitude prescribing them, but not, of course, on the pharmaceutical industry making and selling them. How did we come to this sorry state?

Sixty years ago a researcher, little known outside of academic circles, singlehandedly set us on this path of cholesterol paranoia: Ancel Keys, Ph.D., a proponent of what has become known as the lipid hypothesis, concluded that excess cholesterol caused heart disease. He started out thinking that dietary fat in general drove cholesterol levels up, but as the years went by, he came to believe that saturated fat was the true cholesterol-raising villain. (This idea of saturated fat as villain is so ingrained in the minds of health writers that the words "saturated fat" are almost never written alone but always as "artery-clogging saturated fat.") Which is more or less the basis for the lipid hypothesis: Saturated fat runs up cholesterol levels, and elevated cholesterol leads to heart disease. Nice and simple, but not true. It has never been proven, which is why it is still called the lipid *hypothesis*.

Because of Keys's influence, researchers for the past five decades have been beavering away in labs the world over, desperate to find enough actual proof to convert the lipid hypothesis into the lipid fact. But so far, they've fallen way short. In the process, however, they have vastly expanded our knowledge of the biochemistry and physiology of the cholesterol molecule. Thanks to their efforts, we now know that cholesterol is transported in the blood attached to carrier proteins, and that these protein-cholesterol complexes are called lipoproteins. Their densities now describe these lipoproteins: HDL (high-density lipoprotein), LDL (low-density lipoprotein), VLDL (very-low-density lipoprotein), and a number of others. Some of these lipoproteins are considered good (HDL) and others bad (LDL). And, of course, the drug companies have developed medications purported to increase the former while decreasing the latter.

But they jumped the gun. Researchers have discovered a type of lipoprotein called small, dense (or type B) LDL that may actually end up being a true risk factor for heart disease. Problem is, this small, dense type B LDL is worsened by the very diet those promoting the lipid hypothesis have hailed for decades as the best diet to prevent heart disease: the low-fat, high-carbohydrate diet. Turns out that fat, especially saturated fat, decreases the amount of these small, dense LDL particles while the widely recommended low-fat diet increases their number. The opposite of the small dense LDL are large fluffy LDL particles, which are not only *not* harmful but are actually healthful. But the LDL-lowering drugs lower those, too.

Cracks should have appeared in the firm entrenchment of the lipid hypothesis (that now basically posits that elevated LDL causes heart disease) when a recent study showed that of almost 140,000 patients admitted to the hospital for heart disease, almost half of them had LDL levels *under* 100 mg/dL (100 mg/dL has been the therapeutic target for LDL for the past few years). Instead of stepping back, scratching their heads, and thinking, *Hmmm, maybe we're on the wrong track here*, the authors of this study concluded that maybe a therapeutic level of 100 mg/dL for LDL is still too high and needs to be even lower. Such is their lipo-phobic herd mentality.

Nutritionist Jonny Bowden, Ph.D., and cardiologist Stephen Sinatra, M.D., have teamed up in this book to slash through the tall thicket of misinformation surrounding cholesterol, lipoproteins, and the lipid hypothesis. They wrote their fact-based book using easy-to-understand terminology, and present a much more valid hypothesis of what really causes heart disease and a host of other diseases such as diabetes, high blood pressure, and obesity, which will open your eyes to the emperor's state of undress. If you are worried about your cholesterol level or contemplating taking a cholesterol-lowering drug, we urge you to read this book! This book will put the facts in your hands to make a more informed decision. And we're confident you will enjoy their book as much as we did.

Michael R. Eades, M.D.
Mary Dan Eades, M.D.
May 2012
Incline Village, Nevada

CHAPTER 1

WHY A NEW EDITION OF THIS BOOK WAS NEEDED

A LOT HAS CHANGED IN THE WAY THE MEDICAL ESTABLISHMENT views cholesterol and heart disease since we first came together almost a decade ago to write the original version of *The Great Cholesterol Myth*—and most of those changes have been for the better.

We now have technology that allows us to clearly identify at least thirteen different subtypes of cholesterol, many of which behave in unique ways in the body. Being able to measure cholesterol with much greater specificity than ever before is good news indeed, because it gives us much more information and far greater accuracy when it comes to predicting future cardiovascular events.

The sad news is doctors are mostly still measuring it the old way. Which is equivalent to using a pad and pencil in the age of the smartphone. We'll return to this point throughout the book.

We now have sophisticated lab tests to tease out risk factors that have been hiding in plain sight for decades—factors we now understand are directly and profoundly connected to heart disease.

So the good news is that we have all kinds of cool ways of measuring sophisticated risk factors that most people never heard of a decade or two ago. Ten years ago, for example, few people even knew about (much less understood) the microbiome—a whole ecological system of microbes that lives in our gut and profoundly affects so many areas of our health. Even genetic testing, still in its infancy, is nonetheless light-years ahead of where it was in the early days of 23 and Me. There are now at least a dozen cardiac markers that we can test that influence the likelihood of you getting heart disease. And best of all, many of these risk factors can be strongly modified by our own life choices.

Every year we meet more and more physicians at conferences who are realizing the importance of inflammation and oxidation in making arteries vulnerable to plaque. Every year we meet more and more physicians who have come around to the notion that nutrition and diet—the redheaded stepsister of traditional medical education—can be powerful allies in the fight against heart disease (and not as previously believed, by sticking to a low-fat diet!).

In fact, the connection between diabetes and heart disease—sugar, anyone?—is the central thesis of this book. Insulin resistance is something that nearly always precedes type 2 diabetes, and, as we will argue, is an early warning sign of heart disease.

Understanding insulin resistance—and how to prevent, treat, and even reverse it—is one of the most important things you can do if you want to prevent heart disease. We've all heard of pre-diabetes, but we suggest that "pre-heart disease" is just as real a phenomenon, and that phenomenon is called diabe-tes. We will argue that if you catch the signs of diabetes early enough, you can prevent heart disease—for many, if not most, people. By the end of chapter 12 we hope you will agree with us.

And now for the bad news. Most doctors don't know this. Even worse, most are still prescribing powerful drugs for a condition known as "high cholesterol" that is a lab test, not a disease, and—to add insult to injury—is being measured in an antiquated way.

Unfortunately for all of us a very high percentage of doctors practicing conventional medicine in the United States still think an LDL cholesterol reading of more than 100 is a big problem. They will reach for their prescription pad the moment it creeps north of 129. A very high percentage of doctors practicing conventional medicine in this country also continue to believe that fat and cholesterol clog your arteries, that obesity is caused by eating too much fat, that low-fat diets are generally effective, and that cholesterol causes heart disease.

All of which tells us we've got a heck of a lot more work to do. Many doctors continue to cling to the old technology, an antiquated method of classifying cholesterol into large gross categories of "good" and "bad." Worse, these same doctors are prescribing powerful drugs—statins—based almost entirely on the readout from a test that should have been dumped in the dustbin of out-of-date medical ideas a long time ago.

THE PROMISE OF THIS BOOK

The promise of this book is that we are going to set you straight on the subject of cholesterol and heart disease. We're probably going to anger a lot of the conventional medicine crowd, but we hope we're also going to win over a few converts. Like politics, nutrition and medicine are very polarized. But unlike politics, there is a large group of "independent voters" in the fields of nutrition and medicine, doctors and patients alike, who look for the truth wherever it's to be found and don't cling stubbornly to official talking points. It's those independents that we hope we can win over with our message that it's time to move beyond—way beyond—conventional cholesterol testing and conventional dietary prescriptions for heart disease.

Which, if you haven't already noticed, don't work very well.

We feel the message of this book is so important—and so potentially life-saving—we want you to hear it right now, on the first few pages. Maybe it will prompt a conversation with your doctor, or even motivate you to consider a different approach to the prevention of your own heart disease. If our book has some small part in accomplishing that, we will consider our mission accomplished. Here's what you need to know:

- Cholesterol does not cause heart disease. Cholesterol is involved in heart disease, but not in the way most people think it is. Cholesterol levels—as currently measured—do not even predict heart disease (let alone cause it).
- The cholesterol test your doctor currently gives you— the one for "good" and "bad" cholesterol"—is obsolete. There are at least thirteen identified subtypes of cholesterol—not two—making it all the more mystifying that doctors continue to stick to measuring two.

- Lowering cholesterol does not save lives—and this has been shown in study after study.
- Problematic blood measurements, such as high blood sugar, are actually markers of dysfunction that show up fairly late in the game. By the time these traditional red flags show up on your annual blood test, you could already be well on the road to pre-diabetes. And remember, pre-diabetes *is* diabetes; it's just not official yet. And diabetes *is* pre-heart disease. You cannot ignore the early warning signs of diabetes, and unfortunately, most doctors only look for the ones that show up after the damage has already started.

Fully one-third of those with full-blown diabetes don't know they have it, and the vast majority of those with early signs of diabetes are utterly clueless about their condition and the disaster that may await them further down the path. We'll explain the relationship between diabetes and heart disease throughout the book, but for now just keep in mind that more than 80 percent of diabetics die of cardiovascular disease. Do the math.

Insulin resistance is diabetes' first metabolic footprint, the clue that shows up well before things go deeply south.[1] Insulin resistance syndrome more than doubles the risk of diabetes, which in turn more than doubles the risk of dying of heart disease or stroke.[2] The good news: Insulin resistance itself can be detected many years before an official diagnosis of diabetes or heart disease, which means you can interrupt the path of heart disease for a double-digit percentage of the population.

If this book has one single, actionable takeaway, it's this: Get tested for insulin resistance. There are many ways to test for insulin resistance—we'll discuss them all in chapter 9—but test for it you must. It can reveal problems years, or even decades, before you get a diagnosis of either diabetes or cardiovascular disease.

The best news is that you can stop insulin resistance—and most often reverse it—with diet. Really. You won't need a single pharmaceutical drug to reverse insulin resistance if you get it early enough and make the right dietary changes. And if you do identify insulin resistance early, you can probably prevent it from morphing into a heart attack down the road. Researchers writing in the medical journal *Diabetes Care* said it eloquently: "Insulin resistance is likely the most important single cause of coronary artery disease," adding that in young adults preventing insulin resistance would prevent approximately 42 percent of heart attacks![3]

NOW LET'S TALK ABOUT STATINS

Are you on a statin drug?

If you are, it's almost certainly because your doctor was worried about your LDL cholesterol number being too high. And if you aren't on a statin drug, it's probably because your doctor thought your LDL cholesterol number was just fine, hence no need for preventive treatment.

In both cases, there's an excellent chance that your doctor was dead wrong. This book will explain why.

Remember, the only real importance of the HDL-LDL cholesterol test is to predict an outcome—in this case heart disease. And if the HDL-LDL cholesterol test did in fact predict whether a given patient is likely to get heart disease, there'd be no reason for this discussion.

But it doesn't.

Sorry to be the bearer of bad news, but the test—which, back in the 1960s, was considered state-of-the-art—has become obsolete. Given the far more accurate measures we now have at our disposal, the old-fashioned HDL-LDL test is long past its expiration date. The prescription you got from your doctor to prevent heart disease was very likely based on a test that's just about as useful as a horoscope from *People* magazine.

How do we know this? Because when you plug in the other, far more accurate predictors of heart disease—which we'll talk about throughout this book—it turns out many people with "high LDL" actually have very low risk for heart disease. Conversely, many people with "low LDL" can have a very high risk for a cardiovascular event. (This was true for one of the authors.)

The danger of continuing to rely on this obsolete test cuts both ways—many people who have "high LDL" but are actually at low risk are being over-treated with powerful medications that come with a long list of side effects (see chapter 8). Meanwhile, many people who have "low LDL," but actually have a high risk for an event, are walking around untreated, thinking everything's just fine. And that's tragic.

Think of it this way: Knowing someone's HDL and LDL is like knowing their political party. But political party does not always predict the way someone is going to vote. In fact, on many important issues, if you want to make an accurate prediction on how someone is going to vote, it's far more important to know their age, sex, and whether or not they're married than it is to know whether they're a Republican or a Democrat.

And it's the same thing with heart disease. Except it's far more serious that your predictions be accurate. Make a mistake predicting how someone's going to vote and it's not really a big deal. Make a mistake about whether someone is at risk for heart disease and, well, it's a very big deal—especially if that someone is you or a member of your family.

That is exactly why we want to see the "HDL-LDL" test retired forever, replaced by the far more sophisticated and accurate measures of cardiovascular risk that we now have available. These measures include ApoB, total particle number, and insulin resistance, all of which we will go over during the course of this book.

If you are one of the millions of people who got a clean bill of health because of low LDL, but your total particle number was actually very high, you are at great risk and are going untreated. (This was exactly the case with Jonny.) Similarly, if you're one of the millions of people on a statin because of high LDL but your total particle number is actually very low, you're probably on a medication you don't need and putting up with side effects that you don't have to endure.

Study after study shows us that relying on LDL alone misses an awful lot of heart disease. That's a lot of people dying because they were diagnosed using an obsolete test. Our hope is that this book will change that. It's our mission to see the "good and bad cholesterol" test replaced by measures that do a far better job of accurately predicting cardiovascular disease than "LDL cholesterol."

A GUIDE TO USING THIS BOOK

In this first part of the book, you'll learn exactly what cholesterol is, and what it isn't, and how it really works in the body. (Be prepared to be surprised.) In clear understandable terms you'll learn how atherosclerosis actually develops, and you'll understand the critical role of chronic inflammation and oxidative damage.

Then in part two, we'll introduce the real villain of the heart disease story: sugar. You'll see why sugar got a free pass all these past few decades while fat was blamed for our health woes, and you'll come to see what a huge mistake that was. (And it's still going on.) You'll see the clear lines from sugar and starch intake to diabetes, and the frighteningly short line from diabetes to heart disease. You'll also come to understand the very insignificant role dietary fat plays in all of this. Finally, you'll learn a lot about the real effects of statin drugs and how clever and insidious marketing has made them into the blockbuster drugs they are today.

In part three, we'll tell you the way to combat the real promoters of heart disease—inflammation and insulin resistance. We'll talk about the things you can do to build and maintain a healthy heart for decades and decades: food, supplements, activity, relationships, community. We kiddingly referred to this last section of the book as our "Eat-Play-Love" section, but only half in jest. Both of us—with more than eighty

"WHAT DOES MY CHOLESTEROL TEST MEAN?"

Dr. Jonny: A friend of mine recently brought me his cholesterol test. He showed me four measurements: total cholesterol, HDL, LDL, and triglycerides. He asked me, based on these numbers, to tell him whether or not I thought he was at a risk for an "event."

I explained that, based on these numbers, there was no way to tell.

Let me explain.

Let's say you're playing poker against someone who has two deuces showing. What can you positively say about that hand? Not much, really. You can say for sure that he doesn't have a royal flush or a straight. But without knowing the other three cards, there's no way you can predict whether he has a winning (or losing) hand. You have to decide to bet (or not bet) based on incomplete evidence, which is why poker is ultimately a game of "chance."

But you don't want guessing about heart disease to be a game of chance. And you don't want it to be based on incomplete evidence. HDL and LDL are like the visible two cards in a poker hand. Your doctor is "betting" on whether or not you're going to get heart disease based on this woefully incomplete information.

This is a tragedy for two reasons. One, because whether or not you're at risk for a heart attack is way more consequential than whether or not you have a winning poker hand. And two, because your doctor now has an easily accessible way to check the other three cards so she doesn't have to guess!

years of combined experience in the health field—have firmly and independently concluded that it's not just what you eat and how you exercise that determines your health, though those things certainly matter. But it's also how you love, how you think, how you feel, how you digest, how you manage stress, how you contribute, how you sleep, how you kick back and relax, how you meditate, how you contemplate, and how you play.

They are all related. They all matter. And every one of them has an impact on the health of your heart. A lot more than your cholesterol level does.

Enjoy the journey of discovery that awaits you.

PART ONE

In part one, we tell you how we came together to write the original edition of *The Great Cholesterol Myth*. We'll take you on our own personal journeys of discovery, when our suspicions were (independently) raised about whether we had been told the whole story about fat and cholesterol. You'll see how we went from being true believers in the low-fat diet and in the cholesterol hypothesis, to disrupters and challengers of conventional thinking about heart disease, cholesterol, and statin drugs.

CHAPTER 2

WHY YOU SHOULD BE SKEPTICAL OF LDL AS AN INDICATOR OF HEART DISEASE

THE TWO OF US CAME TOGETHER TO WRITE THIS BOOK because we believe that you have been completely misled, misinformed, and in some cases, directly lied to about cholesterol.

We believe that misinformation, scientifically questionable studies, and corporate greed have created one of the most indestructible and damaging myths in medical history: that cholesterol causes heart disease and that statins are the answer.

The millions of marketing dollars spent on perpetuating this myth have successfully kept us focused on a relatively minor character in the heart disease story—and created a market for cholesterol-lowering drugs worth more than $30 billion a year. The real tragedy is that by putting all of our attention on cholesterol, we've virtually ignored the *real* causes of heart disease: inflammation, oxidation, sugar, and stress.

In fact, as you'll learn in this book, cholesterol numbers as they are now tested—i.e. "HDL" and "LDL"—are a pretty poor predictor of heart disease; up to 70 percent of people hospitalized with heart attacks have perfectly normal cholesterol levels, and about half the people with elevated cholesterol levels have perfectly normal, healthy tickers. (Those numbers might change if doctors used the much more modernized version of cholesterol tests, which we'll talk about throughout the book—but they continue to use the old-fashioned "good" and "bad" test that predicts about as accurately as flipping a coin.)

Many of the general dietary guidelines accepted and promoted by the government and by major health organizations such as the American Heart Association are either directly or indirectly related to cholesterol phobia. These standard guidelines warn us to limit the amount of cholesterol we eat, despite the fact that for at least 95 percent of the population, cholesterol in the *diet* has virtually no effect on cholesterol in the *blood*.

These guidelines warn us of the dangers of saturated fat, despite the fact that the relationship between saturated fat in the diet and heart disease has never been convincingly demonstrated, and despite the fact that research shows that replacing saturated fat in the diet with carbohydrates actually *increases* the risk for heart disease.[1]

Both of us became skeptical of the cholesterol theory at different points in our careers, traveling different pathways to arrive at the same conclusion: Cholesterol does not cause heart disease.

We also believe that, unlike trans fat, for example, saturated fat is *not* the dietary equivalent of Satan's spawn (and we'll show you why). Finally, and most important, we strongly believe that our national obsession with lowering cholesterol has come at a considerable price. Cholesterolmania has caused us to focus all our energy around a fairly innocuous molecule with a marginal relationship to heart disease, while ignoring the *real* causes of heart disease.

We're each going to tell you in our own words how we became cholesterol skeptics and why we fervently believe the information contained in this book could save your life.

DR. JONNY

Before I became a nutritionist and ultimately an author, I was a personal trainer. I worked at Equinox Fitness Clubs in New York City, and the vast majority of my clients were there for one thing: weight loss. It was 1990. Fat was considered dietary enemy number one, and saturated fat was considered *especially* bad because we all "knew" it clogged your arteries, raised your cholesterol, and led to heart disease. So, like most trainers, I put my clients on low-fat diets and encouraged them to do a ton of aerobics plus a little bit of weight training.

Which worked.

*Some*times.

More often than not, the strategy bombed.

Take Al, for example. Al was an incredibly successful, powerful businessman in his early sixties with a huge belly he just couldn't get rid of. He was eating a very low-fat diet, doing a ton of aerobics on the treadmill in his house, and yet his weight was hardly budging. If everything I had been taught as a personal trainer was right, that shouldn't have been happening.

But it was.

Then Al decided to do something I didn't approve of. He went on the Atkins diet.

Remember, those were the days when all of us were taught that fat, especially saturated fat, was pure evil. We had been taught that we "need" carbohydrates for energy and survival. We had been taught that diets such as the Atkins diet were dangerous and damaging, largely because all that saturated fat would clog your arteries, raise your cholesterol, and lead to a heart attack.

So I was pretty sure Al was headed for disaster. Except he wasn't.

Not only did he start shedding weight and losing his substantial "apple-shaped" belly, but he also had more energy and was feeling better than he had in decades. I, meanwhile, was impressed with Al's results, but I was convinced he was paying a huge price and that once he got the blood test results from his annual physical, I would be vindicated.

I wasn't.

Al's triglycerides—a type of fat found in the bloodstream and elsewhere—had dropped, his blood pressure had gone down, and his cholesterol had risen slightly, but his "good" cholesterol (HDL) had gone up more than his "bad" cholesterol (LDL), so overall his doc was pretty happy.

Right around this time, Dr. Barry Sears—the MIT-trained biochemist and creator of the Zone diet—came to give a workshop at Equinox. It was there, thirty years ago, that I first learned this critical lesson: *Food has a hormonal effect.*

When it comes to gaining and losing weight, it's hormones—even more than calories—that control the show.

And hormones are controlled by food.

For example: Carbs in general stimulate hormones that *promote* weight gain; fat does not. Ergo, up the fat in the diet a bit and reduce the carbs a bit. It's a way better approach to hormone management.

But conventional medicine argued that fat would raise your cholesterol, which, of course, would eventually kill you. In the end, the argument against high-fat diets always hinged on cholesterol. Conventional medicine collectively thought that a high-fat diet like the one my client Al was on would produce disastrous results.

Right around this time, a biochemist named Barry Sears came to New York City to give a workshop at Equinox, which, of course, I eagerly attended. Sears, whose Zone diet books have sold millions, had a novel approach that can be summed up in four words: *eat fat, lose weight.* If Sears had been anything but an MIT-trained biochemist, he probably would have been laughed out of the room. But given his credentials and remarkable knowledge of the human body, he was pretty hard to dismiss.

Now Sears wasn't the first one to embrace fat and protein in the diet and recommend that we eat fewer carbs. Atkins, whose original diet was the one Al had tried so successfully, had been saying similar things since 1972. But the whole rap against Atkins was that his diet was high in saturated fat and would therefore likely cause heart disease. So even though many people grudgingly admitted that you could lose weight easily following his program, everyone (including me) believed that the cost would include a hugely increased risk for heart disease.

What If the Whole Theory That Cholesterol Causes Heart Disease Was Wrong in the First Place?

Meanwhile, my eyes were telling me something very different, and it wasn't just because of what I had seen happen with Al. It was happening with other clients as well. Sick of not getting results on low-fat, high-carb diets, they threw caution to the wind and embraced the Atkins diet and the Protein Power diet and other diets that had in common that they limited carbohydrate intake. They were eating more fat—even more saturated fat—but nothing bad was happening at all, unless, of course, you count feeling better and getting slimmer as nothing.

Which got me thinking.

Why weren't we seeing consistent results with our clients who were faithfully following low-fat diets and getting plenty of aerobic exercise? Conversely, why were our clients who were going on low-carb diets getting such high marks on their blood tests and astonishing their doctors? What if everything we'd been told about the danger of saturated fat wasn't exactly correct? And—if what we'd been taught about saturated fat wasn't the complete truth—what about this relationship between fat and cholesterol? Was it really all as simple as I'd been taught?

After all, even back in the early 1990s when people only talked about "good" and "bad" cholesterol, it was still obvious that, overall, saturated fat had a positive effect on Al's cholesterol, as it did on the cholesterol levels of so many of my other clients. Saturated fat raised folks HDL much more than it did their LDL, which, by the standard of the day, was a *good* thing. Could this whole cholesterol issue be a little more complicated than I and everyone else had previously believed?

Eventually, I thought—going way out on a limb here—what if the whole theory that cholesterol causes heart disease was wrong in the first place? If that were the case, the effect of saturated fat on cholesterol would be pretty much irrelevant, wouldn't it?

Then I began reading the studies.

The Lyon Diet Heart Study[2] found that certain dietary and lifestyle changes were able to reduce deaths by 70 percent and reduce cardiovascular deaths by an even more impressive 76 percent, all without making as much as a dent in cholesterol levels. The Nurses' Health Study[3] found that 82 percent of coronary events were attributable to five factors, none of which had anything to do with lowering cholesterol. And that was just the tip of the ever-growing iceberg.

Study after study on high-protein, low-carb diets—including those rich in saturated fat—showed that the blood tests of people on these diets were similar to Al's. Their health actually *improved* on these diets. Triglycerides went down. Other measures that indicated heart disease risk also improved.

In the mid-90s I went back to school for nutrition, ultimately earning a Ph.D. in what was then called "holistic" (integrative) nutrition and a C.N.S. (certified nutrition specialist) certification from the Certification Board for Nutrition Specialists, which is associated with the American College of Nutrition. During my studies, I talked to many other health professionals who shared my concerns, including one of the top lipid biochemists in the country, the late Mary Enig, Ph.D. She did some of the early research on trans fats and fervently believed that it is trans fats, not saturated fats, that are the real villains in the American diet; I wholeheartedly agree.

Enig was hardly alone in thinking that we have been collectively brainwashed on the subject of saturated fat and cholesterol. When Americans were consuming whole, full-fat foods such as cream, butter, pasture-raised meats, raw milk, and other traditional foods, the rate of heart disease was a fraction of what it is now. Many of us began to wonder whether it was a coincidence that the twin global pandemics of obesity and diabetes just happened to occur around the time we collectively banished these foods because of the phobia about cholesterol and saturated fat in the diet and began to replace them with vegetable oils, processed carbs, and, ultimately, trans fats.

Study after study has shown that lowering the risk for heart disease has very little to do with lowering cholesterol. And more and more studies reports were coming out demonstrating that the real initiators of damage in the arteries were oxidation and inflammation. These factors, along with sugar and, were clearly what aged the human body the most. *These* were the culprits we should be focused on.

In my career, I have examined the strategies that seemed to work for the healthiest, longest-living people on earth and found that lowering cholesterol has almost *nothing* to do with reducing heart disease, and definitely nothing to do with extending life. One of the greatest frustrations I experienced was trying to reassure my clients that with a higher-protein, higher-fat diet they'd see significant improvements in their weights *and* the health of their hearts. I was constantly butting heads with my clients' doctors, who completely bought into the myth that saturated fat will kill you by clogging your arteries, raising your cholesterol, and ultimately leading to heart disease. And that anyone who thought otherwise was clearly a whack job or at the very least "anti-science."

Fast-forward to 2010. Fair Winds Press—my publisher for thirteen books over the course of seven years—came to me with an idea. "How about a book on how to lower cholesterol with food and supplements?" they asked.

To which I replied, "I'm probably not the guy to write that one. I don't think lowering cholesterol matters very much."

As you can imagine, that was met with a collective startle. My publishers were more than a little curious. "How can lowering cholesterol *not* be important?" they wanted to know. "Don't doctors believe high cholesterol is the cause of heart disease? Don't they believe that lowering it is the most important thing you can do when it comes to preventing heart attacks?"

"They do indeed," I replied, "and they're wrong."

The book I wanted to write reveals the truth about cholesterol and heart disease. To do it, I joined forces with my friend Steve Sinatra, a board-certified cardiologist, trained psychotherapist, and nutritionist.

DR. SINATRA

Most doctors today will recommend that you take a statin drug—they might even nag you to do so—if your cholesterol numbers are high. They will do so whether or not you have evidence of arterial disease and are a man or woman, and despite your age. In their minds, you prevent heart disease by lowering cholesterol.

Once upon a time I used to believe that, too. It made sense, based on the research and information that was promoted to doctors. I believed it to the extent that I even lectured on behalf of drug makers. I was a paid consultant to some of the biggest manufacturers of statin drugs, lecturing for hefty honorariums. I became a cholesterol choirboy, singing the refrain of high cholesterol as the big, bad villain of heart disease. Beat it down with a drug, and you cut your risks. My thinking changed years ago when I began seeing conflicting evidence among my own patients. I saw, for instance, many patients with low total cholesterol—as low as 150 mg/dL!—develop heart disease.

In those days we pushed patients to undergo angiograms (invasive arterial catheterization imaging) if they had sufficient symptoms of chest pain, border-line exercise tests, and especially cholesterol readings of greater than 280 mg/dL. We did this because our profession believed that all people with high cholesterol were in danger of having a heart attack.

We did the imaging to see how bad their arteries were. And, indeed, sometimes we found diseased arteries. But just as often we didn't. Many arteries were perfectly healthy. These results were telling me something different than the establishment message—that it wasn't just a simple cholesterol story.

Faced with these discrepancies I began questioning and investigating conventional thinking about cholesterol and looking at the cholesterol research more closely. I found other doctors who had made similar discoveries on their own and heard about how study findings were being manipulated. For example, bio-chemist George Mann, M.D., of Vanderbilt University, who participated in the development of the world-famous Framingham Heart Study, later described the cholesterol-as-an-indicator-of-heart-disease hypothesis as "the greatest scam ever perpetrated on the American public."

These and other dissenting voices were drowned out by the cholesterol chorus. To this day, practically all of what has been published—and receives media attention—supports the cholesterol paradigm and appears to have the backing of the pharmaceutical and low-fat industries along with leading regulatory agencies and medical organizations.

However, I stopped being a choirboy for choles-terol. I stopped believing. Here's why:

I found that life can't go on without cholesterol, a basic raw material made by your liver, brain, and almost every cell in your body. Enzymes convert it into vitamin D, steroid hormones (such as our sex hormones—estrogen, progesterone, and testosterone—and stress hormones), and bile salts for digesting and absorbing fats. It makes up a major part of the membranes surrounding cells and the structures within them.

The brain is particularly rich in cholesterol and accounts for about a quarter of all the cholesterol we have in our bodies. The fatty myelin sheath that coats every nerve cell and fiber is about one-fifth cholesterol. Neuronal communication depends on cholesterol. It is not surprising that a connection has been found between naturally occurring cholesterol and mental function. Lower levels are linked to poorer cognitive performance.

I remember one patient—a federal judge I'll call Silvio—who came to see me. He was taking a statin drug and complained that his memory had gone to pot, so much so that he voluntarily took himself off the bench. His LDL level was down to 65 mg/dL. I took him off the statin, told him to eat a lot of organic, cholesterol-rich eggs, and within a month got his LDL level up above 100 mg/dL. His memory came roaring back. (Memory loss is one potential side effect of cholesterol-lowering drugs.)

Some researchers suggest that doctors should be extremely cautious about prescribing statin drugs to the elderly, particularly those who are frail. I totally agree. I have seen frail individuals become even frailer and much more prone to infections. Though that surprised me at the time, it no longer does.

Cholesterol plays a big role in helping fight bacteria and infections. A study that included 100,000 healthy participants in San Francisco over a fifteen-year period found that those with low cholesterol values were much more likely to be admitted to hospitals with infectious diseases.[4]

Life can't go on without cholesterol, a basic raw material made by your liver, brain, and almost every cell in your body. Many such patients told me afterward that their strength, energy, appetite, and vitality returned after going off statin drugs. They obviously needed their cholesterol.

In addition to being a board-certified cardiologist, I've had a lifelong interest in nutrition. I'd been using nutritional supplements in my practice since the early 1980s, particularly coenzyme Q_{10} (CoQ_{10}), an absolutely vital nutrient that is made in every cell in the body and is a major chemical participant in the production of cellular energy. CoQ_{10} is critically important for the strong pumping action of the heart, which gobbles the stuff up. And in the early 1990s I discovered something that shook my belief in statin drugs to the core—they depleted the body of CoQ_{10}.

That fact is widely known now, but it wasn't then. And it certainly gave me pause. How could these miracle drugs that were believed to be the answer to heart disease be good for you in the long run if they depleted the very nutrient upon which the heart depends?

Even today, many doctors aren't aware of the effect that statin drugs have on CoQ_{10} levels. How ironic that the very drug they prescribe to reduce the likelihood of a heart attack actually deprives the heart of the fuel it needs to perform properly? No wonder fatigue, low energy, and muscle pain are such frequent accompaniments to statin drug use.

It wasn't until the mid-1990s that statin drugs really took off, but before then physicians had other go-to drugs for lowering cholesterol. Many research studies were conducted using these drugs, and in 1996 the U.S. Government Accountability Office evaluated these trials in a publication titled *Cholesterol Treatment: A Review of the Clinical Trials Evidence*. The report explained that though some trials showed a reduction in cardiovascular-related deaths (primarily among those who entered the studies with existing heart disease), there was a corresponding *increase* in *non*-cardiovascular-related deaths across the trials. "This finding, that cholesterol treatment has not lowered the number of deaths overall, has been worrisome to many researchers and is at the core of much of the controversy on cholesterol policy," the authors wrote.

It was also quite clear from the report that those who benefited the most from lowering their cholesterol levels were middle-aged men who already had heart disease. "The trials focused predominantly on middle-aged white men considered to be at high risk of coronary heart disease," the report stated. "They provide very little information on women, minority men and women, and elderly men and women."

It's been more than a decade since that report was written, but it remains true that lowering cholesterol has a very limited benefit in populations other than middle-aged men with a history of heart disease. Yet doctors continue to prescribe statin drugs for women and the elderly, and, shockingly, many are arguing for treating children with statins as well.

By now my conversion from cholesterol true believer to cholesterol skeptic is complete. I still prescribe statins—but only on occasion, and almost exclusively to middle-aged men who've already had a first heart attack, coronary intervention (e.g., bypass, stent, angioplasty), or coronary artery disease.

I've come to believe that cholesterol is a minor player in the development of heart disease and that whatever good statin drugs accomplish has very little to do with their cholesterol-lowering ability. (We discuss this at great length in chapter 8.) Statin drugs are anti-inflammatory, and their power to reduce inflammation is much more important than their ability to lower cholesterol. But we can lower inflammation (and the risk for heart disease) with natural supplements, a better diet, and lifestyle changes such as managing stress. Best of all, none of these come with the growing laundry list of troubling symptoms and side effects associated with statin drugs and cholesterol lowering.

LIKE DEAD MEN WALKING

So there you have it. Two individuals with very different journeys arriving at the same conclusion. And because that conclusion may be pretty hard to swallow if you've been brainwashed by the cholesterol establishment—and who hasn't?—it might be helpful to take a moment and talk about a study we alluded to earlier—the Lyon Diet Heart Study.

In the early 1990s, French researchers decided to run an experiment—known as the Lyon Diet Heart Study—to test the effect of different diets on heart disease.[5]

They took 605 men and women who were prime candidates for heart attacks. These folks had every risk factor imaginable. All of them had already survived a first heart attack. Their cholesterol levels were through the roof, they smoked, they ate junk food, they didn't exercise, and they had high levels of stress. People like this give insurance underwriters nightmares. To be frank, these folks were "dead men walking."

The researchers divided the participants into two groups. The first group was counseled (by the research cardiologist and the dietician during a one-hour session) to eat a Mediterranean-type diet that emphasizes fresh fruit and vegetables, whole grains, legumes, nuts, healthy fats such as olive oil, and seafood. The second group was the control group and received no dietary advice from the investigators but was advised, nonetheless, to follow a *prudent diet* by their attending physicians.

What was this prudent diet, you ask? Pretty much the standard (and, as we shall see, useless) diet that doctors have been recommending for decades: Eat no more than 30 percent of your calories from fat, no more than 10 percent from saturated fat, and no more

Lowering cholesterol has a very limited benefit in populations other than middle-aged men with a history of heart disease.

than 300 mg of cholesterol a day (about the amount in two eggs). So what happened with the study?

Actually, it was stopped.

Why? Because the reduction in heart attacks in the Mediterranean diet group was so pronounced that the researchers decided it was unethical to continue. To be precise, the Mediterranean diet group had a whopping 70 percent reduction in deaths and an even more impressive 76 percent reduction in cardiovascular deaths. What's more, angina, pulmonary embolism, heart failure, and stroke were also much lower in the intervention group. A huge victory for the Mediterranean diet and a big dunkin' for the prudent diet.

So what happened to these folks' cholesterol levels? Gosh, you'd imagine they dropped like crazy, because so few of them were dying of heart disease.

Um, not so much. Their levels *didn't budge*.

Let's repeat that one more time: a 76 percent reduction in deaths from heart disease but not a whit of change in cholesterol levels. Neither in their *total* cholesterol levels *nor* in their levels of LDL (the so-called "bad" cholesterol). You'd think this would shake up the cholesterol establishment a bit, wouldn't you?

Think again. The prestigious *New England Journal of Medicine* refused to publish the study. (It was eventually published in another highly regarded journal, *The Lancet*.) We have a hunch that the reason the *New England Journal of Medicine* didn't publish the study was precisely because there was no difference in cholesterol levels between the two groups of people, the ones who did so well and the ones who did not. The American medical establishment is so firmly locked into the notion that cholesterol and fat cause heart disease that any inconvenient evidence to the contrary—and there is a massive amount of it, as you will soon find out—has to be ignored or explained away.

Lower heart disease rates? And no movement in cholesterol numbers?

Something has to be wrong!

Actually something *was* wrong, but not with the study. What was—and is—wrong is the blind belief that cholesterol simply makes a huge difference.

AN INCONVENIENT FACT

Not convinced? Fast-forward to a drug study completed in 2006, the widely publicized ENHANCE trial.[6] If you were following the news in 2008 you couldn't have missed this one, because it made the front pages of the newspapers and all of the television news shows. Here's what happened.

A combination cholesterol-lowering medication called Vytorin had been the subject of a huge research project, the results of which were finally coming to light and receiving an enormous amount of negative attention. One of the many reasons for this negative attention was the fact that the companies jointly making the drug (Merck and Schering-Plough, who've since merged) waited almost two years before releasing it.

No wonder. The results stunk. Which was the *other* reason this drug test made the front pages.

The new "wonder" drug lowered cholesterol just fine. In fact, it lowered it *better* than a standard statin drug. So you'd think everyone would be jumping for joy, right? Lower cholesterol, lower heart disease, let's have a party for the shareholders.

Um, not quite. Although the people taking Vytorin saw their cholesterol levels plummet, they actually had *more* plaque growth than the people taking the standard cholesterol drug. The patients on Vytorin had almost twice as great an increase in the thickness of their arterial walls, a result you definitely don't want to see if you're trying to prevent heart disease.

So their cholesterol was wonderfully lowered and their risk for heart disease went up—shades of "the operation was a success but the patient died."

There are countless other examples, many of which we'll discuss later on, but let's just mention one of them right now. It's known as the Nurses' Health Study, and it's one of the longest-running studies of diet and disease ever undertaken. Conducted by Harvard University, the study has followed more than 120,000 females since the mid-1970s to determine risk factors for cancer and heart disease.[7] In an exhaustive analysis of 84,129 of these women, published in the *New England Journal of Medicine*,[8] five factors were identified that significantly lowered the risk for heart disease. In fact, wrote the authors, "Eighty-two percent of coronary events in the study . . . could be attributed to lack of adherence to (these five factors)."

Are You Ready for the Five Factors?

1. Don't smoke.
2. Drink alcohol in moderation.
3. Engage in moderate-to-vigorous exercise for at least half an hour a day on average.
4. Maintain a healthy weight (BMI under 25).
5. Eat a wholesome, low-glycemic (low-sugar) diet with plenty of omega-3 fats and fiber.

Wait, didn't they miss something? Where's the part about lowering cholesterol?

It's not there. Lowering cholesterol didn't even make the list of the five most important things you can do to prevent heart attacks.

Of course, there's not roughly $30 billion plus a year to be made peddling that advice (a number that the gross revenue from statin drugs alone), and popping a pill is a lot easier than changing your lifestyle, but there it is. The inconvenient fact that lowering cholesterol has almost *no effect* on extending life is simply ignored by the special interests that profit enormously from keeping you in the dark.

As the writer Upton Sinclair said, "It is very difficult to get a man to understand something, when his salary depends upon his not understanding it."

◀ WHAT YOU NEED TO KNOW

- Cholesterol levels are a very poor predictor of heart attacks.
- More than half the people admitted to hospitals for cardiovascular disease have normal cholesterol as it's conventionally measured.
- Lowering cholesterol has extremely limited benefits, does not save lives, and should no longer be the focus of our efforts to prevent heart disease.

CHAPTER 3

CHOLESTEROL IS HARMLESS

NOW LET'S TALK ABOUT *YOU*

Unless you're an information junkie, there's a good chance that you're reading this book because you have something at stake here. Let us guess: You're concerned about *your* cholesterol.

Maybe you're a woman whose doctor has read you the riot act because your cholesterol is approaching 300 mg/dL, and your doc has convinced you that you'll drop dead of a heart attack if you don't go on medication right away.

Maybe you're a middle-aged man who has already had a heart attack, and your doctor is adamant about putting you on a cholesterol-lowering drug.

Or maybe you're a fit guy in your sixties whose cholesterol is 240 mg/dL and whose doctor is "worried" about that number.

Only *one* of the three hypothetical cases listed above has any business being on a cholesterol-lowering drug. Can you guess which one? Don't worry: By the time you finish this book, you'll know the answer. And you'll also know a heck of a lot more about cholesterol than most doctors in the United States. And, no, we don't make that statement lightly.

Okay, so you're concerned about your cholesterol—but you don't want to blindly follow recommendations without doing your own research. If you did, you'd simply follow your doctor's orders and have no interest in reading this book.

To understand the cholesterol myth—and to fully appreciate how the related health advice is obsolete—you'll need to know a lot more about cholesterol than the average person knows. Understanding the full story of cholesterol touches on medicine and research, as well as politics, economics, psychology, and sociology. It's got a cast of characters ranging from the obnoxious and egotistical to the well-meaning and misguided.

Sadly, much to the story has little to do with saving lives, though it may have started out that way. Instead, it involves staggering amounts of money, the politics of publication, and the sociology of belief—i.e., why bad ideas continue to survive past their expiration dates.

We'll also shine a light on the revolving door that exists between government advisory committees and the industries they're supposed to police. For example, when the National Cholesterol Education Program lowered the "optimal" cholesterol levels in 2004, eight out of nine people on the panel had financial ties to the pharmaceutical industry, most of them to the manufacturers of cholesterol-lowering drugs who would subsequently reap immediate benefits from these same recommendations.

THE BIRTH OF THE DIET-HEART HYPOTHESIS

Neither of us buys into the myth that cholesterol is the proper target for the prevention of heart disease. But how, exactly, did cholesterol and saturated fat come to be branded as the twin demons of heart disease in the first place? To answer that question, we need to go back to 1953. And if every story needs a villain, one person in particular has been christened the arch-dietary nemesis of the twentieth century: Ancel Benjamin Keys.

Keys was a public health scientist and is often considered the granddaddy of the low-fat movement. He is best remembered for launching the *Seven Countries Study*—the first major international study investigating links between diet, lifestyle factors, and heart disease. The massive study seemed to confirm a link between saturated fat consumption and cardiovascular disease, and Keys spent the latter part of his career pushing the newfangled (at the time) idea that too much saturated fat in the diet was harming our tickers.

Highly successful by any metric we could imagine, Keys managed to spread his ideas to the public and steer scientific consensus toward saturated fat phobia. But Keys has also been the butt of some serious allegations. Depending on who you ask, the whole Seven Countries Study was a sham because he chose only countries he knew would confirm his hypothesis. Or that he made a famous graph by cherry-picking six countries out of twenty-two countries that had available diet and mortality data, making it look like there was a near-perfect correlation between national fat consumption and heart disease. Or, even better, that

When the National Cholesterol Education Program lowered the "optimal" cholesterol levels in 2004, eight out of nine people on the panel had financial ties to the pharmaceutical industry.

his Seven Countries Study data actually showed that *sugar*, not saturated fat, was the real heart-killer—and he simply ignored those findings and drowned out dissenting voices, like that of his rival nutritionist John Yudkin, in order to preserve his ideology.

Full disclosure: We have been among the Keys-bashers. We've leveled some of these very charges against the guy. We've given him a whole lot of credit for fostering the biggest nutritional experiment in history—the low-fat high-carb diet—and being single-handedly responsible for the epidemics of obesity, diabetes, and heart disease that followed in the wake of the very recommendations he tirelessly promoted.

Today, We're Doing Things A Little Differently.

See, history is rarely as black and white as we'd like to believe—and the Keys debacle is no exception. Many of the claims slung against him, it turns out, are a mix of myth and fact. But, when it comes to getting out of our current health crisis, *none of that really matters*.

That's right. No matter which part of the "villain" narrative is true or false—the fact remains that we got to where we are *somehow*. When all is said and done, the dietary recommendations are the dietary recommendations and the widespread cultural bias against dietary fat is not disappearing anytime soon. That's what we need to live with. That's what we need to combat. What matters is not how we got into this predicament, but that *we're in it*. And now that we're here, it's time to roll up our sleeves and undo the damage.

You want to understand the widespread fear of cholesterol, and you want to make intelligent, science-based, rational choices about diet and lifestyle. You want to know what to eat to prevent heart disease.

So, where do we go next?

First, it's important to understand how nutritional research is actually done—then you will have a far greater understanding of how all the diet "experts" come to their conclusions. And be forewarned: Understanding the studies on which most nutritional advice is based will be like watching sausage made. And we can promise you this: You'll never feel the same way about eating sausage again.

MYTHS AND TRUTHS ABOUT DIET RESEARCH

First things first: Most diet research stinks.

There, we've said it. Now we'll show you why much of the nutrition research you hear about in the news is so misleading, inadequate, often irrelevant, and sometimes truly dangerous.[11] This includes—most especially—the research that claims to show that saturated fat will kill you and that cholesterol categorically causes heart disease.

How to Do a Randomized, Controlled Study

Let's say I'm a drug company, and I want to find out if the new blood pressure drug my company has come up with actually works in humans.

So, I design a study: I take a group of people. I make sure they're as "identical" as people can be—i.e., "30-year-old nonsmoking men from the Northeast with no previous health issues, but moderately high blood pressure."

In other words, I *match* the subjects for age, sex, medical history, and so on—all the things that could possibly skew the results make it hard to determine

THE SNACKWELL PHENOMENON

Low-fat had become the new mantra of the times, something we like to call the "Snackwell Phenomenon." Food companies rushed to create low-fat versions of every food imaginable, all marketed as "heart-healthy," with no cholesterol. (No one seemed to notice that manufacturers replaced the missing fat with tons of sugar and processed carbs, both of which are far more dangerous to our hearts than fat ever was.)

Butter was demonized and replaced with margarine, one of the most supremely stupid nutritional swap-outs in recent memory. Only much later did we discover that the supposedly healthier margarine was laden with trans fats, a really bad kind of fat created by using a kind of turkey baster to inject hydrogen atoms into a liquid (unsaturated) fat, making it more solid and giving it a longer shelf life. (Any time you read "partially hydrogenated oil" or "hydrogenated oil" in a list of ingredients, that means the food in question contains trans fats.) Unlike saturated fats from whole foods such as butter, trans fats (at least the man-made kind) actually do increase the risk for heart disease and strokes!

About 80 percent of trans fats in the American diet come from factory-produced partially hydrogenated vegetable oil.[1] Yet vegetable oils were (and are!) aggressively promoted as the healthy alternative to saturated fats, even though most of these oils are highly processed, pro-inflammatory, and easily damaged when reheated over and over again, which is standard procedure in many restaurants.

Think it's a coincidence that the obesity and diabetes epidemics went into overdrive around the same time that we started pushing low-fat, high-carb diets as an alternative to those containing more fat and protein? We don't.

But by now, fat—and, by extension, cholesterol— had become the new bogeyman of the American diet, defended only by people who clearly had a horse in the race (e.g., the dairy and meat industries). Meanwhile, low-fat had become the new religion of the masses. Now it was left for the science to catch up. The National Institutes of Health (NIH) funded half a dozen studies that were published between 1980 and 1984, hoping it would find persuasive evidence that low-fat diets prolonged lives.

Did they?

Hardly.

In 1986 the NIH held what's called a "consensus conference" to basically justify the dietary recommendations, yet it was anything but a consensus. Several experts pointed to significant defects in the studies and even called into question their accuracy. But you'd never know it from the final report, which made it seem like everyone had unquestioningly hitched their collective stars to the low-fat bandwagon.

Well, not exactly everyone.

Consensus? Not Exactly.

George Mann, M.D., associate professor of biochemistry at Vanderbilt University College of Medicine and a participating researcher in the Framingham Heart Study, was one of the doubters. The diet-heart idea is the "greatest scam" in the history of medicine, he said. "[Researchers] have held repeated press conferences bragging about this cataclysmic breakthrough, which the study directors claim shows that lowering cholesterol lowers the frequency of coronary disease. They have manipulated the data to reach the wrong conclusions."[2]

Mann also declared that NIH managers "used Madison Avenue hype to sell this failed trial in the way that media people sell an underarm deodorant!"[3] Michael Oliver, a highly respected British cardiologist, concurred. "The panel of jurists . . . was selected to include experts who would, predictably, say that . . . all levels of blood cholesterol in the United States are too high and should be lowered. Of course, this is exactly what was said."[4]

But the dissenting voices met with radio silence. With pompous certainty, the committee made clear in its final report that low-fat diets would afford significant protection against coronary heart disease for men, women, and children over two years old. "The evidence justifies . . . the reduction of calories from fat . . . to 30 percent, calories from saturated fat to 10 percent or less, and dietary cholesterol to no more than 250 to 300 mg daily," it declared.[5]

As Dr. Phil might ask, "And how's that workin' for you?"

One study that attempted to answer this hypothetical question was the Women's Health Initiative, the same program that has suggested that hormone therapy after menopause has more risks than benefits. This $415-million NIH study involved close to 49,000 people, aged fifty to seventy-nine, who were followed for eight years in an attempt to answer the question, "Does a low-fat diet reduce the risk of getting heart disease or cancer?"[6]

They got their answer.

"The largest study ever to ask whether a low-fat diet reduces the risk of getting cancer or heart disease has found that the diet has no effect," the *New York Times* reported in 2006.[7]

"These studies are revolutionary," said Jules Hirsch, M.D., physician-in-chief emeritus at the Rockefeller University in New York City and an expert on how diets influence weight and health. The studies "should put a stop to this era of thinking that we have all the information we need to change the whole national diet and make everybody healthy."[8]

Of course, none of these questionable findings stopped the cholesterol-lowering, fat-avoiding juggernaut that went into full swing in the late 1970s and continues, albeit bruised and battered, to this day. And we have to give the misguided researchers kudos for their motives—by reducing cholesterol levels, they sincerely believed they would be reducing heart disease. As Dwight Lundell, M.D., author of *The Cure for Heart Disease*, wryly put it, "They were taking the bull by the horn—but it was the wrong bull."[9]

When we first met about this project, Steve brought to the meeting a series of papers by one of the most respected researchers in the world, Michel de Lorgeril, M.D., a French cardiologist and researcher at the prestigious National Centre for Scientific Research, the largest public organization for scientific research in France.

De Lorgeril has authored dozens of papers in peer-reviewed journals, and he was the lead researcher for the Lyon Diet Heart Study. The following quotation comes from his only book written in English, and it's a perfect way to end this chapter:

"We can summarize . . . in one sentence: Cholesterol is harmless!"[10]

what the drug itself is doing.

I don't really care about how these folks might be different in terms of their television viewing habits, or if they prefer iPhones over Androids, or if they had a really bad haircut in high school. But I *do* want to make sure they're similar on *any measure that could likely affect blood pressure* (which probably doesn't include smartphone preferences or bowl cuts).

Because blood pressure can easily be influenced by factors such as smoking and obesity and lifestyle, I make sure—just to keep things even—that all my subjects are nonsmokers, not overweight, don't have previously existing heart disease, have a similar level of

stress, aren't taking any other medications, and are more or less uniform on all other important health metrics I can think of.

If you're thinking this is pretty hard to do, you're right: It's next to impossible. But it's the research "ideal," and people who get *most* of it right publish better research than those who get *less* of it right.

So, we're trying to "match" our subjects so they're as similar as possible. We're trying to do the human equivalent of an experiment that uses lab rats with identical genes bred in an identical environment. It's the "sameness" of subjects that is important here.

Next, I randomly assign these very similar

subjects to one of two groups. For the length of this ideal clinical study, both groups would eat identical food, sleep identical hours, and live pretty much identical lives, with one notable exception. One group would get the treatment I'm trying to study—in this case, the blood pressure medication—and the other would get a placebo. At the conclusion of the study, we'd measure their average blood pressure and match it against the baseline levels measured before the study began.

(The control group gets a placebo because the very act of getting a pill can influence the results. That's right: Simply *thinking* you're taking medication can be enough to cause some health improvements. If that doesn't attest to the power of the human mind, we don't know what does!)

If, by the end of the study, there were any significant differences between the two matched groups in *actual blood pressure*—like if the *blood pressure medicine group* had significantly lower blood pressure at the end of the study than the *placebo group*—we'd have a darn good reason to assume that the blood pressure drug was the cause, and the stockholders in the company that makes that medicine would be breaking out the champagne and kazoos.

We tested the hypothesis *"this blood pressure medication lowers blood pressure,"* and, in the case of this hypothetical study, we confirmed the hypothesis. The blood pressure medicine did indeed perform as hoped. We can market our drug with a clear conscience and FDA approval!

Wouldn't it be nice if nutrition studies were done like this? The answer is, "Yes, it sure would be!"

Too bad they're not. In fact, most of the nutrition studies you hear about in the media resemble our hypothetical blood pressure drug study about as much as West Virginia resembles West Hollywood.

Enter Epidemiology

Contrary to what alarmist news headlines might suggest, not all studies are created equal—even if when they're published in prestigious peer-reviewed journals. The vast majority of the studies that make it to the mainstream media are *not* rigorously controlled clinical trials (e.g., our hypothetical blood pressure medication). Instead, they are *epidemiological* studies, also known as *observational* studies. These are the kinds of studies that Ancel Keys conducted, and virtually all of the nutrition advice we get from major health organizations around the world comes from studies that are *just* like the Seven Countries Study. They are associational and observational—a type of study that is, by its very design, fundamentally unable to show cause and effect.

Observational studies are exactly what they sound like: Researchers *observe*. They don't intervene, they don't randomize, they don't treat, and they certainly don't manipulate variables. They simply watch large groups of people going about their regular day-to-day lives. Over several years, they collect copious data on what these groups of people do, what they eat, and—eventually—what diseases or deaths befall them. Then the researchers apply sophisticated statistical tools to tease out associations between what those folks were doing and what was happening to their bodies.

Typical findings of these kinds of studies include: "Eating bacon every day is associated with a 21%

increase in cholesterol," or "Eating 1 ounce of nuts a day is associated with lower incidence of heart disease." In short, the goal is to take a lot of data from a lot of people, and then see *which things tend to be found together*. But the fact that two things are found together doesn't mean one caused the others (for example, rain and umbrellas, or firefighters and fires).

You might notice, for example, that in countries where they eat a lot of fiber, there is less incidence of colon cancer. Or that people who have lower levels of vitamin D tend to have higher rates of multiple sclerosis. Or that diabetes incidence exploded upward under the Clinton administration. Or that people who eat more saturated fat have higher total cholesterol.

Whether these correlations matter at all—and what they actually *mean*, if anything—is a topic for a different day. For now we're just talking about the data, not whether that data is clinically important.

The idea that smoking causes lung cancer, for example, came out of epidemiology. And that was a great example of the true value of epidemiology, which is to *generate hypotheses*. Epidemiologists noticed consistently higher levels of lung cancer among smokers, which was an interesting observation—but *only* because this repeated observation led to the *hypothesis* that cigarette smoking *causes* lung cancer. That hypothesis was then tested in a rigorous way, time and time and time again in study after study around which (unlike cholesterol) there is little controversy. And it is now considered to be true that cigarettes wildly increase your risk for lung cancer in a directly causal fashion.

So epidemiology is terrific for observing things, for noticing what's found together, and, most importantly,

for generating *hypotheses*. Epidemiology is like the preliminary detective work one does when gathering up clues at a crime scene, clues that suggest a hypothesis of what might have gone down. But that's just the beginning. No one is convicted of a crime based on clues—you *use* the clues to build a case. In science, that "case" is built with the bricks of randomized, double-blind, placebo-controlled, peer-reviewed research studies. The case isn't built with a few random "clues"—in science, those are the equivalent of circumstantial evidence and would be thrown out of court.

When epidemiology is used as it should be—for generating hypotheses—it's terrific. For example, if two variables keep showing up hand-in-hand across different human populations in multiple epidemiological studies, we can start forming and testing ideas about why that's happening. Does one cause the other? If so, which is cause and which is effect? We can also investigate whether a third, hidden factor drives them both. For example, living in a high-rise building is associated with more frequent bronchitis—but in reality, both those things are due to a third factor common to both—bad air quality.

EPIDEMIOLOGY IS OUR STARTING POINT

When it comes to figuring out links between diet, lifestyle, and disease, epidemiology is our starting point—*not* our final destination. There's a reason all scientists worth their weight in petri dishes abide by the wisdom, *correlation does not equal causation*. As exciting as new findings can be, observational studies rarely give us the full story.

So clearly, epidemiology has its place. The problem is when it's forcibly removed from that place (where it lived happily as a hypotheses generator) and gets inserted somewhere it *really* doesn't belong—such as at the helm of public policy.

Now hold on to your hats, because we're about to show you what sausage-making looks like when it comes to nutritional epidemiology.

You might at this moment be forgiven, for example, for wondering how researchers can observe what thousands—sometimes hundreds of thousands—of people are eating on a daily basis. The answer is: They can't. So, they collect data using a tried-and-true tool known as the food frequency questionnaire (or, in researcher lingo, the notorious FFQ,).

FFQ stands for food frequency questionnaire, and here's how it works. Researchers ask people to fill out a form every three, six, or twelve months, stating what they've been eating by checking boxes that ask things like, "Over the past twelve months, how often did you eat butter on potatoes, cooked vegetables, rice, grains, or beans?"

If that seems like a ridiculous example, here's the scary part: That question comes straight from the NHANES Food Frequency Questionnaire, developed by the National Cancer Institute.[12]

Here's an example of the actual food frequency

National Health and Nutrition Examination Survey (NHANES) FFQ

Over the past 12 months . . .

28. How often did you eat **COOKED greens** (such as spinach, turnip, collard, mustard, chard, or kale?

☐ NEVER
☐ 1-6 times per year   ☐ 2 times per week
☐ 7-11 times per year   ☐ 3-4 times per week
☐ 1 time per month   ☐ 5-6 times per week
☐ 2-3 times per month   ☐ 1 time per day
☐ 1 time per week   ☐ 2 or more times per day

29. How often did you eat **RAW greens** (such as spinach, turnip, collard, mustard, chard, or kale)? (*We'll ask about lettuce later.*)

☐ NEVER
☐ 1-6 times per year   ☐ 2 times per week
☐ 7-11 times per year   ☐ 3-4 times per week
☐ 1 time per month   ☐ 5-6 times per week
☐ 2-3 times per month   ☐ 1 time per day
☐ 1 time per week   ☐ 2 or more times per day

33. How often did you eat **string beans** or **green beans** (fresh, canned, or frozen)?

☐ NEVER
☐ 1-6 times per year   ☐ 2 times per week
☐ 7-11 times per year   ☐ 3-4 times per week
☐ 1 time per month   ☐ 5-6 times per week
☐ 2-3 times per month   ☐ 1 time per day
☐ 1 time per week   ☐ 2 or more times per day

34. How often did you eat **peas** (fresh, canned, or frozen)?

☐ NEVER
☐ 1-6 times per year   ☐ 2 times per week
☐ 7-11 times per year   ☐ 3-4 times per week
☐ 1 time per month   ☐ 5-6 times per week
☐ 2-3 times per month   ☐ 1 time per day
☐ 1 time per week   ☐ 2 or more times per day

questionnaire that was used by NHANES:

You might be thinking, "This is the worst and most unreliable way I can possibly imagine to collect data on what people eat." And guess what? You're right. And everyone knows it.

People's long-term diet recall is notoriously inaccurate. It's also often skewed by wishful thinking: think "Of course I only eat ice cream once a month!" This leads to chronic underreporting of "bad" foods, and sometimes over-reporting of "good" ones.

Scientists themselves have written papers roasting the almighty FFQ for its failures as a data-gathering tool. In an editorial by researchers from the Fred Hutchinson Cancer Research Center in Seattle—tellingly titled, "Is It Time to Abandon the Food Frequency Questionnaire?"—the authors noted that diet and cancer links that showed up loud and clear using dietary biomarkers were totally undetectable when using food frequency questionnaire data.[13] They concluded that it's "possible that epidemiologists have been deluded in their acceptance of food frequency questionnaires."

I can't tell you how many times I've discussed this with researchers, and every single time the verdict is the same: *It's absolutely awful, but it's all we've got.*

And this, dear reader, is the very method that nutritional epidemiology hangs its hat on. See the problem?

Here's what happens when epidemiology is used for studying diet. Data will show that, for example, over a period of twenty-five years, saturated fat consumption went up in a population, and so did cholesterol. Now that should generate a *hypothesis*—i.e., that saturated fat consumption causes cholesterol to rise.

That hypothesis can now be tested clinically in a variety of settings—such as by feeding people controlled diets with different levels of saturated fat, and measuring what happens to their blood lipids.

The point is that the epidemiological observation *generates* something that can then be analyzed in a more controlled manner to determine cause and effect. So, fire up the Bunsen burners!

But testing the hypothesis generated by an epidemiological study is frequently *not* what happens next.

Instead, there is a wildly premature leap to declarations of causation based on nothing but a pile of associations. The media airwaves start filling with "Red meat causes cancer!" "Bacon causes heart attacks!" and other sensationalist claims that haven't even come close to being confirmed (or refuted) by more rigorous, controlled experiments. In turn, the perception of consumers—that's folks like you and me—gets shaped by totally preliminary findings. And, too often, this becomes the basis of public health policy.

Yellow Finger Syndrome

We've seen association studies miss the most obvious connections and fail to account for many other plausible ones. For example, there is a statistically significant positive correlation between a noticeable yellowing on the fingertips and lung cancer. For years, those with a strange yellowing on their fingertips developed lung cancer at a much higher rate than those who did not have yellowish fingertips. Beginning statistics students were taught this association to illustrate the concept of a *confounding variable*. The confounding variable in this case is *smoking*. Smoking causes *both* lung cancer *and* yellow fingers. Yellow fingers don't cause lung cancer, even though they are frequently found together (correlated).

Researchers love to think they're very sophisticated, and have all kinds of statistical magic to perform on the data to rule out this kind of "confounding." We think they're overly optimistic. There's also a good deal of *confirmation bias* in research as well—people frequently find what they look for and find what they *expect* to find, paying close attention to any correlations that support their hypothesis and throwing out the many that don't.

THE FABULOUS PUNCH LINE YOU'VE ALL BEEN WAITING FOR

So, what does all this have to do with the great cholesterol myth? Simple. An observational study—like the Seven Countries Study—notes an association between saturated fat consumption and heart disease. The relationship is assumed to be causal—that is, eating saturated fat *causes* heart disease. This ultimately results in a massive public health effort to get everyone to eschew saturated fat-rich foods and replace them with seed oils (i.e., "vegetable" oil), which is assumed to be far better for us and will result in improved health and longer lifetimes.

At the end of the day, we've made massive, sweeping changes to the American diet (and beyond) based on little more than two variables that happen to show up alongside each other. And as it turns out, some of those changes have made the problem worse, not better.

There are very few writers in the health-and-wellness space that are better than Denise Minger, whom we were delighted to be able to work with on this book.

No one we know of can debunk a study better, all the more remarkable because she does it with the kind of style and wit rarely found in the world of health. And she does all this armed with nothing but absolutely ironclad data, which she is happy to show you.

Take, for example, this graphic illustrating the craziness of making assumptions and health policy from epidemiological, observational studies.

I'll let the graph speak for itself. It looks like perfect evidence that Justin Bieber has been really *good* for cholesterol levels, but Facebook cancelled out his magical statin-like properties. And because we already "know" cholesterol causes heart disease, it seems an open-and-shut prescription:

Wanna wipe out heart disease? Shut down Facebook.

The Fascinating (and Relatively Unknown) Story of Dr. Ivan Frantz

I can think of no better illustration of the difference between associational studies and honest-to-goodness scientifically sound clinical studies than the following story, uncovered by the writer and podcaster Malcolm Gladwell, who generously allowed us to retell it in our own words.

Around the same time that the Seven Countries Study was on its way to becoming the most referenced and revered study in nutritional history, another big observational study was commencing. It was called the National Diet Heart Study, and it involved research teams in six major cities.[14] Ancel Keys himself supervised the Minneapolis arm of the study.

The study concluded that a diet lower in saturated fat and higher in polyunsaturated fat—i.e. "vegetable

Evidence That Facebook Cancelled Out the Cholesterol-Lowering Effects of Justin Bieber

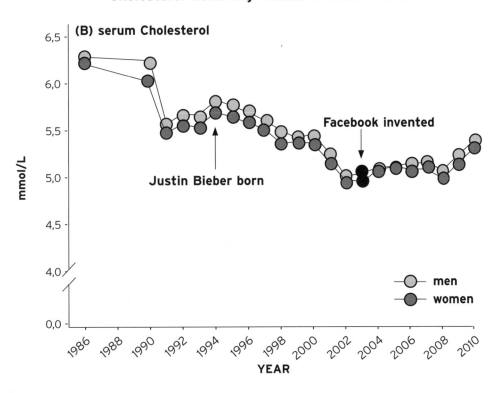

(B) serum Cholesterol

Justin Bieber born

Facebook invented

men
women

YEAR

oil"—was indeed "associated" with a 14 percent reduction in coronary artery disease when compared with a standard diet with higher amounts of saturated fat. The stockholders in the vegetable oil companies broke out the bubbly. If there had been any lingering doubt about the evils of saturated fat and the superiority of vegetable oil, this study erased them. Canola oil for everyone!

Malcolm Gladwell Dug into This Story and Here's What He Found[15]

The researcher in charge of the Faribault, Minnesota, arm of the National Diet Heart Study was a guy

named Ivan Frantz. Frantz was a meticulous researcher and scientist, a medical doctor who was firmly in the camp that believed "it's all about the saturated fat!" This was a man who tested his kids' blood regularly to make sure their cholesterol wasn't too high. In the Frantz household, butter and fatty meat were blacklisted. Frantz, a friend of Keys, was a true believer.

But he was also a serious scientist, and he recognized the second-class citizenship of epidemiology in the scientific world. So, he wanted to do the Faribault, Minnesota, arm of the Diet Heart study differently. He wanted to do a real, *clinical* study, not a mere observational one. That meant creating two matched groups of subjects and controlling exactly what they ate, with one group getting the "saturated fat" diet and one group getting the "vegetable oil" diet. Frantz was—along with most of the medical establishment at the time—convinced that people who substituted margarine for butter and corn oil for lard would live longer, have less heart disease, and generally be healthier on most major indices.

But, Frantz wondered, how am I going to get thousands of people to agree to eat the assigned diet—and how would I even be sure that they stuck to it? In a flash of ingenuity, Frantz got the idea to do his arm of the study in an institutional setting.

He recruited seven institutions that were willing to participate. Patients were separated into matched groups and given either the "saturated fat" diet or the "polyunsaturated fat" (vegetable oil) diet. The only food the patients got was delivered on trays by hospital staff, and Frantz arranged for the two groups to have meals that looked absolutely identical—even though one tray was composed of meals prepared the conventional way, and the other tray was composed of meals in which saturated fat had been replaced with vegetable oil. The study was truly a randomized, double-blind design. Superb.

The study went on from 1968 to 1973, with quite a long period of follow-up. But when the raw data came in, Frantz was—to put it mildly—surprised. The data were equivocal at best. There was no clear advantage for the people who had eaten the diet in which saturated fat had been replaced with vegetable oil. In fact, Frantz thought, the data were kind of weird. Replacing saturated fat with vegetable oil produced zero benefit.

The raw data would have probably remained in Frantz's basement . . . if it hadn't been for Christopher Ramsden. Years after Frantz died and his study had faded from scientific memory, Ramsden—a researcher at the National Institutes of Health—was investigating *linoleic acid*, the primary fat found in vegetable oil. Ramsden wanted to know more about what happens when "vegetable oil"—a "food" product that wasn't even around 100 years earlier—was consumed in the amounts that were now being recommended.

Ramsden wanted to do a clinical study on linoleic acid—the main polyunsaturated fat found in vegetable oil—to help answer the gnawing question, "What *really* happens when you replace natural, traditional saturated fats with vegetable oils?" Ideally, he would have liked to take two matched groups of subjects, feed them the identical diet—same number of calories, same amount of protein, fat, and carbs—except that one group's meals would be prepared with saturated fats and one group's meals would be prepared with vegetable oil.

"But who's going to fund a study like that?" Ramsden probably thought. And then he remembered: That study has already been conducted! It's exactly what Dr. Ivan Frantz had done for his part of the Diet Heart Study!

Ramsden tracked down Ivan Frantz's son, Robert Frantz, a cardiologist at the Mayo Clinic, who agreed to help him. After much searching, they hit pay dirt and Ramsden had the original data from the superbly constructed, randomized control trial that tested the then-current notion that people who replace saturated fat with vegetable fat would be healthier and would live longer.

THE TRANS FAT FACTOR

There's another reason to suspect that vegetable oils and margarines were contributing to the problem of heart disease rather than helping to prevent it: trans fat. Remember that when the dietary and medical powers that be collectively decided that saturated fat was the enemy, they had to replace it with *something*. That something turned out to be hydrogenated vegetable oil, hydrogenated so that it would have a nice long shelf life and remain stable for years. Hydrogenated vegetable oil—also known as trans fat—turned out to be a Frankenfat that some authors (notably our friend, Dr. Steven Masley) have referred to as metabolic embalming fluid.

Trans fat has been implicated as a risk factor in both stroke and heart disease.[16] It was officially "banned" by the U.S. Government in 2015 when the Food and Drug Administration ruled that artificial trans fats were unsafe to eat.[17]

In the study done by Ivan Franz (see text), the margarine they used was almost certainly high in artificial trans fat, though at the time, few scientists knew the dangers associated with that particular substance.

It's also ironic that the food that was so demonized that it had to be replaced on our menu—butter—turns out to have more *mono* unsaturated fat than saturated fat! (Monounsaturated fat is the same kind found in olive oil.)

The margarine fiasco in the late 1980s and '90s is a perfect example of backward medicine and dumb solutions to nonexistent problems. First, make people worried about the saturated fat in butter (even though there's no need to be). Next, solve the "problem" you've just created with a profitable "solution"—margarine loaded with trans fat—that's way worse than the original "problem." Boom! You've got "I can't believe it's not butter"!

He went to work analyzing it. And Frantz had been right: The data *were* kind of weird.

It turned out that not only was there no *advantage* to replacing saturated fat with vegetable oil, there was a distinct *disadvantage*, particularly if you were over sixty-five. Vegetable oil lowered cholesterol just fine—which was what everybody thought would happen. What vegetable oil *didn't* do was save lives. In fact, in people over sixty-five, there was a distinct trend, and not at all in the direction that was expected: *Those who lowered their cholesterol the most had the highest risk of dying.*

Ramsden knew he was about to call into question Ivan Frantz's life's work. What did Ivan Frantz's son, Robert Frantz, have to say? "Publish it." He explained: "My father believed in science, and he believed in truth. He valued those things far more than he did his own 'beliefs.' Publish the data—my father would have wanted you to."

So he did. And here's what Ramsden said when he published it in the British Medical Journal: "Available evidence from randomized controlled trials shows that replacement of saturated fat with linoleic acid effectively lowers serum cholesterol—*but does not support the hypothesis that this translates to a lower risk of death from coronary heart disease*" (emphasis ours). In fact, Ramsden pointed out, the best clinical trials we have reached the exact opposite conclusion.

SO, WHAT DO WE TAKE AWAY FROM ALL THIS?

As Esther Perel once said, "Human beings have a tendency to search for truth in the places where it is easiest to look rather than where it is likely to be found."[18] We might all do well to be less attached to our beliefs and more devoted to the truth.

Our current state of cholesterol confusion isn't simply due to "bad guys doing bad things" through-out nutritional history (i.e., the villainous caricature of Ancel Keys). The problem goes much deeper than any individual researcher or pet theory. It's rooted in our very relationship with science itself—the way we use (and abuse) observational findings; the way the media and policymakers alike confuse correlation for causa-tion; the way the public's dearth of scientific literacy keeps us vulnerable to misleading information.

There's nothing wrong, per se, with epidemiology. We simply need to understand where observational studies land in the hierarchy of scientific research (spoiler alert: pretty low down on the totem pole). We also need to take the necessary steps to determine causation. Sure, conducting controlled trials might be slower, more expensive, and trickier to pull off than running a bunch of food frequency questionnaire answers through a statistical model—but isn't our health worth it?

We need to be much more critical readers of media messages about health. Don't take them at face value. Dig deeper. Do your own research and lis-ten to competing views. The headlines are almost never the whole story.

◀ WHAT YOU NEED TO KNOW

- The theory that fat and cholesterol cause heart disease became widely accepted despite much evidence to the contrary, evidence which continues to accumulate. The case is thankfully being reopened.
- Many doctors did not agree—and *do* not agree—with the cholesterol myth and correctly question the science upon which it was based.
- The adoption of the cholesterol myth by mainstream organizations and the government was not supported by science and had a strong political component to it.

CHAPTER 4

THE REAL DEAL ON CHOLESTEROL

WHEN WE WERE KIDS, DOCTORS STILL MADE HOUSE CALLS.

One of us–Jonny–vividly remembers "Dr. Leo" coming to the house, always dressed in a suit and tie, with black satchel at the ready. He'd take out his trusty tongue depressor, tell you to say "ah," put a flashlight in your eye and a stethoscope on your chest and voilà, he'd pronounce his verdict–a flu, a bug, strep throat. He'd dash off an unreadable prescription and within a day or two the "bug" would be gone.

Now imagine, if you will, that instead of being a boy of ten you are a grown person, age forty-seven, living in Southern California. You have a strange pain, dizziness, and a wicked headache. You definitely don't feel "right." You wonder if you're having a stroke, or possibly a heart attack. You call an ambulance and they take you to Cedars Sinai in Los Angeles, one of the best-equipped and most highly rated hospitals in the country.

They wheel you in past the gleaming high-tech machines that can take a picture of virtually any organ in your body, past the electron microscopes that can measure virtually any metabolic process at the subcellular level, past the Harvard-trained physicians scurrying around with handheld devices that have the computation power of IBM's Big Blue, into the emergency room.

And in walks a doctor with a tongue depressor.

She spends about five minutes with you. She tells you to say "ah," puts a flashlight in your eye, listens to your heart with a device that's essentially the medical version of two tin cans and string, pronounces your diagnosis, writes you a script, and sends you home.

Pretty crazy, right?

Well, the "good" versus "bad" cholesterol test is the tongue depressor of diagnostic tests. It's equivalent to trying to make meaningful decisions about a person's health based on which of two categories of height they fall into—short or tall. In an age when we have access to the entire human genome wouldn't it be pretty ridiculous to diagnose based on "short and tall"? Yet that's exactly what we're doing when we prescribe drugs based on "good and bad" cholesterol?

At this point in our knowledge of heart disease, inflammatory markers, cholesterol fractionization, and genetic markers, the "good" and "bad" cholesterol test is no more useful in predicting outcomes than this month's horoscope. It's an obsolete test, and I'm about to explain why.

CHOLESTEROL 101

This is the real story of what cholesterol is, what it does, how it gets into your bloodstream, and what actually happens once it gets there. Once you see the story in its full Technicolor glory—with all the subtleties and nuances—you will never again accept a prescription for a powerful drug based on nothing more than an outdated test for "good" versus "bad" cholesterol. In fact, you will understand how baffling it is to still be relying on this test in the early decades of the twenty-first century.

So let's get started.

The first and most important thing you need to know about cholesterol is that it cannot travel unaccompanied in the bloodstream. The second thing worth knowing is the astonishing fact that most conventional doctors do *not* know this.

Cholesterol can't travel in the blood because it is *hydrophobic* (hydro=water, phobic=avoiding). Trying to get cholesterol to get from point A to point B in the bloodstream without putting it in some kind of protective container would be like pouring oil in a lake and expecting it to make it to the other side of the lake intact.

Cholesterol *always* has to be contained in a protective structure—the protective container that the body uses to safely transport cholesterol is called a *lipoprotein* (as in "high-density lipoprotein"—HDL—and "low-density lipoprotein"—LDL.) We colloquially call these lipoproteins "cholesterol" but in fact, cholesterol is only a portion of the cargo these lipoprotein "boats" carry around the bloodstream. (For example, lipoproteins also carry triglycerides and protein.)

That is why—as you'll soon see—the single most important metric to know from any test regarding cholesterol is this: How many boats are there in the water. How much cholesterol those boats are carrying is really beside the point. If there are too many boats in the water, the chance of an accident is greater than if there are less boats in the water, regardless of the cargo (cholesterol, protein, triglycerides) those boats happen to be carrying. And there is a simple, widely available test to find out how many "boats" are floating around in your bloodstream, and it's called the NMR particle test. (Much more on the particle test coming—stay tuned!)

If you're beginning to think, "it's all about the lipoproteins," well guess what? You're right. Here's a breakdown of the approximate protein/ cholesterol/ triglyceride content of the basic classes of lipoproteins:

Remember this: *Cholesterol is the cargo and the lipoprotein is the boat.* This is important because what matters is the *boats*–not the cargo!

Lipoprotein Class	Protein	Cholesterol	Triglyceride
VLDL (very low-density) lipoprotein	10%	22%	50%
IDL (intermediate density lipoprotein)	18%	29%	50%
LDL (low-density lipoprotein)	25%	46-50%	31%
HDL (high-density lipoprotein)	33%	30%	4-8%

Though most people–and most doctors–only know about "LDL" and "HDL," the fact is that scientists have now been able to identify at least thirteen different subfractions of cholesterol–HDL2a, HDL2b, LDL IIIa, LDL IIIb, Lp(a), oxLDL, just to name a handful.

The presence (and preponderance) of different subfractions have very different meanings when it comes to risk. For example: HDL2b consists of the largest and most buoyant particles in the HDL "family." Even if your *overall* "HDL" is "normal," a breakdown of the subclasses might reveal that you actually have a very *low* level of large HDL particles, which increases cardiovascular disease (CVD) risk by 1.8 times.

Some subfractions are more likely to promote the formation of plaque. These subfractions are smaller, denser, and more susceptible to inflammation and oxidation (see chapter 5). Some subfractions are *less* likely to be damaged and to therefore become a problem. What's more, researchers can now identify patterns of lipoprotein distribution (i.e., "Pattern A– mostly large, buoyant particles" versus "Pattern B– mostly small, inflammatory particles"). These patterns–independent of anything else–are predictive of cardiometabolic problems such as diabetes, insulin resistance, and metabolic syndrome.

Why Conventional Tests Are Worthless

Here's a great example of the obsolescence of the "good" versus "bad" cholesterol test. The following hypothetical numbers represent what your conventional doc would call a "great" cholesterol test. If you had these numbers, your conventional doc would pronounce your heart in great shape and would be unlikely to write you a script for a statin drug.

TOTAL CHOLESTEROL: 137
LDL: 66
HDL: 42
Triglycerides: 146

If you're wondering how to lower your triglycerides, it's the easiest thing in the world: They drop like a rock on low-carb diets.

Now we should point out that both of us think these test results are problematic, even though conventional docs don't. For one thing, a total cholesterol level of 137 is just *too darn low*—and low cholesterol is associated with a *higher* risk of death from non-heart related issues (like accidents and suicides). And if you're wondering why the heck low cholesterol might be associated with such random things as accidents and suicides, maybe it's because cholesterol is needed for proper brain functioning.

Another thing about those "terrific" cholesterol test numbers above: Most functional medicine and functional nutrition practitioners (like us) think an optimal triglyceride level is under 100, not under 150. We would not be overjoyed with a triglyceride level of 146 even though it's within the "normal" range for most labs.

Triglycerides to HDL Ratio: A Hidden Clue to the State of Your Health

The ratio of triglycerides to HDL is one of the best predictors of both heart disease and insulin resistance (see chapter 9). People with a high triglyceride to HDL ratio have a 16x greater risk of heart disease. That's a 1600 percent increase![1] You want your triglycerides to HDL ratio to be around 2 or less (i.e., 100 triglycerides, 50 HDL). A ratio of 5 (example: 200: 40) increases your risk for cardiovascular events significantly. A ratio of 2 (or less) is wonderful. In other words, if your triglycerides were 100 and your HDL was 50, you'd have the lowest statistical risk for a heart attack.

The triglyceride to HDL ratio in the above test is found by dividing the triglycerides (146) by the HDL (42) which yields a ratio of 3.47—not terrible, but certainly not great. But if this person's triglycerides dropped to 100, the ratio would go immediately down to 2.38 (100:42). That's a huge improvement in risk, and one you could make just by dropping your triglycerides even if your HDL cholesterol remained exactly the same.

But your doc isn't looking at any of this; he or she is looking at a cholesterol test in which all the numbers are "in range" so no problems are assumed. Your doctor is very happy; you have a very low total cholesterol, and a low LDL, everything else (like triglycerides) is "in range" so you're sent home with a

Cholesterol is an essential molecule without which there would be no life, so important that virtually every cell in the body is capable of synthesizing it.

pat on the head, and told that everything is just fine.

But it's really not.

And we haven't even started talking about the number of boats in the water, which is where the real action is.

Enter Modern Cholesterol Testing

So the standard, old-fashioned "good" and "bad" cholesterol test isn't going to give you much good information and, as we saw above, may conceal some important facts. And that's when a more modern cholesterol panel comes in.

The state-of-the-art test for cholesterol, as of this writing, is the NMR particle test, also known as the NMR Lipo-Profile. This test doesn't just tell you how much "HDL" and "LDL" you have, it tells you what *kind* of LDL you have, and, most importantly, how many boats are in the water carrying around cholesterol cargo. These boats—the lipoproteins—are technically called particles, and the NMR test tells you your total number of them. Now *that's* important.

The total number of particles predicts heart disease many times better than simply knowing how much LDL you have. (Remember—the more boats in the water, the more chance of an accident.) The NMR test also identifies how many of those particles are small and dense and atherogenic, and how many are big and fluffy and far less damaging.

The point is that—given the extraordinary range of measurement tools we now have at our disposal to measure the intricacies of blood lipid levels—it is head-shakingly baffling that doctors continue to hold on to a test invented in the 1960s that's about as accurate as a tongue depressor.

HOW DOES ATHEROSCLEROSIS DEVELOP, ANYWAY?

*Arterio*sclerosis literally means "hardening of the arteries." It's the process by which an artery goes from being *compliant*—able to freely expand and contract to accommodate blood flow—to being *firm and stiff*. *Athero*sclerosis involves the development of plaque (discussed below) and is the most common cause of ar*terio*sclerosis. It's also the most likely to kill you.

And it all starts with an irritant.

Now, this irritant could be a toxin from the air. Or it could be—and often is—cigarette smoke. It could be a stray LDL particle (more on that in a moment). Or it could be the stress of high blood pressure, banging up against the inner walls of the arteries and causing distress among the layer of cells that lines them, the *endothelium*.

Endothelial cells are the one-celled line of defense between what's floating around in the blood-stream and the actual artery wall—and when those endothelial cells become damaged and dysfunctional, the condition is called *endothelial dysfunction*. (It's like the artery's version of "leaky gut.") Many modern physicians see endothelial dysfunction as one of the root causes of modern illness. When there's a break in the security of the artery wall—that is, when the endo-thelial layer is damaged—the stage is set for the heart disease version of the Invasion of the Body Snatchers.

First, a rogue molecule—most often a rogue LDL—breaks through the broken and dysfunctional barrier and parks where it doesn't belong. Once that LDL par-ticle gets into that sub-endothelial space, others fol-low, like cockroaches in a New York apartment. They become like "squatters," taking up "illegal residence" in the artery wall. They bind to substances called *pro-teoglycans* in the arterial wall and become a magnet for oxidative forces. This institutes a full-on inflammatory response. Mayhem ensues.

Remember—this process of inflammation and oxidation of rogue LDL particles can all be contained in the artery wall and may not even bulge into the *lumen*, the "inner tube" of the artery. As Dr. Peter Attia points out, this is the reason a person with advanced atherosclerosis can still have a normal angiogram!

As plaque progresses, it can—and usually *does*—eventually start to expand or bulge from the artery wall *into* the lumen, narrowing the passageway. This compromises the delivery of oxygen to the tissues (ischemia) and can lead to the rupturing of plaque and even to a full-on *myocardial infarction*—a heart attack.

The process of atherosclerosis *always*—100 percent of the time—starts with a penetration of the (damaged) artery wall by a rogue lipoprotein. Many things, such as high blood pressure or cigarette smoke, may weaken and damage that artery wall, making it an easy target for penetration. But it's the LDL particle that "does the deed" and actually moves into that "no-parking" zone. It takes up residence, and thus begins the cascade of plaque formation that can lead to a lot more serious stuff.

One of the first things that happens is that the immune system senses something that doesn't belong. It mounts an attack and sends cells called *macrophages*—literally "big eater"—to dispose of the intruder. The macrophages gobble up the illegally parked LDL, like little Pac-Men, and in doing so get so stuffed that they die. Dead macrophages are known as foam cells, because they're stuffed with a fat and

sterol mix that looks like sea foam. This "sea foam" spreads out like a little lake, but it's still very much in the artery wall—specifically, the *tunica intima*, the artery wall's innermost layer.

What happens next is that the smooth muscle cells immediately sense that something is amiss, so they dance a little migration dance over to the tunica intima and they begin building a fibrous cap on the plaque. The fibrous cap—made of proteins like collagen and elastin—is like a protective scab on a wound. As one clever instructor from the Kahn Academy referred to it, the resulting structure is like "fat with a cap."

The smooth muscle cells also get confused by all the dead foam cells and start to think, "maybe we should lay down some bone here!" so they start depositing calcium into the mix. Note to all: Calcium is a great nutrient, but you want it deposited in your *bones*, not your *arteries*.

Meanwhile, the "fat with a cap" is beginning to protrude from the tunica intima (the artery wall) into the artery itself. This creates two conditions. The first is resistance. The radius of the artery has just shrunk a bit to accommodate the intrusion, and that means the artery offers more resistance to blood flow, just as a hose with a kink is more resistant to water flow. The second thing that happens is that the wall of the artery itself becomes stiffer, due partially to all the calcium that's been laid down near and around the fibrous cap.

Now remember, lots of people have plaque, and don't necessarily have problems. What makes plaque a problem is when it ruptures. If it ruptures, you're in trouble. The fibrous cap comes loose and can easily cause a blockage of blood flow which, depending on

LDL particles aren't the problem—LDL particles winding up in the wrong place and then getting attacked by oxidative and inflammatory compounds is the problem.

location, can in turn cause a stroke or a heart attack.

There is now a widely available test, called the Lp-PLA2, that can determine your risk for having plaque ruptured (see page 203). Guess what—it's not on the standard cholesterol test. Quelle surprise. We'd pay a lot more attention to tests like that than we would to LDL tests.

The process of atherosclerosis always involves an errant LDL particle. So maybe you're thinking that lowering the total number of LDL particles with statin drugs does kind of make sense after all. Then there would be less LDL particles around to get into places they don't belong. Sure. But that makes as much sense as trying to reduce forest fires by getting rid of trees.

The LDL particle only lodges in the wrong place *if* there's an irritant or break in the protective arterial wall (the endothelium).

If there's a solution to the problem, it has three essential components: One, we need to reduce our exposure to toxins that create arterial wall injury. Two, we need to keep LDL particles away from where they don't belong. And three, we need to prevent or reduce oxidation and inflammation of those LDL particles and their cholesterol content!

As you can see, this is a complex process that involves a lot more than the general, gross category of "LDL" cholesterol. What's more, LDL cholesterol levels in the blood are highly influenced by receptor activity. There are normal, healthy LDL receptors on

◀ **WHAT YOU NEED TO KNOW**

- Cholesterol travels through the blood in a structure known as a "lipoprotein."
- The lipoproteins are the boats in the water, while cholesterol is one of the passengers.
- The total number of lipoproteins in the blood stream is far more predictive of heart disease than the amount of cholesterol cargo.
- Modern cholesterol testing focuses on the number, size, and patterns of the lipoproteins, not the amount of cholesterol they contain.
- The triglyceride to HDL ratio is one of the most valuable numbers to know when it comes to predicting heart disease (and diabetes!).

cells that will allow LDLs to "park" on the cell and deliver their cargo in a normal, healthy way. But when someone has less LDL receptors, there are less "parking spaces" for the LDL to land in, and hence blood levels of LDL remain higher, regardless of what you eat or how much you exercise.

There is an enzyme that specifically attacks these LDL receptors—it's called PCSK9 (which stands for *Proprotein convertase subtilisin/kexin type 9*, which is why everyone simply refers to it as PCSK9!). Some people have a lot of PCSK9 activity and therefore *less* functioning LDL receptors and therefore *more* LDL traveling in the bloodstream with nowhere to land.

A new class of medicines—PCSK9 inhibitors—are getting a lot of attention since they have been shown to lower LDL.

Whether PCKS9 inhibitors wind up saving lives or just improving LDL lab values remains to be seen. But the very discovery of PCKS9 and the existence of PCKS9 inhibitors demonstrates the lack of simplicity in the relationship between cholesterol and heart disease. It should argue for the retirement of the standard "good" and "bad" cholesterol tests and their replacement with the much more valuable lab tests now available to assess *all* aspects of blood lipids.

EAT THOSE YOLKS! WHY THE CHOLESTEROL YOU EAT DOESN'T MAKE A BIT OF DIFFERENCE TO ANYTHING*

For 99.6 perent of the population, here's the real reason eating cholesterol makes absolutely no difference to your blood test cholesterol.

Cholesterol comes in two forms, unattached and attached. Scientists call cholesterol that has attached itself to another molecule *esterfied*; unattached cholesterol molecules are either *free cholesterol* or, if they were once attached and are now single, *deesterfied cholesterol*.

The body can only use free, or unesterfied, cholesterol. Most of the cholesterol we eat— e.g. in eggs—is esterfied. So in order to be used by the body, we have to first "uncouple" it from whatever it's attached to, a process known as *deesterfication*. And now that deesterfied cholesterol has to compete with the huge amount of ready-to-use *un*esterfied (unattached) cholesterol already being made by your liver and intestines on a daily basis. Which is basically four-fifths of the cholesterol in your body on any given day. Yes, fully 80 percent of the cholesterol in your body does in fact come from your own body—the aforementioned liver being the primary source.

All of which is to say . . . the cholesterol in your diet *just doesn't matter**. And what really rankles about this—and about the fact that most medical doctors don't even *know* it—is that it's been known for decades. For goodness sake, the prime force behind the cholesterol and fat hypothesis, Ancel Keys, knew it all along: *"(T)he cholesterol content, per se, of all natural diets has no significant effect on either the serum cholesterol level or the development of athero-sclerosis in man,"* he wrote in 1954.

Did you hear that? The man who virtually invented the cholesterol theory of heart disease said that the cholesterol you eat doesn't make a whit of difference. And he said it in 1954. We'll let that sink in for a moment.

So if everyone knew eating cholesterol didn't make a whit of difference to blood choles-terol—*"the cholesterol content of all natural diets has no effect,"* said Keys—then why on earth have we been avoiding egg yolks?

The answer is simple. In the opinion of the dietary dictators, making the distinction between cholesterol in the *blood* and cholesterol in the *diet* was just too heavy a lift for the general public, so to simplify the issue for public consumption they demonized cholesterol *in general.*

Better the public should not have to trouble their "pretty little heads" about such compli-cated stuff as the difference between cholesterol *on your plate* and cholesterol *in the blood*, the establishment seemed to be saying. So they told us to avoid all of it.

Or at least they did until 2015. And—like a retraction in the newspapers that's published on page 32 and that nobody reads—the U.S. government quietly noted in the 2015 guidelines that "cholesterol is (no longer) a nutrient of concern for over consumption." (Mention that to your doctor the next time she tells you not to eat eggs!)

*The exception is for the .04 percent of the population with a genetic condition known as familial hypercholesterolemia.

CHAPTER 5

INFLAMMATION AND OXIDATION

INFLAMMATION AND OXIDATION are two of the most vicious processes in the human body. This chapter explains why they are so destructive and what we can do to minimize their damage.

Let's begin with inflammation, which comes in two flavors. We all have experience with *acute* inflammation. It happens every time you stub your toe, bang your knee, or get a splinter in your finger. When you complain about your aching back, an abscess in your mouth, or a rash on your skin, that's acute inflammation. It's visible and uncomfortable, if not downright painful.

The redness on your skin is a result of blood that's rushed to the affected area. The swelling you experience is the result of an army of specialized cells dispatched by the immune system to mend the injured area. The job of these immune system cells is to surround the site of the injury and neutralize nasty invaders such as microbes, preventing the spread of potential infection. The swelling, redness, and soreness you experience as a result of acute inflammation are natural accompaniments to the healing process.

It's the inflammation you're less familiar with that's at the core of heart disease. Acute inflammation hurts, but *chronic* inflammation kills.

Let us explain.

WHY YOU SHOULD CARE ABOUT CHRONIC INFLAMMATION, NOT CHOLESTEROL

Chronic inflammation flies beneath the pain radar. Much like high blood pressure, it has no obvious symptoms. Yet chronic inflammation is a significant component of virtually every single degenerative condition, including Alzheimer's, diabetes, obesity, arthritis, cancer, neurodegenerative diseases, chronic lower respiratory disease, influenza and pneumonia, chronic liver and kidney diseases, and, most especially, heart disease.

When chronic inflammation exists unchecked in the cardiovascular system, it almost always spells big trouble for the heart.

And inflammation is rarely a local phenomenon. For instance, women with rheumatoid arthritis, a highly inflammatory condition that primarily affects the joints, wind up having double the risk of a heart attack when compared to women without it. Microbes that cause problems in one part of the body can easily migrate to other areas and cause inflammatory damage there. An infection that starts in the gums, for example, can easily leak bacteria into the bloodstream; bacteria that may then find fertile ground in a weakened arterial wall and fan the fires of inflammation there.

So how exactly does inflammation happen, and, more importantly, what can we do about it?

OXIDATION: THE FREQUENT INITIATOR OF INFLAMMATION

One of the prime initiators of inflammation is oxidation. If you've ever seen rust on metal, you're familiar with oxidation (also known as oxidative damage), even if you didn't know the technical name for it. You're also familiar with oxidation if you've ever left apple slices out on a picnic table where they were exposed to the air. They turned brown, didn't they? *That's* oxidative damage.

For those of you who don't remember high school chemistry (or would understandably prefer to forget it), electrons travel in pairs and orbit around atoms. Every so often one of those electrons gets "loose," and pandemonium ensues. The atom with the unpaired electron—known as a *free radical*—starts running around like a headless chicken trying to find its head. Free radicals are like college sophomores on spring break—temporarily free from the constraints of dormitory living, they basically go nuts and will "bond" with anyone! Free radicals "hit" on existing, stable pairs of electrons thousands of times a day, trying to find an electron they can pair-bond with, and meanwhile inflicting enormous damage upon your cells and DNA.

The free radicals that come from oxygen (known, not surprisingly, as oxygen free radicals) are the most deadly and damaging kind. *Anti*oxidants are a class of substances, including certain vitamins, minerals, and many plant chemicals, that helps neutralize free radicals, soaking them up like little sponges, thus limiting the damage they can do to your body. The reason cut apple slices don't turn brown so quickly when you squirt lemon juice on them is because lemon juice contains vitamin C, a powerful *anti*oxidant.

Free radicals are so important that in the mid-1950s a scientist named Denham Harman, M.D., Ph.D., put forth a theory called the Free Radical Theory of Aging that remains popular to this day.[1] In it he basically proposes that aging is a kind of "rusting from within," largely due to the damage caused by oxygen free radicals.

Now let's see how inflammation, oxidation, cholesterol, and the arterial walls interact in real life, and how they work together to create a dangerous situation for your heart.

GROUND ZERO FOR DAMAGE: INTRODUCING THE ENDOTHELIUM

The arterial walls are anything but hard and firm. They're composed of smooth muscle that expands and contracts like a mini accordion; they respond to the rhythm of the heart and accommodate the pulsing of the blood. These arteries—far from being a static system of tubes and pipes—are a living, breathing, *very* dynamic organ. And the innermost layer of the artery walls—the "interface," if you will, between the blood inside the arteries and the walls that contain it—is a central player in our little drama.

This layer is called the endothelium—and it's the starting point for the damage that can ultimately lead to a heart attack.

Big word, endothelium, yes, not often bandied about in cocktail party chatter about heart disease, but it's one of the most important places in the arteries for you to know about because *that's* where the damage to your arteries starts. Only always.

The endothelium is just one cell thick, but it's where a tremendous amount of biochemical activity takes place. There's even a name for the pathological state in which damage to that innermost layer exists—it's called *endothelial dysfunction*, and it's a key event in the development of heart disease.

The Good, the Bad, and the Really, Really Ugly!

As of this writing, new research funded by the British Heart Foundation has uncovered still another subtype of LDL cholesterol that is particularly bad. It's called the *MGmin-low-density lipoprotein*, and it's more common in people with type 2 diabetes and in the elderly. It's "stickier" than normal LDL, which makes it much more likely to attach to the walls of the arteries.

This new "ultra-bad" boy is actually created by a process called *glycation*. Glycation happens when there's too much sugar hanging around in the bloodstream. The excess sugar starts gumming up the works, inserting itself in places where it doesn't belong—in this case, the LDL molecule. (We'll have a lot more to say about sugar and its role in heart disease later on in chapter 6. Preview: Sugar is way more of a threat to your heart than fat ever was!)

The point is that there is, indeed, "bad" cholesterol—even "*ultra*-bad" cholesterol—but we're not accomplishing anything by using a shotgun pharmaceutical approach that lowers *total* cholesterol. We need to get into the weeds and figure out what exactly is causing any damage, and we now have sophisticated tools to do just that. The old approach is akin to clipping a hangnail with an axe—and what's more, the old approach has significant unwanted side effects, as we will see in chapter 8.

It's also—as we hope you'll be convinced—an awful lot of effort focused on the wrong molecule. As one of us (Jonny) said on the *Dr. Oz Show* after the first edition of this book came out, "Trying to prevent heart disease by lowering cholesterol is like trying to prevent obesity by taking the lettuce off your whoppers."

WHEN LDL *REALLY* IS BAD FOR YOU: THE SMOKER'S PARADOX

Riddle us this: Why is it that smokers with *normal* LDL (the so-called "bad" cholesterol) levels have a much higher risk of heart disease than nonsmokers with elevated LDL levels?

Sure, we all know how cigarette smoke damages the lungs, and that cigarette smoking significantly increases the odds of getting lung cancer. But, really, what's the connection between smoking and heart disease, or, more specifically, between smoking and LDL cholesterol?

Glad you asked.

Besides the harsh smoke, cigarettes also graciously provide your body with myriad toxic chemicals, all at no extra charge, thank you very much. These chemicals and toxins both constrict the blood vessels and harm the arterial walls. Specifically, they cause your LDL to become oxidized—damaged by the free radicals that are found in abundance in cigarette smoke! (And, by the way, it's not just cigarette smoke that can oxidize LDL. Heavy metals like mercury can do it, as can insecticides, radiation, and all manner of toxins in the environment, the air, and the food supply.)

And listen carefully now: LDL is not really a problem in the body *until* it becomes oxidized. Only oxidized (damaged) LDL gets under the arterial walls starting a whole inflammatory process that ultimately winds up creating plaque while causing further inflammation and injury. It's almost always damaged little oxidized lipoproteins that manage to slip through vulnerable sections of the endothelium, like unruly teenagers sneaking through an unguarded gate to get into a concert.

Once those rogue particles set up residence, they're like a molecular "tent city," creating even more inflammation and oxidation. Meanwhile, non-oxidized LDL is pretty much harmless, just traveling through the bloodstream minding its own business. It's *oxidation*—and its partner in crime, inflammation—that actually initiates the process that culminates in atherosclerosis.

So now it should be clear exactly why smoking turbo-charges the risk for heart disease. Smoking is equivalent to taking a blowtorch to your LDL. A smoker with a low amount of LDL, most of which has been damaged by oxidation, is at far greater risk for heart disease than a *non*smoker with a much *higher* level of LDL, only a tiny percentage of which has been damaged. It's not the LDL that causes the problem—it's *damaged* (oxidized) LDL. And nothing reliably damages your LDL like hot smoke, especially from cigarettes, which—besides nicotine—deliver a vast array of damaging and carcinogenic chemicals.

So LDL floats around in the bloodstream, delivering cholesterol to the cells that need it, and some of this LDL, the LDL that's damaged by oxidation, infiltrates the endothelium. Once the endothelium becomes infiltrated with this damaged LDL, the process of inflammation begins in earnest.

Remember our earlier discussion about harmless "bad" cholesterol (LDL pattern A) and dangerous "bad" cholesterol (LDL pattern B)? Well, one of the reasons *why* pattern B molecules (those BB gun pellet types) are so bad is that *they* are the ones most likely to be damaged and most likely to be oxidized. On top of that, they're small enough to penetrate the arterial walls in the first place. The smaller the particles (and pattern B particles are small indeed), the more inflammatory they are. Oxidized LDL is like "angry" LDL, and the smaller the particle, the angrier it is. So these nasty little damaged LDL particles stick to the endothelium and begin the process of inflammation. In the presence of oxidative damage—or in the presence of high blood sugar, which is such an important initiator of damage that we'll examine it separately in chapter 6—this LDL experiences chemical changes that the immune system perceives as dangerous.

Once the immune system notices this damaged (oxidized) LDL, it sends in the heavy artillery. First, cells known as *monocytes* rush to the scene of the action, releasing chemicals called *cytokines*. Cytokines are essentially chemical messengers that help regulate the immune system response, but many of these cytokines are themselves highly inflammatory. In the presence of some of these cytokines, the lining of the blood vessels (the endothelium) secrete sticky little molecules called *adhesion molecules* that act like molecular glue, grabbing on to the monocytes that have rushed to the scene of the crime to help put out the fire.

Heart surgeon Dwight Lundell, M.D., cleverly refers to this as the "Velcro effect."

Monocytes now convert into a type of cell we like to call "Little Ms. Pac-Man." They're technically called *macrophages*, and their job, much like Ms. Pac-Man in the video game, is to eat up the enemy, in this case the damaged LDL particles and other molecular junk that have caused the problem in the first place. (The word macrophage literally means "big eater.")

The macrophages are like sugar addicts at a pie-eating contest. They have no off button; they'll keep eating, consuming oxidized LDL until they literally choke to death, leaving something called the *lipid core* of plaque. Once they reach a certain size they start to look like foam and actually become what pathologists call "foam cells," living cells that will continue the work of the macrophages, fighting and consuming until the "invader" is gone.

But it isn't an invader that sets them off. It's just plain old LDL experiencing chemical changes from sugar, starches, or oxidation and thus initiating an inflammatory process that can easily become an out-of-control "fire" within your arterial walls. As we've said, without inflammation, it's pretty irrelevant what your cholesterol levels are.

If inflammation isn't halted and if macrophages continue to feast away until they bust, they'll release a whole new set of toxins into the walls of the artery.

"We can see this in surgery as a yellow streak inside the artery wall," said Dwight Lundell, M.D., who has performed more than five thousand heart surgeries. "It is called the 'fatty streak,' and it is the beginning of significant heart disease."[2]

The body tries to contain this fatty streak by building a wall to hold it in—scarring is an example. But the immune system is now on full alert; it sends more soldiers to the front, and they try valiantly to break down the wall (the scar tissue), and the cycle continues—more scarring, more soldiers. Over time, if the body's immune system defenses are good enough, they will weaken the wall of the artery and literally "chew through" the scar tissue. A rupture will occur, resulting in more inflammation, and the potentially deadly cycle continues.

Not good news.

If the cycle is not stopped, the fatty streak grows into what's known as plaque. (Plaque is basically a big old collection of foam cells). Some foam cells will die, and they will release a whole bunch of the accumulated fats (lipids), which in turn develop into the aforementioned lipid core, a soft, yellowy substance that resembles melted butter (but isn't nearly as good for you).

Now if you stop the inflammation at this point in time, the artery heals itself with what's called a *fibrous cap*. The fibrous cap is composed of fibrous scar tissue and will stay nice and stable. (Cardiologists like Steve call this "stable plaque.") Of course, if there's new inflammation, the cycle begins all over again.

So the more inflammation continues, the more foam cells accumulate. This means more macrophages (Ms. Pac-Man), which in turn means more oozy, slimy *lipid core*. This lipid core gets into the bloodstream, where the blood immediately puts out a signal saying, "What the heck is this? Foreign object! Foreign object!" And a blood clot is formed in an attempt to keep this foreign, gooey substance from spreading.

So the blood clot is actually a protective mechanism. It's the blood's—or the body's, if you prefer—way of saying, "Let's contain this threat and keep it from spreading!" But though this strategy makes sense, it has a big downside. That blood clot may block access

◀ WHAT YOU NEED TO KNOW

- Cholesterol is the parent molecule for sex hormones (estrogen, progesterone, and testosterone) as well as for vitamin D and the bile acids needed for digestion. You need cholesterol for life.
- Atherosclerosis begins when a rogue particle of LDL (low-density lipoprotein) gets through a weakened section of the arterial wall and parks itself there, beginning the process of inflammation.
- Inflammation is initiated by damage from rogue molecules known as *free radicals*. This damage is also known as *oxidation* or *oxidative stress*. Antioxidants help fight this damage.
- Cholesterol is only a problem when it's damaged by oxidation and inflammation.
- There are at least thirteen subtypes of LDL ("bad") cholesterol and ten subtypes of HDL ("good") cholesterol.[2] Total particle number is far more important than "LDL."
- A total cholesterol level of 160 mg/dL or less has been linked to depression, aggression, cerebral hemorrhages, and loss of sex drive. So don't be "happy" that your cholesterol is that low.

to the heart muscle, preventing oxygen from getting through. Anytime you deprive cells of oxygen, the tissue they make begins to die. And when that tissue is the muscle of the heart, you're looking at—you guessed it—a heart attack.

So overall, LDL can be likened to trees in a forest. A forest that has tons of trees but gets plenty of rain isn't likely to be the site of a wildfire, but a forest with far fewer trees can be a tinder box just waiting to ignite if all those trees are dried up (damaged) and there's very little rainfall! Getting rid of the trees is surely *one* crude way to prevent forest fires, just as lowering cholesterol indiscriminately might theoretically decrease the risk of a "fire" in your artery walls, but at what cost? Those trees serve a lot of ecological purposes, and removing them is hardly without consequences, both to the environment and to the landscape.

Wouldn't it be better to reduce the conditions under which a fire is likely to break out? That way we could have all the wonderful benefits of trees with none of the side effects of a compromised ecology.

We hope we've convinced you that inflammation, and its main initiator, oxidation, are at the core of heart disease. But inflammation and oxidation aren't the only vicious foot soldiers causing heart disease. Now in chapter 9, we'll lay out the case for why *insulin resistance* is often the earliest sign of impending heart disease and can be picked up way earlier than late-stage signs like elevated markers of inflamma-

WHAT THE FRAMINGHAM HEART STUDY FOUND

Want a much better way to tell whether you're at risk? Look at these two line items on your blood test: triglycerides and HDL (the so-called "good" cholesterol).

Now if you're not too freaked out about doing a bit of math, calculate the ratio of your triglycerides to your HDL. Just divide your triglyceride number by your HDL number. If, for example, your triglycerides are 150 mg/dL and your HDL is 50 mg/dL, you have a ratio of 3 (150:50). If your triglycerides are 100 mg/dL and your HDL is 50 mg/dL, you have a ratio of 2 (100:50).

(If your triglycerides are smaller than your HDL and you get a ratio of less than one, you can pretty much stop reading this book right now. Your risk factor is off-the-charts low.

The triglyceride to HDL ratio is a far better predictor of heart disease than cholesterol ever was. In one study out of Harvard published in *Circulation*, a journal published by the American Heart Association, those who had the highest triglyceride to HDL ratios had a whopping sixteen times the risk of developing heart disease as those with the lowest ratios.[3]

If you have a ratio of around 2, you should be happy, indeed, regardless of your cholesterol levels. (A ratio of 5, however, is problematic.)

tion, elevated blood sugar, and out-of-range blood lipids. Spoiler alert: We'll also tell you how to catch insulin resistance early, and how easy it is to correct without drugs!

But first let's introduce you to a "food" that is a far, far greater risk to your overall health—and specifically to your heart—than fat ever was. This "food"—in all its many forms—is also one of the biggest causes of insulin resistance, which, as you'll see in chapter 6, is the Godfather of the whole operation. We're talking about *sugar.*

FOR MEN ONLY

Note to the men reading this: Endothelial dysfunction has the same acronym (ED) as another condition you may be familiar with or concerned about: erectile dysfunction. They're not unrelated. Our friend Mark Houston, M.D., director of the Hypertension Institute and an associate professor of medicine at Vanderbilt University, wryly commented, "I've never seen someone with a case of ED (erectile dysfunction) that didn't also have ED (endothelial dysfunction)."

Bottom line: A healthy functioning endothelium is essential for . . . well, more things than just the heart!

PART TWO

In part two, we're going tackle three of the most important players on the heart disease playing field: sugar, fat, and statins. We're going to make the case that fat—including saturated fat—has been wrongly demonized by the dietary dictators, while sugar—largely due to the superb efforts of the sugar lobby—has been given a pass. Beginning on page 62 we'll show you compelling evidence from neuroscience that confirm what you may have suspected all along—sugar is indeed addictive. Meanwhile, as we will also show you, that addictive substance is the driving force behind diabetes.

And the thesis of this book is that diabetes is a train stop on the journey to heart disease. Sadly, it's a train most people don't know they're on until it's too late. You can get off that train before it reaches its inevitable destination, but that means looking carefully for signs that you're headed in the wrong direction. One of the most important signs to look for is insulin resistance. (More on that in a moment.)

If you're wondering why we're spending so much time on sugar and fat, it's because sugar has a great press agent. We all love it, accept it as part of the American experience, associated with wonderful things like holidays and birthdays and breakfast cereals and cookies, and it's going to take a lot of work to break through those associations and see the real toll it's taken on our health. Similarly, we've demonized fat for so long that we can barely utter the term "saturated fat" without prefacing it with "artery-clogging." Deconstructing the mythology about fats is no small task, and it's why we tried to make the case we did as meticulously as possible.

Which brings us back to insulin resistance. Once you demystify fat and sugar you can see their actual roles in metabolic dysfunction. Insulin resistance is most frequently the result of too many carbs, specifically sugar and processed grains. It's *not* the result of too much fat. And insulin resistance nearly always leads to pre-diabetes, which leads to diabetes, which leads—as you'll see in chapter 9—to heart disease.

In chapter 9 of this section, we will lay out the case that insulin resistance is the first sign of heart disease and that it "shows up" (i.e., is measurable) as much as a decade before you or your doctor notices that anything is "wrong."

And speaking of something being wrong, part two also discusses statin drugs, the number one medication for high cholesterol. We hope that by the time you finish this section of the book you will be convinced that treating "high cholesterol" is very different from treating heart disease. And that the trend to prescribe statins for large swathes of the population who are unlikely to benefit from them is a foolish strategy that will benefit no one but stockholders in Big Pharma.

Let's begin our story by discussing a substance that—as of this writing—we consume to the tune of an eye-popping 152 pounds of a year, *per person*.[1] That innocent-looking white powder known as sugar.

CHAPTER 6

SUGAR: THE REAL DEMON IN THE DIET

SUGAR—ESPECIALLY IN THE CONTEXT OF THE MODERN INDUSTRIALIZED DIET—is a far greater danger to your heart than fat ever was.

In this chapter, we are going to venture into the labyrinth-like worlds of endocrinology and neuro-science. But relax! We promise not to make your eyes glaze over. And we promise that by the time you finish this chapter you will know more than many doctors do about the common link among heart disease, diabetes, obesity, and hypertension—serious conditions that are of interest to most readers.

And we believe you'll come to the same conclusion we have: The smoking gun points at the hyper-processed, sugar-laden foods that dominate our modern diets'—foods that manipulate our hormones and trick our delicate brains. It's not a conspiracy theory. It's not a *Twilight Zone* episode. It's *science*, plain and simple.

ENDOCRINOLOGY 101: THE HORMONAL EFFECT OF FOOD

Our journey starts with a simple premise: Hormones control almost every metabolic event that goes on in your body. And *you* control some of the most critical hormones through your lifestyle.

But you don't have to be a slave to those hormones; you just have to understand them. Because your lifestyle choices have a profound effect on the secretion of important hormones, and lifestyle choices are under your control (see chapter 12). Nonetheless, at the end of the day, your hormones drive a big part of your behavior. (And almost 100 percent of your cravings!)

Food—along with several key lifestyle factors such as stress—is the trigger that stimulates hormones. Those hormones direct the body to store or burn fat, just as they direct the body to perform a gazillion other metabolic operations. Meanwhile, our brain's reward centers—complex neural systems that tell us to keep doing things that feel good and to stop doing things that feel bad—dictate what it is we even *want* to eat. And certain foods can make those systems go haywire—sugar being one of the most notorious offenders. We'll return to this stuff a bit later.

"Food may be the most powerful drug you will ever encounter because it causes dramatic changes in your hormones that are hundreds of times more powerful than any pharmaceutical," said Barry Sears, Ph.D., the author of *The Zone Diet*. Hormones are the air traffic controllers that determine the fate of whatever flies in (or in our case, "slides" in through the gullet!).

This fact has been conveniently ignored by many mainstream dietitians and doctors. The standard message to overweight people at increased risk for heart disease is to simply reduce calories and saturated fat. But in the real world, it's not so simple. Some foods influence our body's metabolic systems in ways that override our hunger signals and boost levels of hormones that *store* fat. Not coincidentally, our main fat-storing hormone also has some serious consequences for the heart.

The name of that fat-storing hormone? Insulin.

INSULIN: WHAT IT IS AND WHY IT MATTERS

Insulin, a hormone first discovered in 1921, is the star actor in our little hormonal play. It is an anabolic hormone, which means it is responsible for building things up—putting compounds like glucose (sugar and amino acids) inside storage units (such as cells). Its sister hormone, glucagon, is responsible for breaking things down—opening those storage units and releasing their contents as needed. Insulin is responsible for *saving*; glucagon is responsible for *spending*.

Together their main job is to maintain blood sugar levels within the tightly regulated range it needs to be to keep your metabolic machinery running smoothly.

Insulin is at the hub of a significant number of diseases of civilization. When you control insulin, you reduce the risk for heart disease and the risk for hypertension, diabetes, polycystic ovary syndrome, inflammatory diseases, and even, possibly, cancer.

Did that get your attention? We hope so.

Both insulin and glucagon are essential to health. It's almost impossible to overstate the importance of this. Without insulin, blood sugar would skyrocket, and the result would be coma and death: the fate of virtually every type 1 diabetic in the early part of the twentieth century before the discovery of insulin. However, without glucagon, blood sugar would plummet, and the result would be brain dysfunction, coma, and death.

So the body knows what it's doing. This little dance between the force that keeps blood sugar from soaring too *high* (insulin) and the forces that prevent it from going too *low* (glucagon, for one) is essential for survival. It's interesting to note that although insulin is the only hormone responsible for preventing blood sugar from rising too high, there are several other hormones besides glucagon—cortisol, adrenaline, noradrenaline, and human growth hormone—that prevent it from going too low. You could say that insulin is such a powerful hormone that it needs five other hormones just to counterbalance its effects!

In fact, as you'll see a bit later on in the book, when insulin metabolism is off the rails—a condition known as *insulin resistance*—it's an early warning sign that something is going very, very wrong. In chapter 9, we'll explore in great detail the relationship of insulin resistance to heart disease. Spoiler alert: We're going to make the case that insulin resistance is one of the most important—and earliest—signs of coming heart disease.

Let's begin by looking at the stunning example of how insulin influences the cardiovascular system: blood pressure.

Insulin Resistance and High Blood Pressure

High levels of insulin will increase your blood pressure in a couple of ways. For one thing, insulin can narrow the artery walls. Narrower walls translate into higher blood pressure because a harder pumping action is required to get the blood through the narrower passageways.

But there's an even more insidious way in which insulin raises blood pressure.

It talks to the kidneys.

Insulin's message to the kidneys is this: *Hold on to salt.* Insulin makes the kidneys do this even if the kidneys would much prefer not to. Because the body controls sodium within a tight range, as it does sugar, the kidneys figure, "Listen, if we have to hold on to all this salt, we'd better bring on more water to dilute it so that it stays in the safe range." And that's exactly what they do. Increased sodium retention results in increased water retention. More water means more blood volume, and more blood volume means higher blood pressure. Fully 70 percent of people with hypertension (high blood pressure) have insulin resistance.[1]

And this is not just theoretical. Research from Wake Forest Baptist Medical Center[2] demonstrates that insulin resistance is *directly* related to high blood pressure. "We found you can predict who's at higher risk for developing high blood pressure based on their insulin resistance," said lead researcher David Goff Jr., Ph.D., M.D. "The one-third of participants [in our study] with the highest levels of insulin resistance had rates of hypertension that were 35 percent higher than the one-third with the least resistance. These findings point out that *reducing the body's resistance to insulin may help prevent hypertension and cardiovascular disease*"[3] (emphasis ours).

The Insulin-Cholesterol Connection

Interesting factoid: Insulin has a profound effect on cholesterol as well. It turns up the cholesterol-making machinery by turbocharging the activity of the enzyme that actually controls the cholesterol-manufacturing machinery in your body. This enzyme—with the unwieldy name of HMG-CoA reductase—is the very same enzyme that's shut down by cholesterol-lowering drugs! You could probably lower your cholesterol—if you still care about that—by simply lowering your insulin levels. And doing so would have none of the side effects of cholesterol-lowering medication, unless you call a longer life span and better health side effects!

By the way, we're not kidding about the "longer life span and better health" part. A classic 1992 study examined the blood work of healthy centenarians in an effort to find out whether there were any commonalities among the members of this unusually long-lived demographic. It found three: low triglycerides, high HDL cholesterol, and—wait for it—low fasting insulin.[4] Your diet affects two of these blood measures—triglycerides and fasting insulin—and both measures will fall like a rock when you reduce or eliminate sugar and processed carbs in your diet.

Remember—the body makes triglycerides out of excess calories from carbohydrates. It's not important to know how the biochemistry of this works; it's just important to know that too much sugar equals high triglycerides (not to mention high fasting insulin). It's hard to change your HDL, but you can significantly improve two out of three measures of longevity—triglycerides and insulin—just by reducing carbs!

In our opinion, lowering triglycerides is one of the major health benefits of a diet lower in sugar, as high triglycerides are far more of a danger sign for heart disease than high cholesterol is.

Beginning to connect the dots?

"Normally, insulin has some fairly positive effects on the body, such as being anti-inflammatory," says Jeff Volek, Ph.D., R.D., one of the top researchers in the field of diet and health.[5] "But if you're insulin resistant, chronically high insulin levels have the opposite effect. They actually promote inflammation and cardiovascular problems. That's not generally appreciated yet; what is well accepted is that high glucose (blood sugar) will cause problems over time."[6]

So insulin is *anti*-inflammatory in people with normal insulin sensitivity, but it is *highly* inflammatory in those with insulin resistance. Which is more than 50 percent of the population, and that's a conservative estimate based on crude measurements. We suspect that if insulin resistance was measured in a state-of-the-art way, such as with LabCorp's LP-IR test, the number would be significantly higher.

Insulin Resistance and Heart Disease

Having insulin resistance is a tsunami when it comes to developing heart disease. Insulin resistance makes it more likely you'll have hypertension, puts you at significantly greater risk for diabetes, is almost certainly correlated with elevated triglycerides, and is heavily correlated with obesity—all major risk factors for cardiovascular disease. But to add insult to injury, that excess insulin has an inflammatory effect on your system as well. As we've seen, inflammation is a major player in the development of plaque, and a far more important risk factor for heart disease than cholesterol is.

If you have any degree of insulin resistance, controlling your insulin by dietary means may be one of the most effective strategies for reducing the risk of coronary disease. It certainly beats the fairly irrele-

The collection of diseases strongly influenced by insulin resistance has been given the acronym CHAOS: coronary disease, hypertension, adult onset diabetes, obesity, and stroke. They're all related, and what they have in common is insulin resistance.

vant strategy of lowering cholesterol!

"[H]aving chronically elevated insulin levels has harmful effects of its own—heart disease for one," Gary Taubes wrote in the *New York Times*.[7] Elevated insulin increases triglycerides, raises blood pressure, and lowers HDL cholesterol—all making insulin resistance even worse and substantially upping the risk for heart disease.

At this point you may be wondering, "How do I know if I have insulin resistance?" An excellent question. Though there are blood measures to determine this—and we'll discuss those later on—there's also a nice, simple, low-tech way to do it. Stand in front of a wall and walk toward it. If your belly touches the wall before the rest of your body, there's an excellent chance that you're insulin resistant. Men with waist sizes of 40 inches or more are almost certainly insulin resistant, as are women with waist sizes of 35 inches or more.

Although there are, indeed, people with insulin resistance who are rail thin, the vast majority of people with insulin resistance are not. We'll talk about other ways to measure insulin resistance through scientifically validated blood tests later on in this book, but the "walk-into-the-wall" way is a good stand-in for now.

Insulin resistance is reversible. And it's hardly a rare phenomenon. The prevalence of insulin resis-

tance has skyrocketed 61 percent in the past decade alone, according to Daniel Einhorn, M.D., medical director of the Scripps Whittier Diabetes Institute in California.[8] The prevalence of insulin resistance has probably been underestimated from the beginning.

The late great scientist Gerald Reaven of Stanford University—whom you'll be learning more about in chapter 9—did the original work on insulin resistance in the 1980s. Here's how he approximated the number of people who were insulin resistant. He divided his test population—nondiabetic, healthy adults—into quartiles and tested their ability to metabolize sugar and carbohydrates. He found that while the top 25 percent of the population could handle sugar just fine, the bottom 25 percent could not—they had insulin resistance (or, in the parlance of researchers, impaired glucose metabolism). So for a long time, it was thought that the number of people with insulin resistance was one in four (25 percent).

But there's a problem.

What happened to the 50 percent of people *between* those two extremes? It turns out they had neither the terrific glucose metabolism of the top 25 percent nor the full-blown insulin resistance of the bottom 25 percent; instead, they fell somewhere in between.

One could easily argue that because only 25 per-

Stand in front of a wall and walk toward it.
If your belly touches the wall before the rest of your body,
there's an excellent chance that you're insulin resistant.

cent of the population had flawless glucose metabolism, the rest of us—up to 75 percent of the population—had *some* degree of insulin resistance! Also, Reaven used young, healthy adults as subjects, and their numbers were definitely not representative of the population as a whole—the fact is, sensitivity to insulin actually *decreases* (and insulin resistance *increases*) as you get older.

The take-home point: Insulin resistance isn't just something that happens to other people. The American Association of Clinical Endocrinologists has estimated that one in three Americans is insulin resistant,[9] and a fair amount of emerging research indicates that the number is quite a bit higher, as you'll see later in the book.

Back in chapter 4 we mentioned that calculating your ratio of triglycerides to HDL cholesterol is a much better way to predict heart disease than by assessing cholesterol levels. (Just so you don't have to go back and look it up: You calculate your ratio by simply looking at two line items on your blood test—triglycerides and HDL cholesterol. If, for example, your triglycerides are 150 mg/dL and your HDL cholesterol is 30 mg/dL, your ratio is 150 divided by 30, or five.) As it turns out, this same ratio is an excellent predictor of insulin resistance. In one study, a ratio of three or greater was a reliable predictor of insulin resistance.[10]

The higher your triglycerides, the greater the chance that you're insulin resistant. This in turn means that insulin is contributing mightily to the very inflammation that damages LDL cholesterol in the first place and starts the whole cycle of plaque formation. The take-home point: Reduce your triglycerides (and raise your HDL), and you reduce your risk of heart disease.

Lowering your sugar intake probably won't affect your HDL level, but it will dramatically affect triglycerides and fasting insulin. And both of these will certainly drop when you lower the amount of sugar and processed carbs you're eating (or drinking).

The bottom line here is that changing your diet can really change your life. No kidding. This is not just theoretical or pie-in-the-sky. A change in diet and a few important lifestyle changes—as outlined in part three of this book—can make the difference between a life of energy, vigor, and health, and a life of constant doctor appointments, weight problems, and diabetes medications.

THE TWINKIE PARADOX

In 2010, Mark Haub—a nutrition professor from Kansas State University—made headlines with what seemed like a kamikaze diet experiment: He spent ten weeks eating a steady stream of Twinkies—one every three hours, to be exact—along with Oreos, Doritos, sugary cereals, and a variety of Little Debbie's snack cakes. To make the diet somewhat less death defying, he also threw in a multivitamin supplement, a daily protein shake, and the odd can of green beans or celery stalks.

The only stipulation was a cap on his calorie intake—1800 a day.

Given what you've learned in this book so far, you might suspect the results were disastrous. Surely his triglycerides shot through the stratosphere. And if he somehow didn't gain weight, he certainly didn't lose any. That tidal wave of sugar probably exhausted his pancreas and turned him insulin resistant in record speed!

But that's not what happened.

In what came to be known as the "Twinkie diet," Haub dropped 27 pounds, raised his HDL by 20 percent, slashed his LDL by 20 percent, lowered his triglycerides by 39 percent, and reduced his body fat from over 33 percent to just shy of 25 percent.

In other words, he seemed—on paper—to have gotten healthier.

Eating a diet literally made of sugary junk food.

The very stuff we've been telling you to avoid like the plague.

In attempt to explain these shocking results, dieticians near and far chimed in. "A calorie is a calorie!" roared the conventional wisdom devotees. The take-home message, many believed, was that it's all about calories in versus calories out. Whether your calories come from a grilled chicken salad or a cream-filled pastry doesn't matter, as long as you're burning off more than you eat each day, or so claim the advo-

cates of the "energy balance" theory.

But is that really the case?

This brings us to one of the biggest problems with weight-loss studies of any sort—especially ones that simultaneously try to assess the effects of sugar. For most people, shedding pounds alone is enough to improve their blood lipids. And the reasons for that are plentiful. For one, losing weight inevitably causes some fat loss from the organs—and once enough fat slurps out of the pancreas and liver, insulin sensitivity improves and a whole host of benefits quickly follow.

A fascinating study from 2015 found that losing less than *one gram* of fat from the pancreas was enough to reverse type 2 diabetes.[11] On top of that, staying in a negative energy balance—that is, consuming fewer calories than you burn each day—ensures liver and glycogen stores get a chance to empty out, which *also* boosts insulin sensitivity.

If you're starting to sense a theme here, you're right. Spoiler alert: Notice that just about everything that *reduces* risk for cardiovascular events also *reduces* insulin resistance, and anything that *increases* risk for cardiovascular events also seems to *increase* insulin resistance. We'll look at this connection—possibly the most important take-home point in the book—in much greater detail when we get to chapter 9.

Researchers have also discovered that weight loss significantly raises our circulating levels of *adiponectin*—a protein hormone that helps regulate our blood sugar and improves lipid metabolism, which can improve the numbers on our blood test and our ability to handle high-carb foods.

In other words, weight loss—when we have some to lose—can improve a number of health markers, regardless of what we're eating.

And that means we can't trust weight-loss studies to tell us about the effects of sugar during non-weight-loss situations. Indeed, the *real* issue is what happens when we stop dropping pounds and try to maintain what we've got. If Haub kept up his Twinkie diet after he was done losing weight, the results, most assuredly, would have been much different.

An aside: One of us—Jonny—was a personal trainer on staff at Equinox Fitness Clubs for many years during the 1990s. During that time, he saw a lot of people lose weight successfully on what trainers then privately referred to as "the model's diet: cocaine, coffee, and an occasional salad." Weight loss in the short term is not a good measure of overall health, and certainly isn't a good predictor of long-term success, or else everyone would just eat Twinkies for a month like Haub did and be just fine. Jonny had an exercise physiology professor in graduate school who used to say: "Losing weight by itself is easy. I can take any client in the world and put them in a closet for a month with just a tube for water. I guarantee they'll lose weight. But so what?"

That said, some folks—especially those in the "everything in moderation" camp—have argued that if we just keep a tight lockdown on our calories, then sugary foods can be a harmless addition to a "well-balanced diet." Such proponents often point to examples like Mr. Haub and his Twinkies as evidence that all calories are more or less equal; we can just count them and be on our merry way.

But there's a problem here. You see, the whole thing's a perverse Catch-22: Sugar might be somewhat less harmful if we strictly moderate our intake (and better yet, are losing weight at the same time), but sugar also makes it just about impossible to actually *do* that. And the reason has to do with what's going on in your noggin.

MEANWHILE, UP IN THE BRAIN . . .

We've covered plenty on the endocrinology front so far. (Hopefully we kept our promise and your eyes didn't glaze over.) But sugar's effects don't end with its effect on hormones. The flip side of sugar's impact on our hormones is its impact on our brain.

If you'll recall, our bodies come equipped with a reward system—a feedback network that tells us what we do or don't like. As far as survival is concerned, this reward system does us all sorts of favors: It tells us to seek out food (because eating feels good), to reproduce (because sex feels good), to form connections in our community (because socializing feels good), and so on.

The problem is that our modern environment—especially our modern food environment—exposes us to all sorts of stuff our delicate reward centers aren't equipped to handle. This includes many substances unanimously deemed addictive—tobacco and opiates, for example—but research is increasingly showing that it also includes certain foods. And guess what? Of all the "foods" with addictive potential, sugar is number one with a bullet.

Hyperpalatability: When Food Becomes a Drug

You've probably heard the phrase "let food be thy medicine," credited to our ancient Greek friend Hippocrates—but what about "let food be thy hopelessly addictive drug"?

It turns out, that second phrase isn't far from the truth. At least when it comes to stuff chemically designed to get us hooked. For decades, food industry scientists have been engineering foods to be "hyper-palatable"—that is, they've been purposefully designed to trigger your brain's reward centers in ways that surpass anything a peach, an egg, or chuck roast could ever accomplish. (For a superb and detailed explanation of how the food industry accomplishes this, read Pulitzer Prize-winning journalist Michael Moss's excellent book, *Salt Sugar Fat: How the Food Giants Hooked Us*.)

By mixing together more salt, more fat, more fla-vorings, and—importantly—more sugar than any food in nature could possibly produce, they've created products that virtually light up the dopamine and opi-oid pathways in our brain. Those are the very same pathways activated by recreational drugs. Indeed, some research has shown that sugary foods have an even more intense effect on the brain's reward path-ways than cocaine.

Certain combinations of ingredients signal our brains to eat, and eat, and eat some more. This isn't the same as a food being delicious and flavorful, by the way: you can feel compelled to overeat on foods you don't even like all that much, but be perfectly content in moderating foods you love. That's why you can relish a perfectly seasoned salmon filet and stop when you're full, but might find yourself unwrapping bar after bar of cheap Halloween candy until you have a stomachache.

Reams of studies have confirmed the addictive nature of sugar. In animals, sporadic access to sugary mixtures results in behaviors resembling that of drug addiction—binging, withdrawal (including anxiety and depression), and cravings.[12]

Recently, scientists have discovered that our reward systems contain glucose-sensing neurons that respond to sugar intake. While a naturally sweet food, like an apple or melon, creates a healthy level of "reward" stimulation, foods with hyper-condensed sweetness—say, a piece of candy—send our reward path-ways into a tizzy, triggering biological compensations that, over time, result in tolerance. Eventually, we need to eat *more* just to feel the same level of pleasure.[13]

Here's where it gets even more fascinating. On its own, sugar isn't a particularly "rewarding" food. Think about it: When was the last time you ripped opened a bag of pure sugar and went to town with nothing other than a spoon and your appetite? Unless you lost a bet, you've probably never even been tempted. Part of the confusion surrounding sugar's addictive properties is the fact that it's a much different animal when it's flying solo than it is when it's hanging out with the wrong crowd. Straight out of the bag—sans flavorings, fat, starches, or salt—sugar doesn't trip our reward pathways as intensely as when we add it to something else. But once we mix it with other tasty items—fat and salt, for example—all bets are off.

As a result, sugar has long been the food indus-try's secret weapon for getting us hooked.

Bottom line? Don't let anyone trick you into think-ing sugar is fine as long as you don't eat too much. "Just a little sugar" might not do as much damage as eating a ton of it—but the caveat is, most of us can't ever stop at "just a little." And for that, we have our brains to thank.

SUGAR: CAUGHT AT THE SCENE OF THE CRIME

We're pretty sure that if you asked a random sampling of ordinary people what part of their diet is most dangerous to their heart, the majority of them would say "fat."

They'd be wrong.

A far more powerful contributor to heart disease is sugar. (And, of course, the insulin resistance that can results from eating too much of it!) Diets that are lower in sugar and processed carbs will reduce inflammation, blood sugar, insulin, insulin resistance, *and* triglycerides. And lowering triglycerides automatically improves that all-important ratio of triglycerides to HDL. (If your triglycerides were 150 mg/dL and your HDL was 50 mg/dL, you'd have a ratio of three, but if you brought your triglycerides down to 100 mg/dL, the ratio would automatically drop to two, or 100:50. Neat, huh?)

Sugar is directly responsible for one of the most damaging processes in the body, something called *glycation*. Here's how it works. Glycation is what happens when sticky sugar molecules glom onto structures and get stuck where they don't belong, essentially gumming up the works.

You see, sugar is sticky—think cotton candy and maple syrup. Proteins, on the other hand, are smooth and slippery—think egg whites, which are pure protein. The slippery nature of proteins lets them slide around easily in the cells and do their jobs effectively. But when you've got a lot of excess sugar in your system, it keeps bumping into proteins, ultimately getting stuck onto the protein molecules. Such proteins are now said to have become *glycated*.

Glycated proteins are too big and sticky to get through small blood vessels and capillaries, including the small vessels in the kidneys, eyes, and feet, which is why so many diabetics are at risk for kidney disease, vision problems, and amputations of toes, feet, and even legs. The sugar-coated proteins become toxic and make the cell machinery run less efficiently. They damage the body and exhaust the immune system. Scientists have given these sticky proteins the acronym AGEs—which stands for *advanced glycation end products*—partially because these proteins are so involved in aging the body.

What does this have to do with cholesterol and heart disease? Actually, everything. Remember LDL cholesterol is a far greater problem once it becomes damaged. And one primary way in which LDL cholesterol gets damaged is through oxidative stress generated by free radicals.

Can you guess the other way it gets damaged? Glycation.

So now you have sugar at the scene of several crimes, all related to heart disease. "High blood sugar causes the lining cells of the arteries to be inflamed, changes LDL cholesterol, and causes sugar to be attached to a variety of proteins, which changes their normal function," says Dwight Lundell, M.D., author of *The Cure for Heart Disease*. High sugar intake, as we saw, also trains our brain's reward centers to make us eat more and more of it—leading to a buildup of fat around the pancreas and subsequently insulin resistance, the central player in every condition we've examined that is intimately connected to heart disease: diabetes, obesity, high blood pressure, and metabolic syndrome.

Is it any surprise that we think reducing sugar is far more important than reducing fat or cholesterol? And by the way, we're hardly the first people to say so.

The Voice of Dissent: Introducing John Yudkin

By 1970, Ancel Keys's research indicting saturated fat in heart disease had been published and was being picked up by the media; the low- or no-cholesterol brigade was gearing up for an assault on the consciousness of the American public. Then in 1972, Robert Atkins published *Diet Revolution*, which became the de facto poster child for the low-carb movement two decades later. Atkins advocated an approach completely opposite to the one promoted by Keys: He said that insulin and carbohydrates, not fat and cholesterol, were the problem in the American diet.

Because his high-fat, high-protein, low-carb diet went so dramatically against the conventional wisdom of the times, Atkins was attacked mercilessly in the press and vilified by the medical mainstream, which turned him into a pariah in the medical community. But in the same year that Atkins published his book, an English doctor named John Yudkin was making waves by politely and reasonably suggesting to the medical establishment that perhaps its emperor, while indeed cholesterol-free and low-fat, was nonetheless naked as a jaybird.

A professor of nutrition at Queen Elizabeth College, University of London, Yudkin was a highly respected scientist and nutritionist who had dozens of published papers in such renowned peer-reviewed journals as *The Lancet*, the *British Medical Journal*, the *Archives of Internal Medicine*, the *American Journal of Clinical Nutrition*, and *Nature*.

Yudkin was typically portrayed by his detractors as a wild-eyed fanatic who blamed sugar as the cause of heart disease, but in fact he was nothing of the sort. In his 1972 book, *Sweet and Dangerous*, he was the embodiment of reason when he called for a reexamination of the data—which he considered highly flawed—that led to the hypothesis that fat causes heart disease. (He's since been proven right—many times!)

In the 1960s, Yudkin did a series of animal experiments in which he fed sugar and starch to a variety of critters, including chickens, rabbits, pigs, and college students. Invariably he found that the levels of triglycerides in all these subjects were raised. (Remember, high triglycerides are a major risk factor for heart disease, and triglycerides rise like an air balloon when you eat a lot of sugar and starch.) In Yudkin's experiments, sugar also raised insulin, linking sugar to type 2 diabetes, which, as you now know, is intimately related to heart disease as well.[14]

Yudkin was one of the many who pointed out that statistics for heart disease and fat consumption existed for many more countries than those referred to by Keys, and that these other figures didn't fit into the "more fat, more heart disease" relationship that was evident when only the seven selected countries were considered. He pointed out that there was a better and truer relationship between *sugar consumption* and heart disease, and he said that "there is a sizable minority—of which I am one—that believes that coronary disease is *not* largely due to fat in the diet."

Three decades later, Dr. George Mann, an associate director of the Framingham Heart Study, arrived at the same conclusion and assembled a distinguished group of scientists and doctors to study the evidence that fat and cholesterol cause heart disease, a concept he later called "the greatest health scam of the century."[15]

Though Yudkin did not write a low-carb diet book per se, he was one of the most influential voices of the time to put forth the position that sugar was responsible for far more health problems than fat was. His book called attention to countries in which the correlation between heart disease and sugar intake was far more striking than the correlation between heart disease and *fat*. And he pointed to a number of studies—most dramatically of the Masai in Kenya and Tanzania—in which people consumed copious amounts of milk and fat and yet had virtually no heart disease. Interestingly, these people also consumed almost no sugar.[16]

The Sweetening of America

To be clear, Yudkin never said that sugar *causes* the diseases of modern civilization, just that a case could easily be made that it deserved attention and study, certainly as much as, if not more than, fat consumption. Heart disease is associated with a number of indicators, including fat consumption, being overweight, cigarette smoking, a sedentary lifestyle, television viewing, and a high intake of sugar. Yudkin himself did several interesting studies on sugar consumption and coronary heart disease. In one he found that the median sugar intake of a group of coronary patients was 147 g, twice as much as it was in two different groups of control subjects that didn't have coronary disease; these groups consumed only 67 g and 74 g, respectively.[17]

"Many of the key observations cited to argue that dietary fat caused heart disease actually support the sugar theory as well," Taubes wrote. "During the Korean War, pathologists doing autopsies on American soldiers killed in battle noticed that many had significant plaques in their arteries, even those who were still teenagers, while the Koreans killed in battle did not. The atherosclerotic plaques in the Americans were attributed to the fact that they ate high-fat diets and the Koreans ate low-fat. But the Americans were also eating high-sugar diets, while the Koreans, like the Japanese, were not."

As Yudkin put it, "It may turn out that [many factors, including sugar] ultimately have the same effect on metabolism and so produce coronary disease by the same mechanism." What is that mechanism? Fingers are beginning to point suspiciously to an *overload of insulin* as a common culprit at the root of at least some of these metabolic and negative health effects, such as heart disease.

As you will soon see, there are now compelling reasons to believe that there is a causal relationship between insulin resistance and heart disease, and, since insulin resistance is eminently treatable, that early testing for insulin resistance could prevent a significant number of heart attacks from ever happening in the first place. We'll outline that case in chapter 9.

Controlling insulin was the main purpose of the original Atkins diet and has become the raison d'être of the low-carb approach to living. Though the Atkins diet is certainly not the only way to control insulin, Atkins—who was after all a cardiologist—is to be commended for being prescient when it comes to identifying carbohydrates and insulin resistance as causative factors in diabetes, obesity, hypertension, and, you guessed it, heart disease.

Cholesterol Insanity

Yudkin's warnings against sugar and Atkins's early low-carb approach to weight loss were mere whispers lost in the roar of anti-fat mania. By the mid-1980s, fat had been utterly and completely demonized, and fat phobia was in full bloom, with hundreds of cholesterol-free foods being foisted on a gullible public.[18] In November 1985, the National Heart, Lung, and Blood Institute launched the National Cholesterol Education Program with the stated goal of "reducing illness and death from coronary heart disease in the United States by *reducing the percent of Americans with high blood cholesterol* [italics ours]."[19]

In 1976, Nathan Pritikin opened his Pritikin Longevity Center in Santa Barbara, California, and for the next decade preached the super-low-fat dogma to all who would listen, which included most of the country. Pritikin died in 1985, but his mantle was quickly taken up by Dr. Dean Ornish. Ornish's reputation—and much of the public's faith in the low-fat diet approach—was fueled by his famous five-year intervention study, the Lifestyle Heart Trial, which demonstrated that intensive lifestyle changes may lead to regression of coronary heart disease. Ornish took forty-eight middle-aged white men with moderate-to-severe coronary heart disease and assigned them to two groups. One group received "usual care," and the other group received a special, intensive, five-part lifestyle intervention consisting of (1) aerobic exercise, (2) stress-management training, (3) smoking cessation, (4) group psychological support, and (5) a strict vegetarian, high-fiber diet with 10 percent of the calories coming from fat.

When Ornish's study showed some reversal of atherosclerosis and fewer cardiac events in the twenty men who completed the five-year study, the public perception—reinforced by Ornish himself—was that the results largely stemmed from the low-fat diet. This conclusion is an incredible leap that is in no way supported by his research. The fact is that *there's no way to know* whether the results were because of the low-fat diet portion of the experiment (highly unlikely in our view), the high fiber, the whole foods, the lack of sugar, or some combination of the interventions. It is entirely possible that Ornish would have gotten the same or better results with a program of exercise, stress management, smoking cessation, and group therapy plus a whole foods diet high in protein and fiber and low in sugar.

Yet low-fat eating managed to remain the dietary prescription of every major mainstream health organization. This recommendation was built on a foundation of two basic beliefs: that low-fat diets will reduce cholesterol, and that reducing cholesterol will actually reduce heart disease and extend life.

Although some studies have shown that low-fat diets do reduce overall cholesterol, many—most, in fact—have shown nothing of the sort. When you replace fat in the diet with carbohydrates, which is exactly what low-fat diets do, you wind up with *higher* triglycerides and *lower* HDL cholesterol.

Bad news indeed. Higher triglycerides are an independent risk factor for heart disease—and raising them while lowering HDL cholesterol at the same time is a double whammy, a really bad "side effect" of the supposedly heart-healthy low-fat diet. Not only do you raise one important independent risk factor for heart disease (triglycerides) while at the same time lowering one *protective* measure (HDL cholesterol), but you *also* change the all-important ratio of triglycerides to HDL cholesterol in the worst way possible. A higher triglycerides number and a lower HDL cholesterol number mean a much *higher* ratio of triglycerides to HDL. As we've seen, you want your ratio to be *low*, not high; low-fat, high-carbohydrate diets make the ratio *higher*.

THE SUGAR LOBBY IN ACTION

So how did fat get demonized while sugar got a "get out of jail free" card?

Well, there's no political lobby for "fat," but there's a powerful one for sugar.

In 2003, the World Health Organization (WHO)—not exactly a bunch of wide-eyed radicals—published a conservative, eminently reasonable report called *Diet, Nutrition and the Prevention of Chronic Diseases*.[20] In it, the WHO made the unremarkable statement that it would be a good idea for people to derive no more than 10 percent of their daily calories from added sugars. The report suggested that people could lower their risk of obesity, diabetes, and heart disease simply by curbing some of the sugar they were consuming. A completely mainstream, noncontroversial, "vanilla" recommendation if ever there was one. Who could possibly object, you might think?

Well, the U.S. sugar industry, for one.

"Hoping to block the report . . . the Sugar Association threatened to lobby Congress to cut off the $406 million the United States gives annually to the WHO," reported Juliet Eilperin in the *Washington Post*.[21] The *Post* quoted an April 14, 2003, letter from the Sugar Association's president, Andrew Briscoe, to the general director of WHO in which he stated, "We will exercise every avenue available to expose the dubious nature of the *Diet, Nutrition and the Prevention of Chronic Diseases* report."

Two senators wrote a letter to then Health and Human Services Secretary Tommy G. Thompson, urging him to squelch the report. Soon afterward, the U.S. Department of Health and Human Services submitted comments on the report, stating that "evidence that soft drinks are associated with obesity is not compelling."

Oh, really? Shades of the tobacco industry's defense of cigarettes.

But our story doesn't end there. In fact, the sugar industry's backlash against the 2003 WHO report was far from its first rodeo, as far as manipulating public perception goes. In fact, it's been playing that game for longer than some readers have been alive.

Want proof of the fix? In 2016, the smoking gun we'd all been waiting for fell from the sky and landed in the pages of *JAMA Internal Medicine*.[22] No, it wasn't a brand new study. In fact, the fuss was over a very old one. Back in 1967, Harvard scientists had conducted a massive review of all the sugar and heart disease studies available at the time. (One of those researchers was none other than Mark Hegsted, better known for his role in drafting the 1977 Dietary Goals for the United States—the committee report that helped shape America's catastrophic nutritional guidelines.)

After assessing study after study in humans and animals alike, Hegsted et al. published a paper in the prestigious *New England Journal of Medicine* claiming that sugar didn't play any convincing role in heart disease. The evidence, the paper claimed, showed there was "only one avenue" by which diet could influence heart disease: that avenue was blood lipids, and the only dietary players of import were fat and cholesterol.[22] Any benefits of reducing sugar, the researchers concluded, were so puny compared to those of reducing fat that "in our opinion they have no practical importance."[23]

At a time when diet and heart disease research was in its fledgling stage, a single well-respected review could shape consensus and steer the direction of future research. And that's exactly what this paper did. With sugar declared innocent (by fancy Harvard scientists, no less), anti-fat-and-cholesterol research took center stage, dominating the scientific discourse for decades to come. Meanwhile, sugar research dwindled to near oblivion. Why would anyone waste grant money chasing a sugar and heart disease hypothesis that had been confirmed DOA?

There was just one problem.

Unbeknownst to anyone other than industry insiders, the review had been secretly funded, designed, and directed by the Sugar Research Foundation—a Washington, D.C.-based trade group dedicated to defending sugar's honor. And no one would've been the wiser if not for the sleuthing work of Cristin Kearns, a former dentist from Colorado who cracked the case herself.

Years earlier, Kearns had stumbled upon what turned out to be the find of a lifetime. Tucked away in the University of Illinois archives were reams of papers from Roger Adams—an organic chemistry professor who'd served on the Sugar Research Foundation's scientific advisory board. Those papers encompassed over a decade of correspondence—spanning 1959 to 1971—between Adams and the foundation, totaling a whopping 1551 pages from 319 different documents.

What Kearns found in that treasure trove was shocking. For one, it turned out that in 1965—right after the *Annals of Internal Medicine* had published some articles linking sugar to heart disease—the Sugar Research Foundation had struck a deal with Harvard researchers Mark Hegsted and Robert McGandy, paying them $6,500 (the equivalent of over $50,000 today) to do some damage control: The foundation asked them to write a review article of "several papers which find some special metabolic peril in sucrose," with the implication that sugar needed to look good—or at least, not look *bad*. Those internal documents showed ongoing back-and-forths between Hegsted and the foundation's vice president throughout the whole review process, concluding with a word of praise from the VP that the article—with its anti-fat, sugar-neutral conclusion—was up to snuff: "Let me assure you this is quite what we had in mind and we look forward to its appearance in print," he wrote to Hegsted.

When the review was finally published, there wasn't a peep about the Sugar Research Foundation's involvement—despite declarations of other industry funding.

Now, let's jump back to what that 1967 *New England Journal of Medicine* review actually found. If we look closely, we can see how painstakingly the researchers tried to downplay sugar's harmful effects, which were hard to ignore even then. For example, the paper conceded that sugar versus complex carbs could play a "slightly significant role" in regulating blood lipids, and that "these effects are somewhat more pronounced when diets low in fat are consumed." But the researchers then threw us a logical curve ball: "Since diets low in fat and high in sugar are rarely taken, we conclude that the practical significance of differences in dietary carbohydrate is minimal in comparison to those related to dietary fat and cholesterol."[24]

Did you hear that noise? That was the sound of a thousand "someone's pulling a fast one on us" alarm bells going off. Even in a review paper designed to pardon sugar, researchers couldn't get around the fact that sugar behaved *especially* bad when it came to low-fat diets. And tragically, the "low in fat, high in sugar" diet the researchers cited as problematic was the very one they helped steer Americans toward.

How's that for a cruel twist of fate?

The implications of Kearns's sugar industry findings can't be overstated. Not only did Big Sugar *try* to control the public and scientific narrative about its product, but it actually *succeeded*. Scientists stopped pouring their time and brainpower into potentially life-saving sugar research, instead turning their focus squarely on fat and cholesterol. As Kearns wrote in a 2012 *Mother Jones* article she co-authored with Gary Taubes, "Research on the suspected links between sugar and chronic disease largely ground to a halt by the late 1980s, and scientists came to view such pursuits as a career dead end."[25]

What's more, Kearns and Taubes continued, "So effective were the Sugar Association's efforts that, to this day, no consensus exists about sugar's potential dangers."

And it was true. In a 2005 report by the Institute of Medicine, the authors acknowledged that there was a ton of evidence suggesting that sugar consumption could increase the risk of heart disease and diabetes—and that it could even raise LDL ("bad") cholesterol. The problem was they couldn't say that the research was definitive. "There was enough ambiguity, they concluded, that they couldn't even set an upper limit on how much sugar constitutes too much," Taubes wrote.

This dovetailed nicely with the last assessment of sugar by the Food and Drug Administration (FDA) back in 1986 that basically said "no conclusive evidence on sugars demonstrates a hazard to the general public when sugars are consumed at the levels that are now current."

"This is another way of saying that the evidence by no means refuted the [charges against sugar], just that it wasn't definitive or unambiguous," Taubes said. It's also worth noting that at the time, we were consuming approximately 40 pounds per year of "added sugars," meaning sugar beyond what we might naturally obtain from fruits and vegetables. (That comes to about two hundred extra sugar calories a day, about a can and a half of Coke.)

That doesn't sound so bad, really, and if that were all the sugar we were consuming, most nutritionists in America would be pretty happy. The problem was it wasn't 40 pounds a year. Even back then the Department of Agriculture said we were consuming 75 pounds a year, and by the early 2000s it was up to 90 pounds. As of late 2011, we were up to 156 pounds a year. That's the equivalent of thirty-one 5-pound bags for every man, woman, and child in America.[26]

Now, back to our story. It turned out there was more—*much* more—in Kearns's food industry exposé.

From 1967 to 1971, the Sugar Research Foundation funded a series of animal experiments—officially titled "Project 259: Dietary Carbohydrate and Blood Lipids in Germ-Free Rats"—designed to evaluate the effects of sugar on heart disease risk. The results were both fascinating and disturbing: There was evidence that gut bacteria could influence how sugar affected triglycerides. Not only that, but compared to starch, sugar seemed to promote high levels of beta-glucuronidase—an enzyme known, even back then, to be associated with bladder cancer and potentially atherosclerosis.

That's right: A study from *half a century* ago was already incriminating sugar as a heart-harmer and potential carcinogen.

If you're wondering why you haven't heard about this before, the reason is simple: Project 259 never saw the peer-reviewed light of day. The Sugar Research Foundation made sure of it. Instead of publishing what would have been game-changing information for the nutrition field (and human health at large), the foundation axed the project and buried its findings deep underground—quietly letting the scientific community continue its misguided witch-hunt against fat.[27]

The sugar industry, it turned out, also tried to distract the public from sugar's link with tooth decay. An analysis of the Roger Adams papers showed that the sugar industry was well aware that sugar caused cavities—the scientific evidence, even then, was overwhelming. But instead of informing the public they should eat less sugar, the Sugar Research Foundation decided to spend its dollars promoting health interventions that would reduce sugar's harmful effects—including funding research on enzymes to break up dental plaque, getting chummy with scientists from

the National Institute of Dental Research, and developing questionable vaccines against tooth decay (we couldn't make this stuff up if we tried).[28]

And the list goes on. Buried amidst those industry documents was a copy of a 1954 speech from the Sugar Research Foundation's president, discussing a strategic opportunity to get Americans to eat more sugar by pushing a low-fat diet—thanks to preliminary research at the time linking fat and cholesterol to heart problems. Another document, an internal memo from the group's vice president in 1964, proposed that the foundation should start funding research to "refute our detractors," as well as embark on a deliberate program to counteract "negative attitudes toward sugar"—including the ideas presented by John Yudkin.[29]

And if you're tempted to think, *"but all that happened a million years ago,"* please don't. It was precisely this subterranean effort—funded by deep-pocketed lobbyist groups. Aided and abetted by sympathetic researchers who, for a price, were willing to produce scientific cover for the sugar industry and "manufacture doubt"—they produced the food environment in which we live today. (For a fascinating account of how industry "buys" science to create a narrative that supports their financial interests, read *Merchants of Doubt* by historians Naomi Oreskes and Erik Conway, or watch the 2014 film based on it.)

The narrative set in motion by the sugar industry back in the day continues to this very day. Fat and cholesterol are demonized in mainstream medicine while sugar gets a handy-dandy "get out of jail" card. That narrative fits well with the philosophy "a calorie is just a calorie," implying that the only problem with sugar is empty calories.

In fact, in terms of metabolic and heart health, the notion that "a calorie is just a calorie" is . . . well, fake news. But it's a wonderful cover story for the sugar-soaked industry known as processed food.

In case there was any doubt that the sugar industry not only *knew* about the perils of sugar, but actively tried to suppress that knowledge from public awareness, this should kick that to the curb. The Sugar Research Foundation papers not only confirmed what we've all suspected, but made it clear that the rabbit hole went much deeper than anyone could've guessed.

And now, with that depressing history in mind, let's return to our chapter's science lesson: the nitty gritty of sugar's effects on our bodies.

What's So Bad about a Little Sugar?

The way in which sugar damages the heart is directly related to insulin resistance. Ordinary table sugar, known technically as *sucrose*, is actually composed of equal parts glucose and fructose, two *monosaccharides* (simple sugars) that are anything but metabolically equal. Glucose can be used by any cell in the body. Fructose, on the other hand, is metabolic poison—at least at the levels in which it's currently consumed. It's the fructose in our sweetened foods—usually in the form of high-fructose corn syrup—that we should fear the most.

But before you point the finger of blame exclusively at high-fructose corn syrup (HFCS), an additive that's made it into virtually every processed food on the market, consider the following:

- Regular sugar (sucrose) is 50 percent glucose and 50 percent fructose.
- High-fructose corn syrup is 55 percent fructose and 45 percent glucose, a difference that just doesn't matter very much.

So sugar and high-fructose corn syrup are *essentially* the same thing.

Because high-fructose corn syrup has gotten so much heat in the press, some food manufacturers now proudly advertise that their products contain none of it and are instead sweetened with "natural" sugar (meaning ordinary sucrose). Meanwhile, the Corn Refiners Association has claimed that high-fructose corn syrup is being unjustly targeted and is no worse than "regular" sugar.

Sadly, the association is technically right. Fructose is the damaging part of sugar, and whether you get that fructose from regular sugar or from HFCS doesn't make a whit of difference. That doesn't absolve HFCS at all; it just means that "regular" sugar is virtually *just as bad* as HFCS. It's the fructose in each of them that's causing the damage, and here's why.

Fructose and glucose are metabolized in the body in completely different ways. They are *not* identical. Glucose goes right into the bloodstream and then into the cells, but fructose goes right to the liver. Research has shown that fructose is seven times more likely to form the previously mentioned artery-damaging AGEs (advanced glycation end products). Fructose is metabolized by the body like fat, and it turns into fat (triglycerides) almost immediately. "When you consume fructose, you're not consuming carbs," says Robert Lustig, M.D., professor of pediatrics at the University of California, San Francisco. "You're consuming fat."

Fructose is the major cause of fat accumulation in the liver, a condition known technically as *hepatic steatosis* but which most of us know as fatty liver. And there is a direct link between fatty liver and our old friend, insulin resistance.

A top researcher in the field of insulin resistance, Varman Samuel of the Yale School of Medicine, told the *New York Times* that the correlation between fat in the liver (fatty liver) and insulin resistance is remarkably strong. "When you deposit fat in the liver, that's when you become insulin resistant," he said.[30]

And all together now, class: What causes fat to accumulate in the liver? Fructose.

If you want to watch a bunch of lab animals become insulin resistant, all you have to do is feed them fructose. Feed them enough fructose and, sure enough, the liver converts it to fat, which then accumulates in the liver—with insulin resistance right behind it. This can take place in as little as a week if the animals are fed enough fructose, whereas it might take a few months at the levels we humans normally consume. Studies conducted by Luc Tappy, M.D., in Switzerland revealed that feeding human subjects a daily dose of fructose equal to the amount found in eight to ten cans of soda produced insulin resistance and elevated triglycerides within a few days.[31]

Fructose found in whole foods such as fruits, however, is a different story. There's not all that much fructose in, for example, an apple, and the apple comes with a hefty dose of fiber, which slows the rate of carbohydrate absorption and reduces insulin response. But fructose extracted from fruit, concentrated into a syrup, and then inserted into practically every food we buy at the supermarket—from bread and hamburger buns to pretzels and cereals—well, that's a whole different animal.

High-fructose corn syrup was first invented in Japan in the 1960s and made it into the American food supply around the mid-1970s. It had two advantages over regular sugar, from the point of view of food manufacturers. Number one, it was sweeter, so theoretically you could use less of it. Number two, it was much cheaper than sugar. Low-fat products could be made "palatable" by the addition of HFCS, and before long, manufacturers were adding the stuff to everything. (Doubt us? Take a field trip to your local supermarket and start reading labels. See if you can find any processed foods that don't contain it.)

The result is that our fructose consumption has skyrocketed. Twenty-five percent of adolescents today consume 15 percent of their calories from fructose alone! As Robert Lustig points out in a brilliant lecture, "Sugar: The Bitter Truth" (available on YouTube), the percentage of calories from fat in the American diet has gone down at the same time that fructose consumption has skyrocketed, along with heart disease, diabetes, obesity, and hypertension. Coincidence? Lustig doesn't think so, and neither do we.

Remember our mention of metabolic syndrome? It's a collection of symptoms—high triglycerides, abdominal fat, hypertension, and insulin resistance—that seriously increases the risk for heart disease. Well, rodents consuming large amounts of fructose rapidly develop it.[32] In humans, a high-fructose diet raises triglycerides almost instantly; the rest of the symptoms associated with metabolic syndrome take a little longer to develop in humans than they do in rats, but develop they do.[33] Fructose also raises uric acid levels in the bloodstream. Excess uric acid is well known as the defining feature of gout, but did you know that it also predicts future obesity and high blood pressure?

Fructose and glucose behave very differently in the brain as well, as research from Johns Hopkins has suggested. Glucose decreases food intake while fructose increases it. If your appetite increases, you eat more, thus making obesity, and an increased risk for heart disease, far more likely. "Take a kid to McDonald's and give him a Coke," Lustig said. "Does he eat less? Or does he eat more?"

M. Daniel Lane, Ph.D., of the Johns Hopkins University School of Medicine stated, "We feel that [the findings on fructose and appetite] may have particular relevance to the massive increase in the use of high-fructose sweeteners (both high-fructose corn syrup and table sugar) in virtually all sweetened foods, most notably soft drinks. The per capita consumption of these sweeteners in the USA is about 145 lbs./year and is probably much higher in teenagers/youth that have a high level of consumption of soft drinks."[34]

All told, the case for fructose being a major contributor to heart disease is way stronger than the case against fat. In fact, it's not even close. It's also worth pointing out that every single bad thing that fructose does to increase our risk for heart disease—and it does a lot—has virtually nothing to do with elevated cholesterol.

The fact is that sugar is far more damaging to the heart than either fat or cholesterol. But that has never stopped the diet establishment from continuing to stick to its number one talking point: *Fat and cholesterol are what we ought to be worried about.*

As the old journalistic maxim goes, "Never let the facts get in the way of a good story." Unfortunately, this story is long past its expiration date. Sticking to it in the face of all evidence continues to make many people very sick indeed.

◀ WHAT YOU NEED TO KNOW

- Sugar is the missing link among diabetes, obesity, and heart disease. It overrides our body's natural hunger regulation, making it very easy to overeat. It is also a major contributor to inflammation in the artery walls.
- Hypertension, high triglycerides, and a high ratio of triglycerides to HDL are all better predictors of heart disease than cholesterol. Sugar, or more specifically fructose, raises every single one them.
- High levels of both sugar and insulin damage LDL particles in the blood, making them far more likely to end up incorporated into arterial plaque.
- When sugar in the bloodstream sticks to proteins, it creates damaging and toxic molecules called *advanced glycation end products*, or AGEs.

CHAPTER 7

THE TRUTH ABOUT FAT: IT'S NOT WHAT YOU THINK

YOU CAN'T TALK ABOUT CHOLESTEROL WITHOUT ALSO TALKING ABOUT FAT, which is convenient, because it's exactly what we're going to discuss in this chapter.

When you're done reading it, you may have an entirely different perspective on fat and a much more accurate notion of what the terms "good fat" and "bad fat" mean. And no, we're not just going to tell you the stuff you've heard a million times, such as "fat from fish is good" (completely true) and "saturated fat is bad" (very far from always true).

But let's not get ahead of ourselves.

According to conventional wisdom, fat and cholesterol are the twin demons of heart disease, linked together in our minds as firmly as Hell and Damnation or Bonnie and Clyde. We've been admonished to lower our cholesterol and stop eating saturated fat. These two mandates are the basis of the diet-heart hypothesis, which has guided national health policy on healthy eating for decades and basically holds that fat and cholesterol in the diet are a direct and significant cause of heart disease.

Okay, so fat and cholesterol (whether they show up in your diet or in your bloodstream) are pretty much kissing cousins.

We've discussed cholesterol in the previous chapters, so let's clear up some misconceptions about fat—what it is, what it does, what it doesn't do—and why all this matters in the first place. Once we've done that, we'll be able to look at the relationship among heart disease, fat in the diet, and cholesterol in the blood with completely new eyes.

Let's get to work!

WHAT EXACTLY IS FAT, ANYWAY?

Fat is the collective shorthand name given to any big collection of smaller units called fatty acids. You can think of "fat" and "fatty acids" as analogous to paper money and a bunch of coins. The dollar bill is the "fat" and the coins are the "fatty acids." Just as a dollar can comprise different combinations of coins—one hundred pennies, four quarters, ten dimes, twenty nickels, and so forth—a "fat" comprises different combinations of fatty acids.

There are more fatty acids in a stick of butter than there are in a spoonful of butter, just as there are more coins in $5 than there are in $1. But whether you're dealing with a splash of olive oil, a tub of lard, or a tablespoon of fish oil, all fat on earth is composed of fatty acids. The only difference between the fat in olive oil and the fat in lard is that if you looked at them under a microscope, you'd see that each is made up of a different mix of fatty acids (i.e., nickels, dimes, quarters, etc.).

There are three families of fatty acids: saturated fatty acids, monounsaturated fatty acids, and polyunsaturated fatty acids. (There's actually a fourth class of fatty acids called trans fats, a kind of "Franken-fat," but we'll address that later.) The difference between all these fat types has to do with the number of chemical double bonds that exist in the fatty acid's molecular chain. Monounsaturated fats have one double bond, polyunsaturated fats have more than one, and saturated fats have none.

In this section we'll concentrate primarily on saturated fat, but keep a place on your dance card for two members of the polyunsaturated family called *omega-3 fatty acids* and *omega-6 fatty acids*. They're of special importance, and we'll be talking about them in depth later on.

Now a word of complete candor from your authors. We wrote this book for our families. We wanted the average intelligent person who didn't have a background in science to be able to follow the basic arguments and have a clear sense of the takeaway messages. We wanted the discussions within the book to be simple enough that they could be easily grasped by nonmedical people. And, frankly, fat is complicated.

So this is the part of the book where we could easily slip into a short course on the biochemistry of fats. It's interesting to write about, it fills a lot of pages—and it's deadly dull for readers. Don't worry, we're not going to write sprawling essays about the chemical structure of fat and give you a pop quiz at the end. And as much as we enjoy talking about this stuff and would be happy to chat about it if you met us at a cocktail party, the truth is it causes many people's eyes to glaze over pretty quickly.

So if you're interested in reading the Full Monty about how double bonds, saturation, chain length, and other cool biochemical stuff affects us at a molecular level, please, by all means, be our guest! That information is widely available. It's not controversial, it's not debated, and it's not really germane to our story. So, mercifully, we've decided to minimize the "in the weeds" lectures here and instead give you the essentials—what you really need to know about saturated, polyunsaturated, and monounsaturated fats. The technical bits we'll cover are only there because they're really, really important.

Saturated Fat 101: Everything We Learned Was Wrong!

Saturated fats are primarily found in animal foods (meat, cheese, butter, eggs) and, less often, in certain plant foods, such as coconut, coconut oil, cocoa butter, and palm oil. They tend to be solid at room temperature (think butter) and soften when warm.

Here's the part they don't tell you. Just as polyunsaturated fats aren't a singular entity—they include both omega-3 and omega-6 fats, which have wildly different health effects—saturated fat, too, is actually a collection of different fatty acids. And those different saturated fatty acids have diverse effects on your cholesterol levels, metabolism, and overall health.

That's why, when we talk about "saturated fat," we also have to ask: *Which* saturated fat? And it's also why we can't use a study on coconut oil to tell us about the health effects of cheese, or a study on egg yolks to tell us about the health effects of steak—even when scientists wave their magical statistical wands trying to predict such things. Saturated fat isn't a singular entity, and neither are the foods that contain it.

Importantly, no matter which saturated fat we're talking about, the news is *not* as bad as we've been told—full stop. What's more, certain saturated fats are uniquely beneficial, as has been born out in study after study. How's that for some juicy fine print to the "saturated fat is bad" hoo-ha?

They also have a few other characteristics worth mentioning. Saturated fats are very stable. They're tough—when exposed to high heat they don't "mutate" or "damage" as easily as their more delicate cousins, the unsaturated (especially polyunsaturated) fats do. That's one reason why lard (with its high con-

centration of saturated fatty acids) is actually a better choice for frying than the cheap, processed, polyunsaturated vegetable oils that gradually replaced it as restaurants tried to be more "health" conscious.

The problem with vegetable oils is that they're nowhere near as resistant to damage as saturated fats are. When you heat and reheat them for frying, as virtually every restaurant in America does, it causes the formation of all sorts of noxious compounds, including carcinogens. Those multiple double bonds we mentioned earlier? They're woefully vulnerable to chemical attack. Compared to saturated fat, the unsaturated fatty acids in vegetable oils are much more easily damaged by high heat and more susceptible to oxidation and the production of free radicals. Those vegetable oils transform into all sorts of mutant molecules under the stress of high heat and reheating, but when high heat is applied to saturated fat, it behaves like the strong, silent uncle at the family gathering; everyone else is going nuts, but he's calm and serene!

Even when heat isn't in the picture, polyunsaturated fats are fragile flowers, so to speak. Mere exposure to oxygen and sunlight will cause an open bottle of soybean oil to go rancid on the counter, while an open jar of coconut oil will sit there for eons without oxidizing. (We'll talk about some of the other problems with the overuse of vegetable oils in our diet later on.)

Now let us ask you a question, and please answer honestly: Did you shudder in horror when we implied a few sentences ago that using lard for cooking might actually be a good idea? You probably thought to yourself, "Now they've gone too far. Did they really say lard

DR. JONNY

When I was in fifth grade back in Queens, New York, there was a kid named A.J. who was always, and I mean *always*, getting in trouble. But it was for the most minor stuff: coming in a couple of minutes late from recess, whispering in class, or, worst case scenario, throwing a spitball. There could be five other kids doing the same thing, but A.J. would always be the one to get caught. Singled out, reprimanded, parents called in to school, the whole humiliating deal.

But there were a couple of other kids in the class who were real pieces of work. One kid, Gilbert, compulsively lit firecrackers, scaring everyone to death, and then disappeared before he could be caught at the scene of the crime. Another kid named Howie took delight in breaking people's windows with rocks. A third one, Corky, was a bully. And yet none of them ever managed to get caught. Rarely did any of these kids even get a stern talking-to. The role of the "bad kid" in the class was played by A.J., who would have to serve detention, sit in the corner, and be yelled at in front of the class, all for fairly meaningless infractions, while the kids who were doing all the really bad stuff got off scot-free.

Now it's not that old A.J. didn't do anything wrong. But unlike the other kids, he never beat anyone up, he never did anything mean, he never destroyed anyone's property—and yet whenever there was trouble, he was always the scapegoat.

I think saturated fat is like that kid A.J. It's not that it's perfect. It's just that it's far less important than the stuff we ignore—such as high intakes of omega-6 fatty acids, low intakes of omega-3s, and obscene intakes of sugar and processed carbs.

Is saturated fat so wonderful that we should all resolve to melt a ton of butter and add it to our smoothies right this minute? No, of course not. Saturated fat has some negatives. It is mildly inflammatory. It may contribute to insulin resistance.

If the dietary dictocrats are going to warn us against inflammatory food components, why choose saturated fat, a relatively minor factor in inflammation compared to the omega-6 to omega-3 ratio? If they're going to warn us about saturated fat because of its purported connection to insulin resistance, why do they continue to promote ridiculously high carbohydrate intakes, which are demonstrably worse?

Saturated fat is a lot like A.J. Not perfect, but it doesn't deserve to get beat up. And the irony is that while everyone's pushing him around and blaming him for everything bad that happens, the real culprits are getting away.

is better to fry with than canola oil? That's nuts!"

We'd be surprised if you didn't recoil in horror. Most people would do just that—and it's because most people have totally bought into the idea that saturated fat is the worst thing on the planet.

The idea that lard—with its high content of saturated fat—could ever be a better choice than those high omega-6 vegetable oils that are continually pushed on us is in direct opposition to fat theology, the deeply held belief that saturated fat and cholesterol are the root of all heart disease evil. That notion has been the prevailing dogma about saturated fat, cholesterol, and heart disease for decades. By now you're more than familiar with this notion, known as the diet-heart hypothesis—it's the mantra that has guided public policy on diet and heart disease for virtually every major governmental and mainstream health organization, such as the American Heart Association.

There's only one problem. It isn't true.

Despite its horrible reputation, saturated fat is far from a dietary demon. More and more health profes-

A WORD ABOUT META-ANALYSES AND WHY THEY'RE IMPORTANT

A little backstory about meta-analyses and why people do them. Say you want to learn about the sex habits of college students. There are probably a couple dozen relevant studies you could look at, but as with any other area of research, there's no guarantee that all the studies will reach the same conclusions. In fact, it's almost certain that they won't. One study might find, for example, that college kids are having more sex, while another study might find that they're actually having less. (A critical look at these two studies might uncover the fact that researchers in the two studies used slightly different definitions of the term "sex" when they surveyed the students, something that might account for the difference in results.)

Sometimes researchers overlook an obvious variable that could skew the results. Although researchers always try to control for these variables (such as age, sex, and smoking) and generally "match" subjects by the most important criteria, they don't—they can't—always control for every variable that might make a difference (and this is particularly true in diet research). The point is, if you look at anything worth studying you're going to find a whole bunch of research on it, and among those research studies you're almost guaranteed to encounter conflicting findings and areas of disagreement about how to interpret those findings.

Even something that now seems as clearly connected as the link between smoking and cancer started out as a hypothesis and had to be tested in all sorts of populations under all sorts of conditions. Studies can and do reach different conclusions depending on the statistical

sionals, researchers, scientists, doctors, and nutritionists are beginning to reexamine the case against saturated fat, and they're finding that it's based on very little solid evidence (and a lot of guilt by association). Not only that, but different types of saturated fat—from different dietary sources—have such diverse impacts on our health, it's hard to make blanket statements about saturated fat on the whole. As we'll see, some saturated fatty acids are not only non-harmful, but we might be better off eating *more* of them rather than less.

SATURATED FAT AND HEART DISEASE: WHERE'S THE EVIDENCE?

Look, there is no shortage of studies pointing to an association between increased saturated fat intake and cardiovascular risk, but there are a few things to know about those studies.

Number one, the associations are far weaker than one might suspect, given how entrenched the belief is that saturated fat clogs your arteries. In many of these studies, the major "risk" examined was cholesterol, so we wind up with a circular argument in which

measures used, the populations studied, and even the definition of terms. (Is a "smoker" defined as anyone who has even one cigarette a week? Or is a "smoker" defined as someone who smokes at least half a pack a day?)

Which brings us, finally, back to meta-analysis.

Sometimes researchers gather up a whole bunch of these individual studies whose results are clustered all over the place like pins on CNN's election maps. Then they'll ask, "What do these studies, taken together as a whole, really tell us about what's going on?" They'll gather up all the studies on, say, smoking and cancer, college students and sex, or saturated fat and heart disease. They'll examine them scrupulously, tossing out any studies whose methods, designs, or data don't meet the highest standards of research excellence. (Meta-analyses typically exclude small pilot studies, unblinded studies, studies with too few participants, or studies that do not collect data on something the researchers consider important.)

Once the "best-of-the-best" studies are selected for inclusion (and lesser studies are eliminated), the researchers go to work and apply every statistical manipulation you can imagine to tease out the real relationships from the mass of accumulated data. They look at the findings of the individual studies and compare them. They pool the subjects from all the studies. They look for trends, directions, statistical significance, and hidden relationships. And though meta-analyses themselves are not infallible, they're a great way to look at the big picture to gauge what's really going on.

higher saturated fat intake increases the risk for heart disease, but *only* if you accept the use of cholesterol levels as a stand-in for heart disease. Studies that measure the effect of saturated fat on heart disease and mortality *directly*—rather than indirectly by measuring its effect on cholesterol—are few and far between. But there are some important ones, which we'll discuss in a moment.

Number two, as scientists have looked more carefully at the association between saturated fat in the diet and levels of cholesterol in the blood, they are beginning to see that even here the relationship is murky. As we'll explain shortly, not all saturated fatty acids have the same impact on your cholesterol levels—making it hard to make any single, overarching blanket statements about saturated fat as a whole. What's more, the stuff saturated fat seems to do depends a whole lot on what we're comparing it to (unsaturated fats? Carbs? Protein?), who's eating it (a lean twenty-something, or an obese middle-ager with diabetes?), the overall dietary context (an energy-surplus Standard Western Diet, or a ketogenic weight-loss diet?), among plenty of other factors that add nuance and caveats to the saturated fat story.

And the kicker: Even when all saturated fats are lumped together in studies (which is most of the time), the collective effect is still more positive than negative. Even those who still believe in the conventional division of cholesterol into "good and bad" cholesterol division have to face the (well-documented) fact that saturated fat usually causes HDL ("good" cholesterol) to go up more than LDL ("bad" cholesterol). Even by conventional standards that's a net gain.

One of the basic tenets of fat theology is that saturated fat increases the risk of heart disease. In the scientific literature, this issue is as far from being settled as you might think from listening to CNN. In 2012, Patty Siri-Tarino, Ph.D., and Ronald Krauss, M.D., of the Children's Hospital Oakland Research Institute together with Frank B. Hu, M.D., Ph.D., of Harvard, decided to do a meta-analysis—a study of studies. In this case, they looked at all previously published studies whose purpose was to investigate the relationship of saturated fat to coronary heart disease (CHD), stroke, or cardiovascular disease (CVD). Note that this is one of those hard-to-find studies we mentioned earlier: a study of the *direct effect* of saturated fat on health. The researchers weren't just interested in the effect saturated fat had on *cholesterol*—they wanted to know the effect saturated fat had on *heart disease*. (Remember, they are *not* the same thing!)

Twenty-one studies qualified for inclusion in their meta-analysis, meaning these studies met the criteria for being well designed and reliable. All in all, the twenty-one studies included 347,747 subjects who were followed for between five and twenty-three years. Over this period of time, 11,006 of the subjects developed coronary heart disease (CHD) or stroke.

Ready for the findings? How much saturated fat people ate predicted absolutely nothing about their risk for cardiovascular disease. In the researchers' own words, "Intake of saturated fat was not associated with an increased risk of coronary heart disease (CHD) or stroke, nor was it associated with an increased risk of cardiovascular disease (CVD)." Those folks consuming the highest amount of saturated fat were statistically identical to those consuming the least amount when it came to the probability of CHD, stroke, or CVD. Even when the researchers factored in age, sex, and study quality, it didn't change the results. Saturated fat did *bupkis*—it didn't increase or decrease risk in any meaningful way. Period.

"There is no significant evidence for concluding that dietary saturated fat is associated with an increased risk of CHD or CVD," the researchers concluded.[1]

Now—and this is a very important point—it's not that there's no evidence that saturated fat doesn't raise cholesterol. There is, and we'll examine that more in a moment. But the above meta-analysis didn't just look at cholesterol levels; it looked at what we *really* care about—heart disease and dying. So never mind whether saturated fat raises my cholesterol level. What I really want to know is, does eating saturated fat increase my chances of getting a heart attack or not? The meta-analysis looked at exactly that real-life endpoint we truly care about, and on that all-important metric, the verdict was clear. Saturated fat in the diet has virtually no effect on your risk of dying from a heart attack.

That meta-analysis is hardly the only study that has found saturated fat innocent of any direct involvement in cardiovascular disease. In the fall of 2011, a new study came out in the *Netherlands Journal of Medicine* titled "Saturated Fat, Carbohydrates, and Cardiovascular Disease." Like the above-discussed meta-analysis, its purpose was to examine the current scientific data on the effects of saturated fat, looking at all the controversies as well as the potential mechanisms for the role of saturated fat in cardiovascular disease.

Here's what the researchers wrote: "The dietary intake of saturated fatty acids is associated with a modest increase in serum total cholesterol, but *not* associated with cardiovascular disease [italics ours]."[2]

And it doesn't end there. In 2014, another wave-making study was published in the *Annals of Internal Medicine* examining the associations between various dietary, circulating, and supplementary fatty acids and subsequent heart disease risk.[3] This meta-analysis included thirty-two studies of fatty acid intake from people's diets, seventeen studies of fatty acid level biomarkers (standing in as indicators of dietary intake), and twenty-seven randomized, controlled trials of fatty acids consumed as supplements. In contrast to the entrenched "saturated fat causes heart disease" dogma, the results showed *no* increased risk of heart disease from eating saturated fat—as well as no association with saturated fat biomarkers. (What's more, increasing polyunsaturated fat intake, the long-standing battle cry of mainstream nutrition, didn't show any clear benefit for heart health.)

In the researchers' own words: "Current evidence does not clearly support cardiovascular guidelines that encourage high consumption of polyunsaturated fatty acids and low consumption of total saturated fats."

Still not convinced? A 2015 meta-analysis published in the *British Medical Journal* found that "Saturated fats are not associated with all-cause mortality CVD, CHD, ischemic stroke, or type 2 diabetes." All-cause mortality means dying from anything—accidents to cancer. Another way to say it is "total deaths from anything you can think of."[4] A 2016 re-evaluation of Minnesota Coronary Experiment data found that "replacement of saturated fat in the diet with linoleic acid effectively lowers serum cholesterol," but that evidence from available trials "does not support the hypothesis that this translates to a lower risk of death from coronary heart disease or all causes."[5] And a 2017 meta-analysis of randomized controlled trials determined that "Available evidence from adequately controlled randomized controlled trials suggest replacing SFA with mostly n-6 PUFA is unlikely to reduce CHD events, CHD mortality or total mortality"—and what's more, the whole reason very early meta-analyses seemed to incriminate saturated fat was because they included poorly controlled trials.[6] And most recently, a meta-analysis of cohort studies, conducted by researchers in China, found that—when comparing the lowest levels intake to the highest ones—there was no increased risk of cardiovascular disease from eating saturated fat.

The picture should be pretty clear by now.

As we've been saying throughout this book, cholesterol is only used as a marker. (In other words, it's a stand-in answer for what we *really* want to know—namely, what is the likelihood of developing heart disease?) But if you're looking for a metric to predict who is and isn't going to get heart disease, cholesterol—as we've seen in this book—is a lousy choice for a marker. If cholesterol *really* predicted heart disease (wrong belief number one), and if saturated fat *really* did terrible things to your cholesterol (wrong belief number two), then that might be reason to eliminate saturated fat from your diet.

But it turns out neither of those two things is true. Let's take those two notions one by one, because they are the bedrock beliefs of fat theology.

FAT THEOLOGY: TWO MAIN TENETS DEBUNKED

Researchers in Japan examined the first of those beliefs—that cholesterol is a good predictor of heart disease—with another meta-analysis. They searched for all studies that had examined the relationship of cholesterol to mortality, excluding any done before 1995 and any that had fewer than five thousand subjects. Nine studies met the criteria, but four had incomplete data and so were excluded. The researchers then performed a meta-analysis on the remaining five studies, which together involved more than 150,000 people followed for approximately five years.

The researchers placed everyone into one of four groups depending on their cholesterol levels: less than 160 mg/dL, 160 to 199 mg/dL, 200 to 239 mg/dL, and higher than 240 mg/dL. (These categories mirror the American Heart Association guidelines, which state that 200 mg/dL or lower is "desirable," 200 to 239 mg/dL is "borderline high," and higher than 240 mg/dL is bad news indeed.)

Which group do you think would have the worst possible outcomes? According to everything we've heard from the cholesterol zealots, the answer is simple: Those whose cholesterol readings were the highest (240 mg/dL and over), and even those with cholesterol readings in the "borderline" category (200 to 239 mg/dL), should be expected to die at a higher rate than those with a cholesterol level of 160 to 199 mg/dL. And those in the under 160 mg/dL category should live longest of all!

That is precisely and exactly what did *not* happen.

In fact, the group with the *lowest* cholesterol levels died at the *highest* rate.

In scientific terms, the risk for dying from any cause whatsoever (called "all-cause mortality") was highest in the group with low cholesterol. Compared with the reference group (160 to 199 mg/dL), the risk of dying from any cause whatsoever was significantly decreased in the group having "borderline high" cholesterol of 200 to 239 mg/dL and even further decreased in the group having "high" (greater than 240 mg/dL) cholesterol. In contrast, your risk of dying from any cause was the highest of all if your cholesterol was under 160 mg/dL![7]

So *high* cholesterol is associated with a *reduced* risk of death? Not exactly what you might expect but exactly what the study found. Total cholesterol is so irrelevant as a metric that in 2007 the Japan Atherosclerosis Society stopped using it in any tables related to the diagnosis or treatment criteria in its guidelines.[8] It's not that the society abandoned the cholesterol theory, mind you. It just now relies entirely on LDL levels to determine who should be classified as having "high cholesterol," reasoning that if total cholesterol is high simply because you've got a terrifically high HDL level, that shouldn't be counted as a bad thing. Many American doctors—even the most conservative ones—would probably agree that the LDL number is the important one, even if they don't fully embrace the notion that it is the *type* of LDL—not the LDL number—that matters the most.

But is the LDL level a better predicator of heart disease or mortality than the total cholesterol level?

Once again, let's go to the video. Researchers in Japan set out to answer this question in something

called the Isehara Study.[9] The Isehara Study was based on data collected from annual checkups of residents in Isehara, a smallish city (population: 100,000) located in the central Kanagawa Prefecture in Japan. A database of 8,340 men (average age sixty-four) and 13,591 women (average age sixty-one) was mined for cholesterol readings, and the 21,931 people were divided into seven groups ranked from lowest to highest LDL cholesterol levels (in mg/dL): <80, 80 to 99, 100 to 119, 120 to 139 (reference group), 140 to 159, 160 to 179, and >180. In both men and women, overall mortality was significantly *higher* in the group with the lowest LDL cholesterol levels (under 80 mg/dL).

Although it's true that in this study mortality from heart disease was greater in the group with the highest LDL levels (over 180 mg/dL), this was only true in men. In women the opposite was so—fewer women died of heart disease in the group with the highest LDL levels. In any case, this increase in heart disease in the high LDL group of men was apparently more than offset by the increase in deaths from other causes.

Okay, hopefully this information will get you, and your doctor, to at least question the notion that cholesterol is an important marker or predictor of heart disease. But let's say for the sake of argument that you, or your doctor, is not quite willing to throw out the cholesterol theory. Fine, no problem. After all, you, like most of us, have been indoctrinated with the idea that anything that raises your cholesterol is bad news, and that's a hard thing to let go of, especially when you've been hearing it for your entire adult life.

But before you go back to demonizing saturated fat, let's examine the second belief that constitutes the bedrock of fat theology, the idea that saturated fat does really bad things to your cholesterol.

When cholesterol was assessed in the old-fashioned way—"total," "good," and "bad"—this idea might have made sense, because a number of studies show that saturated fat does raise total cholesterol and LDL cholesterol. And if you bought into the theory that cholesterol is a big cause of heart disease, this would be a good enough reason to give up the butter.

But this where it stops being so simple. You see, saturated fat isn't one single nutrient. Literally dozens of unique saturated fatty acids exist—and, the kicker, they all have different effects on your cholesterol and health. Some raise LDL; some don't. Some raise HDL; some don't. Some are associated with heart disease in observational studies; some are statistically inno-cent. Given all the fuss made—and rightfully so—about the differences between omega-3 and omega-6 poly-unsaturated fats, it's curious the Dietary Powers That Be are so tight-lipped when it comes to differentiating between various saturated fats. It's kind of a big deal. Let's look at why.

THE DEVIL'S IN THE DETAILS: THE DIFFERENT TYPES OF SATURATED FAT

Here's the stuff you won't read in media headlines. Far from being one "thing," saturated fatty acids can be grouped into three categories, all based on the number of carbon atoms in their chain (don't worry—this is as technical as we'll get!). Long-chain saturated fats are, no surprise, long: They have fourteen to twenty carbon atoms. Medium-chain saturated fats have between six and thirteen carbon atoms. Short-chain saturated fatty acids have less than six carbon atoms.

That wasn't too painful, right?

As few studies as there are looking directly at the effects of saturated on heart disease, even fewer break down those effects by saturated fat subtype. So, until the research world conspires in our favor to answer our most pressing questions (hint: they're not usually the same questions grant money goes to fund), here's what we have to work with: a bunch of studies looking at individual saturated fatty acids and blood cholesterol. It's not perfect, but the findings—as we'll see next—are enough to make it abundantly clear that talking about "saturated fat" as a single nutrient is like talking about "Africa" as a travel destination. Just as Cape Town is a far cry from the Sahara Desert, short- and medium-chain saturated fats are a whole different beast than their long-chain brethren.

In a 2018 systematic review and meta-analysis, Australian researchers set out to investigate how medium-chain saturated fats versus long-chain satu-rated fats affected people's cholesterol levels.[10] (For reference: Medium-chain fats—also known as medium-chain triglycerides or MCTs—are, as of this writing, wildly popular as a supplement. MCTs are abundant in coconut oil, while long-chain saturated fats are abun-dant in dairy fat, tallow, and lard.) After identifying a dozen eligible trials in humans, the researchers found that diets enriched with medium-chain fatty acids sig-nificantly raised HDL levels, without impacting LDL. But while medium-chain saturated fats *raised* HDL, long-chain saturated fats had almost no effect on HDL. Even the famed Nurses' Health Study found that medium-chain or short-chain saturated fats were *not* associated with increased heart disease risk, even though long-chain saturated fats were (bearing in mind, yet again, that correlation isn't causation).[11]

Medium-chain saturated fats deserve some special mention here. Although mainstream nutrition still gives it the side-eye, coconut oil rose to superfood status due to its high concentration of these special fats—in particular, lauric acid, a twelve-carbon fatty acid—which have benefits far beyond the realm of heart health. Their shorter length allows them to head straight to the liver for energy, reducing the potential for fat storage. Possibly even more exciting, these fats have been shown to benefit a number of neurological conditions, including epilepsy, Alzheimer's disease, and autism, while also having antimicrobial properties. And while coconut oil alone supplies plenty of medium-chain fats, an even more concentrated source—MCT oil—has recently hit the scene as a popular supplement. MCT oil is typically extracted from coconut oil, and may have an even greater capacity than its parent oil to raise HDL without impacting (or even lowering) LDL.

In one 16-week trial comparing high intakes of MCT oil to olive oil, MCT oil-consuming participants actually saw a significant *drop* in their LDL levels.[12]

Short-chain saturated fats have also been studied for their unusual health benefits. This group of fats—the tiniest of the bunch—are produced when bacteria in your colon ferment certain fibers, and that's where we get the majority of them. But here's where dairy earns its stripes: Butter, especially the grass-fed variety, is one of our few dietary sources of *butyric acid*—one of the most beneficial short-chain saturated fats out there. Butyric acid not only independently reduces cholesterol levels, it also serves as food for colon cells, helps protect against colon cancer, fights oxidative stress, and reduces inflammation.

In sum, although the research isn't totally consistent—and it rarely is in the field of nutrition—here's what the science typically shows when it comes to individual saturated fatty acids:

- Stearic acid (long-chain): Mainly found in beef, butter, lard, mutton, coconut, palm kernel oil, and cocoa butter. It has a neutral effect on LDL in general, and compared to other saturated fats, slightly *lowers* LDL. Your body can also convert a small amount of stearic acid into oleic acid—the same monounsaturated fat abundant in olive oil.

- Palmitic acid (long-chain): The most common form of saturated fat in most people's diets. It's extremely abundant in palm oil, but is also found in red meat, dairy, salmon, and egg yolks. It can significantly raise LDL levels without impacting HDL.

- Myristic acid (long-chain): Found in coconut oil, dairy products, palm oil, and palm kernel oil. This form of saturated fat has the greatest LDL-raising effect out of all the saturated fats, without raising HDL.

- Lauric acid (medium-chain): Highest in coconut oil and palm kernel oil, making up almost half the fat in each of those oils. It has a small LDL-raising effect, but raises HDL significantly—in fact, it's the most powerful HDL-raiser out of any saturated fat!

- Capric acid, caprylic acid, and caproic acid (all medium-chain): Found in coconut oil, palm kernel oil, and the now-popular MCT oil. Due to their short length, they're rapidly broken down and absorbed rapidly, getting directly transported to the liver for energy. They tend to raise HDL cholesterol and lower triglycerides.

- Butyric acid (short-chain): Highest in butter, and also produced in the colon when bacteria ferment certain fibers. Butyrate can help suppress cholesterol synthesis in the body and lower LDL levels—on top of improving insulin sensitivity and blood sugar control, which (as you'll see in chapter 9 or as you saw in chapter6), may be one of the most important factors in the development of heart disease.

Looking at this list, you might notice a bit of a problem. Most of the foods here contain more than one type of saturated fat. And sometimes—like in the case of coconut oil, those different saturated fats have seemingly opposite effects on cholesterol. In coconut oil, for example, one of the fats—lauric acid—raises HDL cholesterol. Another—stearic acid—has no impact at all on cholesterol. What happens when both of those saturated fatty acids join forces within one food? Does one clearly dominate? Do their effects cancel out? Do they play "rock, paper, scissors" to figure out a winner?

Often, the only way to tell is by studying each food directly. For an example of how this pans out in the real world, we can look at a recent randomized trial testing the blood lipid effects of eating different fats—two saturated, and one monounsaturated. In this study, ninety-four healthy men and women were assigned to consume 50 grams daily of extra-virgin coconut oil, butter, or extra-virgin olive oil for a total of four weeks.[13]

The results? Compared to baseline, the coconut oil significantly raised participants' HDL levels, but didn't touch their LDL. Meanwhile, butter had a small HDL-raising effect while dramatically raising LDL. (In case you're wondering, the olive oil raised HDL about as much as butter and didn't impact LDL one way or the other.)

Amusingly, the researchers called the results "somewhat surprising," due to coconut oil's high content of saturated fat—which, in their words, "is generally held to have an adverse effect on blood lipids by increasing blood LDL-C concentrations." The different *composition* of these fats—rather than their overall saturated fat content—was responsible for their specific effects on blood cholesterol.

Does this mean we should swap out butter for coconut oil to fill our culinary needs? Not so fast! Even if we go out on that long, ever-weakening limb that asserts our blood cholesterol directly and significantly raises heart disease risk, recall that butter is one of our only dietary sources of butyric acid—that special little fat with a whole slew of health benefits. Butter might raise LDL more so than it does HDL, but it does so alongside some pretty impressive health perks.

Can you see why trying to study the effects of saturated fat as a single, all-encompassing category is an exercise in futility?

A Word on Dairy

Dairy: Is it good for your bones? Bad for your heart? Is butter an artery-clogging killer, or falsely accused? And what about the French—with their historically low heart disease rates and famously cheese-rich cuisine?

It turns out, there's a reason the science is so confusing (and often contradictory) when it comes to dairy—and it has to do with something called *milk fat globule membrane*. Most milk fat comes in the form of tiny droplets surrounded by a thin membrane made of lipids, proteins, and enzymes, and that membrane happens to be chock-full of compounds that affect everything from brain function to gut health to immune defense, and even gene expression.

In dairy products made from less processed milk—think cream and cheese—milk fat globule membrane remains intact. During processing methods like homogenization, though, fat globules get broken down and the structure of their membrane gets altered, losing its bioactive properties. This could be why studies tend to be inconsistent when looking at high-fat dairy products: Less refined, fat globule membrane-containing items like cheese, cream, and yogurt tend to have a negligible impact on LDL, while butter—which has much lower levels of milk fat globule membrane, as a result of the churning process transferring the membrane to the buttermilk fraction—tends to raise LDL significantly. Studying high-fat dairy products as a whole misses this important nuance!

In 2015, a fascinating randomized trial was published in the *American Journal of Clinical Nutrition* looking at the impact of milk fat globule membrane on blood lipids and cholesterol metabolism.[14] In it, Swedish researchers placed fifty-seven overweight adults on one of two diets, each with the same number of calories, for eight weeks total: one diet containing 40 g per day of milk fat as whipping cream (containing milk fat globule membrane), and the other containing the same amount of milk fat, but in the form of butter oil (*without* intact milk fat globule membrane).

Despite containing the exact same amount of milk fat, the two diets produced wildly different results. Whereas the diet with butter oil increased total and LDL cholesterol, the diet containing milk fat globule membrane didn't alter the participants' lipid profiles. The researchers suspected this was due to milk fat globule protein suppressing the expression of certain genes related to cholesterol metabolism.

When it comes to dairy, of course, the important question isn't how it impacts cholesterol levels, but how it impacts *actual disease and mortality outcomes*. Even here, the scientific literature isn't totally clear. A review of eighteen observational studies found that milk, cheese, and yogurt tended to be *negatively* associated with cardiovascular disease, whereas butter had mixed results—raising the risk in some studies, and having a neutral effect in others.[15]

THE CARBOHYDRATE SWAP

For decades, most health professionals have told us that we'd be doing ourselves a huge favor if we just cut out saturated fat and replaced it with carbohydrates. And that's exactly what most people did. After all, this idea fit nicely with the prevailing ethos: Saturated fat is bad, and "complex" carbohydrates are good. If we just swap 'em, everyone will go home happy, and all will be right with the world.

So, as our old friend Dr. Phil might've said, "How's that working for you?"

The answer is, "Not so well."

One important study shed light on the whole "carbs for saturated fat" swap but raised a lot of eyebrows because of its unexpected results. The study, titled "Dietary Fats, Carbohydrate, and the Progression of Coronary Atherosclerosis in

DR. SINATRA: THE CASE AGAINST CANOLA OIL

Back in 1997, I wrote an article for *Connecticut Medicine* about oxidized LDL and free radicals. I was very gung ho about canola oil at the time—as were most of my colleagues—and I was emphatic in my recommendation of it.

But the paper was rejected.

A Yale professor of medicine who was on the peer-review board—a biochemist, in fact—reviewed the paper and nixed it for publication. But he was kind enough to suggest some review articles on canola oil in the literature.

I read them.

My reaction: "What have I been smoking all these years?"

The success of canola oil and its reputation as the healthiest of oils is a triumph of marketing over science. It's a terrible oil. It's typically extracted and refined using very high heat and petroleum solvents (such as hexane). Then it undergoes a process of refining, degumming, bleaching, and—because it stinks—deodorization using even more chemicals. The only kind of canola oil that could possibly be okay is organic, cold-pressed, unrefined canola oil, and hardly anyone is using that.

Our friend Fred Pescatore, M.D., best-selling author of *The Hamptons Diet* and former medical director of the Atkins Center, is something of a cooking oil expert. Here's what he had to say about canola oil: "I would never use this stuff!"

If you'd like to read more about the dark side of canola oil, check out the definitive paper by lipid biochemist Mary Enig and Weston A. Price Foundation president Sally Fallon. Widely available online, it's called, tellingly, "The Great Con-Ola."

As for my 1997 paper, I revised it, removing the recommendation to use canola oil. The paper was accepted and published.

Post-menopausal Women," was conducted by the distinguished researcher Dariush Mozaffarian and his associates from Harvard Medical School.[16]

As the study title suggests, Mozaffarian set out to investigate how various fats—saturated, polyunsaturated, and monounsaturated—influenced the progression of heart disease in postmenopausal women who ate a relatively low-fat diet. Noting that standard dietary advice has always been to eat less saturated fat, the researchers wondered exactly what terrific things would happen if you replaced terrible saturated fat with other food substances. According to the standard advice, replacing saturated fat with good stuff (e.g., carbs or "good fats" such as vegetable oils)

DR. JONNY: GOOD CARBS, BAD CARBS

Whenever I give a talk about healthy eating and I mention that a diet very high in carbohydrates is problematic for most people, I'm very careful to add the caveat: "I'm not talking about fruits and vegetables!" So here's a quick cheat sheet on "good" versus "bad" carbs.

Good carbs include the following foods:

- Fruits
- Vegetables
- Beans and legumes

Bad carbs, which cover almost all carbs that come in a box with a bar code*, include:

- Cereals
- White rice
- Pasta
- Breads
- Cookies

- Pastries
- Snack foods
- Sodas
- Juice drinks
- Crackers

*There are exceptions in the categories of cereal and bread, but they are few and far between. Oatmeal is one example (but not the instant kind). Ezekiel 4:9 bread is another. But by and large if you stay away from most of the foods on the above list—or keep them to an absolute minimum—you'll be much better off.

should substantially reduce your risk for heart disease.

Except that it didn't. "Greater saturated fat intake is associated with *less* progression of coronary atherosclerosis, whereas carbohydrate intake is associated with a *greater* progression [italics ours]," the authors concluded. "Women with higher saturated fat intakes had less progression of coronary atherosclerosis."

Greater saturated fat intake was also associated with higher HDL levels, higher HDL-2 cholesterol levels, lower triglycerides, and an improved total cholesterol to HDL ratio. Saturated fat, at least in this study, was

hardly the dietary demon it's been made out to be.

And if this were not a knockout punch by itself, consider what was associated with a greater progression of coronary atherosclerosis.

Are you sitting down? Carbohydrates.

Especially the high-glycemic, processed variety of carbohydrates, which is exactly what we tend to eat when we replace saturated fat in the diet with so-called "complex" carbs such as breads, pasta, rice, and cereal.

"The findings also suggest," wrote the researchers, "that carbohydrate intake may increase atherosclerotic progression, especially when refined carbohydrates replace saturated or monounsaturated fats."

"Wait a minute," you might well say. "When I take the saturated fat out of my diet and replace it with high-glycemic carbohydrates I'm actually *increasing* my risk for heart disease?"

Um, yes.

By the way, Mozaffarian and his research team didn't just look at cholesterol. They looked at actual clinical events, such as heart attacks and deaths, from any type of cardiovascular disease. They also looked at lesser known metrics that only your doctor will appreciate (such as coronary revascularization and unstable angina).

Bottom line: Greater saturated fat intake didn't increase the risk for any of them.

VEGETABLE OILS: MYTHS AND MYTH-CONCEPTIONS

The researchers also tested what happens when you replace saturated fat with polyunsaturated fat (such as vegetable oils), the conventional dietary advice given by just about every major health organization. Maybe high-sugar carbs aren't so good for us after all, but what about the much-touted vegetable oils, which contain the "healthy fat" our doctors keep telling us about? Swapping saturated fat for a nice helping of healthy vegetable fat has got to be just the ticket to heart health, right?

So the researchers looked at the effect of replacing saturated fat with polyunsaturated fat. Just for fun, they also took a look at what happens when you swap carbs for polyunsaturated fat. When carbs were replaced with polyunsaturated fat there was no change in atherosclerotic progression—in terms of heart disease risk, it was a wash. But when saturated fat was replaced with polyunsaturated fat, there was a big change—but not in the expected direction. Replacing saturated fat with polyunsaturated fat actually led to an *increase* in the progression of coronary atherosclerosis![17]

(This seemingly crazy finding will make a lot more sense when we discuss those special classes of polyunsaturated fat mentioned earlier in the chapter, omega-3s and omega-6s. Stay tuned.)

If you're confused by these findings, you're hardly alone. The *American Journal of Clinical Nutrition* devoted an entire editorial to the findings titled "Saturated Fat Prevents Coronary Artery Disease? An American Paradox."[18] But it's only a paradox if we refuse to question the bedrock belief of fat theology that saturated fat consumption increases the risk for heart disease. The research is showing that it does not.

We worry deeply about the wholesale, unqualified recommendation to reduce saturated fat at all costs, because it invariably means that people will replace it with processed carbohydrates. That switcheroo is just about guaranteed to both reduce HDLs and increase triglycerides, and if you're trying to prevent heart disease, those are very bad outcomes indeed.[19] In the Nurses' Health Study, for example, refined carbohydrates and their high glycemic load were independently shown to be associated with an increased risk for coronary heart disease.[20]

Now don't misunderstand us. If you wanted to swap some saturated fat out of your diet and trade it for some low-sugar, high-fiber, nutrient-rich carbohydrates, such as Brussels sprouts or kale, no one would complain. Substituting saturated fat with low-glycemic carbs such as vegetables doesn't increase the risk of heart attacks at all, but substitution of saturated fat with high-glycemic carbs does—by a fair amount, actually. A study in the *American Journal of Clinical Nutrition* found that replacing saturated fats with high-glycemic index carbs was associated with a 33 percent increase in heart attack risk.[21] Because most people replace saturated fat with exactly these kinds of processed, high-glycemic (high-sugar) carbs (e.g., breads, cereals, and pasta), the conventional wisdom to cut out saturated fat and consume lots of carbs instead is starting to look like an increasingly bone-headed notion.

Although it's not perfect, saturated fat does a number of good things in the body. Its wholesale replacement by the worst kind of carbohydrates is turning out to be a cure far worse than the disease.[22] A recent Dutch study added to the list of accumulating research showing that when you substitute high-glycemic carbohydrates for saturated fat you actually increase cardiovascular risk.[23] But the Dutch researchers had an interesting take on this, one that appreciates that an accumulation of saturated fat in the body is not necessarily the best thing in the world.

They pointed out that eating a high amount of carbs causes your body to hold on to the saturated fatty acids that you're also consuming—and those saturated fats get preserved, stored in your body rather than burned for energy. Meanwhile, all those extra carbs you're eating get converted into more saturated fatty acids in the liver. Now you've got a serious excess of saturated fatty acids—you're holding on to

GLYCEMIC INDEX AND GLYCEMIC LOAD

Glycemic index is a measure of how quickly a given amount of food raises your blood sugar (and keeps it elevated). Glycemic load is a related (and more accurate) measure of the same thing. High-glycemic foods—such as most white breads, white rice, and cereals—are simply those that send your blood sugar on a roller-coaster ride. Low-glycemic foods include most fruits and vegetables as well as beans and legumes.

the ones you're eating, and your liver is creating even more of them, fueled by the carbs you're consuming. Because large amounts of saturated fat can lessen the anti-inflammatory actions of HDL cholesterol,[24] this isn't a good situation.

However, the Dutch researchers correctly noted that cutting saturated fat out of the diet is not the most effective way to combat the accumulation of saturated fatty acids in the body. It's far better, they suggested, to reduce dietary carbohydrates. This way, your body makes fewer saturated fatty acids, and its tendency to hold on to those you do eat is reduced. "Attention should be shifted from the harmful effects of dietary saturated fat per se to the prevention of the accumulation of saturated fatty acids (in the body)," the authors wrote. "This shift would emphasize the importance of reducing dietary carbs, especially carbs with a high glycemic index, rather than reducing dietary saturated fat."[25]

FAT IN THE DIET: OUR PERSPECTIVE

We want to propose a different way of looking at fat intake. We think what we are about to suggest goes a long way toward explaining the contradictory findings, or apparently contradictory findings, on saturated fat, diet, fat reduction, and cardiovascular disease.

To do this, we have to briefly introduce the other two categories of fats besides saturated: monounsaturated fats and polyunsaturated fats. (Remember, all fatty acids fall into one of these three broad categories.)*

Monounsaturated fat is the fat that's predominant in olive oil (as well as in nuts, avocados, and nut oils, such as macadamia nut oil). Its health benefits have been well documented and are noncontroversial. Monounsaturated fat is the primary fat consumed in the highly touted Mediterranean diet, and it's generally accepted that this kind of fat is perfectly healthy. For that reason, we won't spend much time on it, because it is pretty irrelevant at this point to the case we're about to make.

The real action is with polyunsaturated fats. Remember, polyunsaturated fats, which are primarily found in vegetable oils, are the very ones we've been admonished to include more of in our diets. When lard was slammed back in the early part of the twentieth century, the health dictocrats started their cheerleading effort for vegetable fats. (The first major beneficiary of this all-out campaign to make vegetable fats synonymous with "healthy" fat was actually the

* Trans fats are a special category.

trans fat-laden Crisco, the most popular vegetable shortening of its time.) Even now, most people believe that substituting vegetable oil for animal fats is universally a good thing.

But is it always?

Let's, as they say, go to the video. Polyunsaturated fats as a whole are divided into two subcategories: omega-3 fatty acids and omega-6 fatty acids. (For those who've always wondered what the heck an "omega" is anyway, you can think of the terms *omega-6* and *omega-3* as real estate terms; they're simply descriptions of the location of certain chemical structures—called double bonds—within the fatty acid. An omega-3 has its first double bond at the third carbon atom in the chain, while omega-6 has its first double bond at the sixth carbon atom in the chain. Now, for our purposes, you can promptly forget all that and just concentrate on what these two types of fatty acids—omega-3s and omega-6s—actually do in the body.)

Omega-6s, as mentioned, are found primarily in vegetable oils and some plant foods. Omega-3s are found primarily in fish, such as salmon, and certain animal foods, such as grass-fed beef, as well as in some plant foods, such as flax and flaxseed oil. So far, so good.

Here's where it gets tricky.

Both inflammatory and anti-inflammatory hormones, known as *eicosanoids,* are made in the body from polyunsaturated fats. (And to answer the inevitable question, yes, we actually need both. Inflammatory compounds are a necessary part of the immune system and play a big part in the healing process when you have a wound or other type of injury.)

Omega-6s are the precursors to the inflammatory compounds in our body—they're the building blocks the body uses to make these inflammatory hormones (specifically *series 2 prostaglandins*). And omega-3s have the opposite function: The body uses omega-3s as building blocks for the anti-inflammatory compounds (known as *series 1 prostaglandins* and *series 3 prostaglandins*).

A ton of research has established that the ideal ratio of omega-6s to omega-3s in the human diet is somewhere between 1:1 and 4:1. This seems to be the best balance to keep inflammation in check and everything running smoothly. It's the ratio found in the diets of both hunter-gatherers and healthy indigenous societies where heart disease is rare.[26]

But the ratio of omega-6s to omega-3s in Western diets is anywhere from an astonishing 15:1 to an even more astonishing 20:1 in favor of omega-6s.[27] If you think of the inflammatory and anti-inflammatory hormones as two armies that work together to create balance in the body, that means we're overfunding the inflammation army by 1,500 to 2,000 percent!

THE LAW OF UNINTENDED CONSEQUENCES

Our extraordinarily high intake of vegetable oil has another unintended consequence, and one that may have a profound effect on cardiovascular health. To understand it, though, you have to take a short excursion into the world of omega-3 fatty acids. (Trust us, it's a short and easy trip.) You see, there are actually three omega-3 fatty acids—ALA (*alpha-linolenic acid*), EPA (*eicosapentaenoic acid*), and DHA (*docosahexaenoic acid*). The only one that is "essential" in the diet

is ALA, which is found in green, leafy vegetables and in flaxseeds, chia seeds, perilla seeds, and walnuts. That doesn't mean the other two aren't important. In terms of their overall effects on human health, the other two are probably *more* important than ALA. The reason the other two—EPA and DHA—aren't considered "essential" is that scientists use the word *essential* in a different way than regular people use it in ordinary conversation. In this context, *essential* simply means that it's something the body can't make, so you have to get it from your diet. Your body can make EPA and DHA, so technically they're not classed as "essential." Because the body can't make ALA, however, it's considered an "essential" omega-3.

But the fact that the body can make EPA and DHA from ALA doesn't mean it does a particularly good job of it. It converts the ALA from the diet into EPA and DHA using enzymes and a complicated series of operations known as *elongation* and *desaturation*, the success of which is influenced by many different factors, including the amount of inflammatory omega-6's in the diet. Even under the best of circumstances, only a small amount of ALA successfully gets converted into the very critical EPA and DHA.

Omega-6s and omega-3s compete for the same enzymes, and when omega-6 intake is very high, it wins the competition by default. A high intake of omega-6 reduces the conversion of ALA into EPA and DHA, which might be another reason why high omega-6 diets contribute to heart disease.[28] So not only are those omega-6 fatty acids pro-inflammatory on their own, but they also reduce the body's ability to produce two of the most anti-inflammatory substances on the planet: the omega-3s EPA and DHA.

It's a double whammy, and your heart is the loser.

No, the omega-6s that have been the darling of the high-carb, low-fat movement, the vegetable oils we've been told to use instead of animal fats—the very vegetable oils that "saturate" (no pun intended) our diet through their incorporation into virtually every baked, fried, and processed food available in the supermarket, the very vegetable oils that restaurants proudly boast of using because they're so "healthy"— are actually turning out to be as bad as, or worse than, the original saturated fats (such as lard) that they replaced, just as margarine turned out to be far worse than butter.

For example, the primary omega-6 fatty acid— linoleic acid—has been shown to increase the oxidation of LDL cholesterol, thus increasing the severity of coronary atherosclerosis.[29] One research study showed that a diet enriched with linoleic acid increased the oxidation of the small, nasty LDL particles, precisely the cholesterol particles that are most dangerous and most involved in the formation of arterial plaque.[30] Omega-6s even inhibit your body's ability to fully incorporate the EPA you get from fish or fish oil supplements into the cell membranes, which is meaningful because EPA is the omega-3 that has the most profound effect on the heart.[31]

Published values for omega-6 intake closely track observed coronary heart disease death rates for all sorts of populations worldwide.[32] And in the famous MRFIT study, subjects with the lowest ratio of omega-6 to omega-3 (i.e., those with the lowest intakes of omega-6 relative to their omega-3 intakes) had the lowest death rate.[33]

THE PARADOX OF THE ULTRA-LOW-FAT DIET

At this point you may well be wondering why low-fat, high-carb diets work at all when they do work. If saturated fat is not the bad guy we thought it was, and if carbohydrates aren't always the good guys, why is it that some of these high-carb, super-low-fat programs seem to work sometimes?

Glad you asked, because we have a theory about that.

Although many people may believe that extremely low-fat diets work because they cut out saturated fat, we suspect a bigger benefit comes from reducing omega-6s. Omega-6 is the predominant fat we consume, and as we've seen, we consume way too much of it. When we follow a very low-fat diet we consume less of it, which automatically lowers the pro-inflammatory to anti-inflammatory ratio. The fact that saturated fat is lowered is actually incidental.

In addition, those famous low-fat, high-carb diets, such as those promoted by McDougall, Ornish, and Esselstyn, are remarkably low in sugar. The carb content may be high, but they're not the carbs most people are gorging on. The carbs in these high-carb diets tend to be vegetables, fruits, and minimally processed starches, such as beans and brown rice. And although some of the starches may be high-glycemic (such as potatoes), they're high in fiber (a boon for gut health and short-chain fatty acid production in the colon) and they don't contain a ton of fructose (as do most processed carbs and virtually all packaged goods). Fructose is the most metabolically dangerous of the sugars, and it is a very minor player in any of the low-fat, high-carb diets that are successful.

We suspect that when very low-fat, high-carb diets work at all—and they frequently don't—they work because of these four dietary factors: fewer inflammatory omega-6s, fewer high-glycemic carbs, more dietary fiber, and much less fructose or sugar. We believe that whatever benefits might sometimes accrue from extremely low-fat, high-carb diets could be easily achieved by simply reducing sugar and processed carbs, eliminating trans fats, *in*creasing omega-3s, and *de*creasing omega-6s. Reducing saturated fat and dietary cholesterol intakes has virtually nothing to do with it.

Besides, what is the mechanism by which saturated fat could cause heart disease? In 2008, the distinguished biochemist Bill Lands attempted to answer this and other related questions about conventional dietary advice in a closely argued review (complete with 231 scientific references) that was published in the scientific journal *Progress in Lipid Research*.

Here's what Lands had to say about saturated fat and heart disease:

"Advice to replace saturated fat with unsaturated fat stimulated my early experiments in lipid research. It made me ask by what mechanisms could saturated fats be 'bad' and unsaturated fats 'good' . . . Fifty years later, I still cannot cite a definite mechanism or mediator by which saturated fat is shown to kill people . . . The current advice to the public needs to identify logical causal mechanisms and mediators so we can focus logically on what food choices to avoid."[34]

When it comes to the theory that saturated fat kills people, Lands was essentially challenging his researcher colleagues to "prove it."

And they haven't.

◀ WHAT YOU NEED TO KNOW

- "Saturated fat" actually refers to a family of fatty acids, each with different health effects—some good, some bad, some neutral. It isn't a single nutrient—it's a family containing many different fatty acids, each with different health effects.
- Saturated fat has been wrongfully demonized. Several recent studies have shown that saturated fat is *not* associated with a greater risk of heart disease.[35]
- The balance between dietary intake of omega-6 and omega-3 is far more important than dietary intake of saturated fat.

CHAPTER 8

THE STATIN DECEPTION

STEPHANIE SENEFF ALWAYS WANTED TO BE A BIOLOGIST.

For as long as she can remember, she has been fascinated by how things work, particularly how living things work. She wanted to know how frogs jump, how grasshoppers breathe, how cells communicate, how the heart talks to the brain, all of which scientists study in detail, frequently by spending hours a day peering into a microscope. She was interested in systems, and to her the human body was the most fascinating system of all. So she was more than a little delighted when, after high school, she was accepted into the biology program at MIT.

After completing her B.S. in biophysics, she entered the MIT Ph.D. program and spent a year working under Professor Harvey Lodish in the laboratory headed by future Nobel Prize winner David Baltimore.

But there was a problem. After a year in Baltimore's lab, Seneff realized two things. One, she wasn't really cut out for the isolation required by a life in the lab, and two, she wanted to start a family. So she quit the Ph.D. program.

But she didn't quit MIT. "In those days," she told us, "you could get a job as a programmer with no prior experience. I got a job at MIT Lincoln Laboratory, where I lucked into a group of pioneers in the fledging field of computer speech processing."

Voilà. Seneff found a home, a perfect blend of her two great interests—biology and computer dialogue systems. She went on to earn a Ph.D. in electrical engineering from MIT, ultimately publishing more than 170 papers and becoming one of the world's leading experts in blending biological systems with computer intelligence. (It was her pioneering work in the field of voice recognition and computer systems that led to commercial applications such as SIRI, the virtual assistant built into the iPhone.)

Then something happened: Seneff's husband was diagnosed with heart disease.

His doctor put him on a high-dose statin—four times the usual dose—and told him it was imperative that he stay on it. "If you go off this, or even reduce the dosage, I can no longer be your doctor," his physician told him.

Almost immediately, the side effects started. He developed debilitating shoulder problems; muscle aches and weakness (he could no longer open drawers or jars); cognitive and memory problems; and depression, something he had never experienced before.

We all know what we do when we first get a diagnosis, or are prescribed a medication we're not familiar with, or begin having a bunch of unexplained symptoms or side effects: We ask Dr. Google, which is exactly what Seneff did.

Except Seneff, as you can probably imagine, is no ordinary Googler. She applied her not inconsiderable,

methodologically precise skills as a researcher to the task at hand and proceeded to try to learn everything there was to learn about cholesterol, heart disease, and statin drugs. Understand, now, that she had not spent four years in medical school being subtly influenced by the drug companies, had not been a consultant to the pharmaceutical industry, had not been visited daily by a charming crew of pharmaceutical reps spinning industry-funded studies touting the benefits of their products. And she had not been paid hefty fees by those same pharmaceutical companies (the way Dr. Sinatra had been) to give "educational" lectures on behalf of their products (lectures that are little more than marketing tools disguised as scholarship).

She had no agenda—other than to help her husband get well. Basically, she wasn't bought or influenced by or beholden to anyone in the heart disease-cholesterol-statin drug establishment. She had no preconceived ideas, either positive or negative, about what she'd find. Her research was motivated only by a desire to get her husband well, and by her lifelong interest in biology and nutrition.

And let's remember that we're talking about someone who has a world-class ability to understand systems, theory, statistics, interpretation, experimental bias, confounding variables, and all the rest of the esoterica associated with evaluating studies.

Here's what Seneff told us about statin drugs when we contacted her for this book: *Statin drugs are toxic. I liken them to arsenic, which will slowly poison you over time."* (P.S.: Seneff's husband terminated his statin therapy, and all of his symptoms disappeared. Needless to say, he also changed doctors.)

THE NEXT MEDICAL TRAGEDY?

Seneff has become one of the most respected and outspoken critics of the cholesterol hypothesis, and she is quite vocal about her opposition to statin drugs, which she believes are the next medical tragedy waiting to happen.

Let's be clear: Although Seneff and other independent researchers are pretty unequivocal in their negative appraisal of statin drugs, we are not—we're a little more moderate. Neither of us believes that statin drugs are all bad. As mentioned earlier, Steve still prescribes them very occasionally, in certain limited circumstances (i.e. to middle-aged men who have had a previous heart attack and are at high risk for a second). Even Duane Graveline, M.D., perhaps the most outspoken critic of statins on the planet and author of *Lipitor: Thief of Memory,* lists low-dose statin therapy as one possible option for "high-risk" people.

Statin drugs do some good in some circumstances, but their benefits, and the circumstances in which they are appropriate, are much more limited than the pharmaceutical companies—and the doctors who buy into their talking points—would have us believe. Furthermore, any good they may accomplish has almost nothing to do with cholesterol lowering, as you will soon see.

Here's what's good about statin drugs. One, they're mildly anti-inflammatory. They lower C-reactive protein (a protein in the blood that's an excellent measure of systemic inflammation). And two, they decrease blood viscosity (making the blood less like ketchup and more like red wine). Any of the benefits seen with statins are almost surely related to these other actions of the drug, not to its fairly mean-ingless ability to lower cholesterol. In fact, that's why statins occasionally show up as beneficial for conditions that have absolutely nothing to do with cholesterol—including gum disease[1] and sepsis,[2] a complex inflammatory syndrome.

(When you finish reading this section, you may find that you agree with a growing number of health professionals who think that statin drugs would be even *more* effective if they *didn't* lower cholesterol. But we digress.)

If you still doubt that the cholesterol-lowering effect of statins is the least important thing they do, put on your detective thinking hat for a moment, do a thought exercise with us, and consider the following: Before the introduction of statin drugs in the 1990s, there were a number of studies done in which cholesterol was successfully lowered by other drugs, notably the class of drugs known as *fibrates*, the go-to treatment for high cholesterol before the near-universal switch to statins in the last decade of the twentieth century.** These drugs actually lowered cholesterol quite well, thank you very much. If lowering cholesterol does in fact prevent heart attacks or strokes, then we should see a significant reduction in heart attacks and strokes anytime we successfully lower it, regardless of the particular drug (or diet) used to accomplish this.

But investigations of the cholesterol-lowering studies before the mainstream use of statin drugs showed quite the opposite. And there's proof, all cataloged, collected, and assembled in one place, thanks to a man named Russell Smith.

** Mevacor, a statin drug, was actually introduced in 1987, but statins didn't become popular until the 1990s.

"DYING WITH CORRECTED CHOLESTEROL IS NOT A SUCCESSFUL OUTCOME"

Back in the late 1980s, Russell Smith, Ph.D., an American experimental psychologist with a strong background in physiology, math, and engineering, decided to write the most comprehensive and critical review of the diet-heart disease literature yet seen. Published in two volumes that spanned more than 600 pages and contained 3,000 references, it was titled *Diet, Blood Cholesterol, and Coronary Heart Disease: A Critical Review of the Literature*.

In the vast majority of studies reviewed, there was no difference in the number of deaths between the group that lowered its cholesterol and the group that didn't.

Then in 1991, together with Edward Pinckney, M.D., an editor of four medical journals and former co-editor of the *Journal of the American Medical Association*, Smith published a summary of this massive work in a book called *The Cholesterol Conspiracy*.

Among many other things, Smith and Pinckney reviewed all of the cholesterol-lowering trials that had been done before 1991. The studies found that using drugs to lower cholesterol was quite effective—at lowering cholesterol. The problem was that they weren't much good for anything else—for example, saving lives. If cholesterol lowering was in fact the holy grail of preventing heart disease and death, then we would expect the research to show a reduction in heart attacks, strokes, and deaths when cholesterol was effectively lowered, wouldn't we?

Here's what Smith and Pinckney concluded:

In the vast majority of the studies reviewed, there was no difference in the number of deaths between the group that lowered its cholesterol and the group that didn't. In fact, in a few cases, more people died in the group that lowered its cholesterol.

Okay, so we've talked about ten out of those twelve cholesterol-lowering trials—pretty dismal results. But what about the remaining two trials?

In these two trials, there were fewer deaths in the group treated with cholesterol-lowering drugs than in the control group. These two studies, accounting for only a sixth of the total number of drug studies conducted, were exactly the ones the cholesterol establishment seized on as "proof" of the link between cholesterol and heart disease. "However," reported Smith and Pinckney, "one of these trials was conducted by a pharmaceutical company, which evaluated its own cholesterol-lowering drug.[3] The second trial involved an estrogen drug that produced more harm than good in three other trials.[4] Therefore, both of these trials are suspect."

Scorecard: Out of twelve studies, ten showed no benefit; the two that did were both somewhat questionable.

Choosing one or two studies that show a positive result and burying the ones that don't is a well- documented tactic of the pharmaceutical industry. It's akin to finding two white checkers in a bucket of black ones and then holding up the white ones claiming that's proof that all checkers are white.

So let's review. Before the introduction of statin drugs, it was overwhelmingly clear that lowering cholesterol by itself did virtually nothing to prevent a single death or even to affect coronary heart disease in any meaningful way. Zip, nada, zilch. Therefore, if any *positive* effects were to be seen in statin drug studies, these beneficial effects couldn't possibly be due to lowered cholesterol.

As Smith and Pinckney conclusively demonstrate, all thirty or so studies completed before 1990 showed that you could lower cholesterol to your heart's content without adding a single day to your life. John Abramson, M.D., a professor of medicine at Harvard Medical School and the author of *Overdosed America*, summed up the problem perfectly in the medical journal *The Lancet*: "You can lower cholesterol with a drug, yet provide no health benefits whatsoever. And dying with corrected cholesterol is not a successful outcome."

STATIN DRUGS: RISKS VERSUS BENEFITS

Let's review: Lowering cholesterol, as the thirty-some odd studies before 1990 showed, accomplished nothing (except, of course, to lower cholesterol). So if there's a benefit to statin drugs at all, that benefit *has* to be coming from something *other* than their ability to lower cholesterol.

Now, one might reasonably argue, *so what?* Suppose you're right that the ability of statin drugs to lower cholesterol is irrelevant, but suppose they do a lot of good anyway? Why not just use them for their other benefits?

Good question. But to answer it, we need to know two things: One, just how great a benefit are we actually talking about? And two, what are the side effects?

In simple terms, we'd want to know the same things we'd want to know about a financial investment: What are we risking versus what are we getting?

With that in mind, let's take a look at the side effects of statin drugs you probably don't know about. (No surprise—this is not exactly data that manufacturers of these drugs are dying to publicize.)

The Dark Side of Statin Drugs

Besides being far less effective than you've been led to believe, statins have myriad unpleasant, and in some cases acute—or even fatal—side effects, such as many of those Seneff's husband experienced. These include muscle pain, weakness, fatigue, memory and cognition problems, and—for a large number of people—very serious problems with sexual functioning.

Statin drugs cut off cholesterol production in the body. That's pretty obvious, right? But to understand why the side effects of this seemingly "innocent" action are so severe and troubling, you have to understand exactly *how* statin drugs cut down on the body's production of cholesterol. When you do, you'll see that cutting off cholesterol production in the way that statin drugs do is like trying to kill a branch at the top of a tree by starving the roots. The "side effect" of starving the roots is that you don't just kill the branch, you destroy the tree. And the irony is that there was no need to remove the branch in the first place.

Besides being far less effective than you've been led to believe, statins have myriad unpleasant, and in some cases acute—or even fatal—side effects.

Let us explain.

Statin Drugs and Your Brain: Memory, Thinking, and Alzheimer's

There are a number of unintended consequences of statin drugs you ought to know about. For one thing,

Note to parents: The fact that some groups are currently advocating statin drugs for children, whose brains aren't even fully developed until they're twenty-five, should be as utterly frightening to you as it is to us.

statin drugs don't stop at just lowering cholesterol in the blood–they *also* lower it in the brain. And that's *not* good news.

Why? Because the brain absolutely depends on cholesterol to function at its best. Although the brain makes up only about 2 percent of the total weight of the body, it contains 25 percent of the body's cholesterol. Cholesterol is a vital part of cell membranes in the brain, and it plays a critical role in the transmission of neurotransmitters. Without cholesterol, brain cells can't effectively "talk" to each other, cellular communication is impaired, and cognition and memory are significantly affected, usually not in a good way! (See the sidebar, "SpaceDoc: The Strange Case of the Missing Memory," on page 112.)

Cognitive and memory problems are one of the most dramatic and frequent side effects of statin drugs, and a 2009 study from Iowa State University demonstrates why. Yeon-Kyun Shin, Ph.D., a biophysics professor in the department of biochemistry, biophysics, and molecular biology at Iowa State, tested the whole neurotransmitter machinery of brain cells in a novel experiment. (Neurotransmitters affect data-processing and memory functions in the brain.) He measured how the system released neurotransmitters when cholesterol was removed from the cells and compared that with how the system functioned when cholesterol was put back in.

Cholesterol increased protein function fivefold. "Our study shows there is a direct link between cholesterol and neurotransmitter release," said Shin. "Cholesterol changes the shape of the protein to stimulate thinking and memory."[5] In other words–how smart you are and how well you remember things.[6]

Adults should be no less sanguine. Speaking at a luncheon discussion put on by Project A.L.S.–a nonprofit dedicated to raising money for brain research and the understanding of Lou Gehrig's disease–the vice chairman of medicine at New York Presbyterian Hospital, Orli Eingin, M.D., had this to say regarding the number-one-selling statin drug in the world, Lipitor: "This drug makes women stupid."[7]

STATIN DRUGS AND YOUR ENERGY

Here is one noncontroversial and incontrovertible fact: Statin drugs significantly deplete your body's stores of coenzyme Q_{10} (CoQ_{10}).

If you don't already know what CoQ_{10} is, this would be a great time to become familiar with it. Once you understand the importance of CoQ_{10} to human health, you'll immediately appreciate why the depletion of CoQ_{10} by statin drugs is such a big deal. The depletion of CoQ_{10} is one of the most important negative effects of statins, and the one that is pretty much responsible for a host of common side effects involving muscle pain, weakness, and loss of energy.

CoQ_{10} is a vitamin-like compound found in virtually every cell in the human body, and when your CoQ_{10} levels fall, so does your general health. CoQ_{10} is used in the energy-producing metabolic pathways of every cell. It's a powerful antioxidant, combating oxidative damage from free radicals and protecting your cell membranes, proteins, and DNA. In a previous book, Dr. Sinatra has referred to CoQ_{10} as "the spark of life," and Dr. Jonny has written about it at length in *The Most Effective Natural Cures on Earth*.

Without CoQ_{10}, our bodies simply can't survive. The production of CoQ_{10} happens in one of the branches of the mevalonate pathway tree that is blocked by the action of statin drugs. When cholesterol production is interfered with in this way, so is the production of CoQ_{10}. Interestingly, the most important muscle in the body—the heart—contains the greatest concentration of CoQ_{10}. The severe reduction in CoQ_{10} caused by statin drugs damages not only the heart but also the skeletal muscles that rely on CoQ_{10} for energy production. How ironic that a drug given to prevent heart disease—which it barely does, and then only in extremely limited circumstances—substantially weakens the very organ it's meant to protect!

The fact that statin drugs cause depletion of CoQ_{10} levels has been known for decades. Merck, the manufacturer of Zocor (one of the best-selling statin drugs), has had a patent on a combination statin-CoQ_{10} drug since around 1990 but never manufactured it. Although no one knows for sure why, it's widely believed that Merck never produced this drug because there was no real economic incentive to alerting the public to the CoQ_{10} problem and then "solving" it with a combo drug. No one else was doing it, so why should Merck bother?

As we age, we make less CoQ_{10}, so keeping what we have is even more important during our middle-age and older years, when statin drugs are prescribed the most. Lower CoQ_{10} means less energy production for the heart and muscles. Stephanie Seneff and her associates at MIT collected a large number of subjective reports by patients on various drugs. They gathered more than 8,400 online reviews by patients on statin drugs and compared them for mentions of side effects with the same number of age-matched reviews randomly sampled from a broad spectrum of other drugs.

To this day, many doctors are completely clueless about the CoQ_{10} connection and are unaware of its significance. One of us, Dr. Jonny, played tennis for years with a terrific eighty-year-old named Marty. Although in great shape, Marty was always winded, had trouble catching his breath, and frequently experienced muscle pain and fatigue, which he (and his doc) attributed to "getting older." It turns out that Marty's doctor had put him on a statin drug for his cholesterol; his symptoms marked a classic case of CoQ_{10} depletion. When Dr. Jonny pointed this out to him and suggested he immediately start supplementing with CoQ_{10}, Marty said, "I'll ask my doctor about that!"

The doctor barely knew what CoQ_{10} was, was utterly clueless about its importance, and was completely unaware of this critically important side effect of the drug he had prescribed—a drug that was especially unnecessary in Marty's case, because high cholesterol is actually protective for older people.

This, folks, is just one example of what we like to

call "cholesterol madness."

If you are on a statin drug and need to remain on one for whatever reason, don't spend one more day without supplementing with CoQ_{10}. Run, don't walk, to your nearest pharmacy or health food store and pick some up. We recommend a minimum of 100 mg twice a day of a highly bioavailable ubiquinone, or you can use the ubiquinol varietal.

STATIN DRUGS AND YOUR GUT BUGS

We've long known that antibiotics alter our gut microbiome (the massive, and incredibly important, collection of microbes inhabiting our colon)—hence the age-old advice to eat live-cultured yogurt or take *acidophilus* tablets after a course of antibiotics. More recently, though, researchers have started exploring the effects of *other* drugs on our gut critters. One of those drugs is statins. So far, the news isn't good.

The reason? Cholesterol is a precursor for bile acid production in our bodies, and taking statins is a sure-fire way to alter the size and composition of our bile acid pool. And it just so happens that bile acids play a big role in shaping the gut microbiome. In mice, twelve weeks of treatment with either pravastatin (Pravachol) or atorvastatin (Lipitor) significantly changed the animals' bile acid levels and reduced their diversity of gut bacteria (an indicator of disease), reduced levels of butyrate (a short-chain fatty acid produced by fiber fermentation in the gut, and which plays a vital role in protecting against colon cancer), and overall changed the gut microbiome to resemble patterns similar to what we see with diet-induced obesity.[9] In another study, treatment with Lipitor raised levels of the harmful microbe

Desulfovibrio, often associated with inflammatory bowel disease.[10]

Although research on the effects of statins and gut bacteria in humans is still in its infancy, we suspect future findings will confirm that impaired or dysfunctional gut health is yet another causality of statin drugs.

STATIN DRUGS AND IMMUNITY (NF-KB)

As mentioned earlier, one of the good things about statin drugs is that they are anti-inflammatory. This is important and probably one of the main reasons statins show any of the benefit they sometimes do. Inflammation, as you learned in chapter 5, is one of four major contributors to heart disease.

We want our anti-inflammatory arsenal to be as powerful as possible, because inflammation is a major component of every degenerative disease known to humankind. Anti-inflammatory foods, supplements, drugs? Bring 'em on!

So the fact that statins are anti-inflammatory is a good thing. But the way they accomplish this anti-inflammatory action may not be without problems. They suppress chemicals in the body (such as NF-kB) based on the idea that these chemicals are bad actors that are associated with inflammation. (The thinking seems to be "let's round those suckers up and march 'em the heck outta here.") But the problem is that those chemicals aren't always bad! Like most of the humans we know, chemicals like NF-kB have bad sides *and* good sides. NF-kB, for example, helps protect against salmonella and e Coli. That's a neat little benefit you don't want to lose just to get a

SPACEDOC: THE STRANGE CASE OF THE MISSING MEMORY

In 2006, magician and performance artist David Blaine decided to do a stunt in which he was immersed in water for seven days. To prepare for this grueling event, he decided to train with a man named Duane Graveline.

Graveline has a particularly interesting resume: He's both an M.D. and an astronaut, one of six scientists selected by NASA for the Apollo program. He's also a renowned expert in the field of zero gravity deconditioning research. The reason Blaine chose him as a consultant was because Graveline himself had once spent seven days immersed in water as part of his own zero gravity conditioning program.

Ask Graveline how terrifying it was to be immersed in water for seven days, and he'd probably tell you it was a walk in the park compared to what he went through when he suddenly lost his memory.

Graveline's story began in 1999, when he took his annual astronaut physical. The doctors said his cholesterol was too high and prescribed Lipitor, the biggest selling drug in the history of medicine. But shortly after starting the medication, Graveline experienced a six-hour episode of transient global amnesia (TGA). TGA is the medical term for a rare phenomenon that can last anywhere from fifteen minutes to twelve hours. TGA sufferers suddenly lose the ability to retain new memory and often fail to recognize familiar surroundings. Often they can't even identify members of their own family, and they frequently become confused and disoriented. People experiencing TGA will literally regress in time—hours, days, weeks, or even years—and not have any memory of their life after the time they've regressed to.

Following the episode, Graveline discontinued the statin. But during his next physical a year

---

mild anti-inflammatory effect that you could probably easily achieve by other methods (like taking fish oil, for example).

And the impact of dramatically lowering cholesterol on the immune system is hardly limited to NF-kB. Research has shown that human LDL itself (the so-called "bad" cholesterol) is able to inactivate more than 90 percent of the worst and most toxic bacterial products.[11]

STATIN DRUGS AND YOUR SEX LIFE

And now for the part that no one is talking about. The dirty little secret about statin drugs. Please don't shoot the messengers. Ready?

Statin drugs have an uncanny ability to completely mess up your sex life. No kidding.

later, he was persuaded to restart the statin at half the previous dose. Two months after doing so, he experienced another episode of TGA. This time it lasted for twelve hours. His awareness was tossed back fifty-six years to when he was thirteen years old—he knew the names of every teacher and kid in his classes, but he had no memory of his subsequent life. He didn't even recognize his wife, who was with him when the incident occurred. Decades had been erased from his mind as if they had never happened.

Fortunately, the amnesia lifted, and his memory reverted back to normal. He stopped taking the statin again, too—this time for good.

Graveline began his own personal search for the facts about statins, and what he found was more than a little disturbing. He learned that TGA had befallen hundreds of other patients taking statin drugs. He also discovered that the side effects of statin drugs in general were both potentially serious and vastly underreported—they included elevated liver enzymes, muscle wasting, sexual dysfunction, and fatigue. He began digging a little deeper into the whole issue of statin drugs and heart disease. He started questioning some of the accepted notions about cholesterol, ideas he himself had once embraced wholeheartedly: for example, the idea that cholesterol causes heart disease and the idea that lowering cholesterol is one of the most important things you can do to protect your heart.

"I came to realize that cholesterol was in no way the heinous foe we had been led to believe it was," he wrote. "Instead, I realized that cholesterol was the most important substance within our bodies, a substance without which life as we know it would simply cease to exist. That billions of dollars have been spent in an all-out war on a substance that is so fundamentally important to our health is undoubtedly one of the great scientific travesties of our era."[8]

Not only is this a common side effect of cholesterol lowering, but it's also vastly underreported. And worst of all, many people who experience sexual dysfunction, especially men, have no idea that it might very well be related to the drug they're taking to lower their cholesterol.

Erectile dysfunction affects more than half of all men between the ages of forty and seventy years.[13]

We've already seen how lowering cholesterol can have serious consequences for memory, thinking, and mood. Just as the brain needs cholesterol for neurotransmitters to properly function, the gonads need it to produce the hormonal fuel to keep our sex lives humming. All the major sex hormones—testosterone, progesterone, and estrogen—come from cholesterol. It's utterly preposterous to assume that lowering cho-

STATINS FOR CHILDREN?

Dr. Sinatra will frequently prescribe a low-dose statin drug for people in this specific population: middle-aged men who have already had a heart attack or have documented coronary artery disease. Both of us believe there is no other good use for statin drugs*. There is virtually no good evidence to support their use in women,[12] they do not need to be prescribed for people who have not had a heart attack, and they definitely—emphatically, positively—should not be prescribed for children.

We want to clarify this position once again, partly to help counteract the enormous lobbying efforts of the pharmaceutical companies, which, as of this writing, are working tirelessly to expand the market for statin drugs to include children, one of the worst ideas in history. In *The End of Illness*, author David Agus, M.D., recommends that everyone in the country be on a statin drug. Agus is well-meaning but completely wrong. His idea, if accepted, may be the next medical disaster just waiting to happen.

So a middle-aged man who has already had a first heart attack may indeed find that a statin drug, along with coenzyme Q_{10} and fish oil, fits into his overall treatment plan. Remember, the antioxidant and blood-thinning effects of a low-dose statin may afford some degree of protection in extremely vulnerable men who have had a previous heart attack or moderate-to-severe coronary disease.

For anyone else, proceed with caution!

* Recently, a case has been made for low-dose statin therapy in cases of extremely elevated particle number

lesterol, which is tantamount to downsizing your body's own sex hormone factory, is not going to have a profound effect on sexual functioning.

Of course it is. And it does.

Several studies have shown beyond any doubt that statin drugs lead to a reduction in sex hormones, most notably testosterone.[14] And this is a very big deal indeed.

Remember, low testosterone is not just a male problem—women also make testosterone (albeit much less of it), and it's increasingly clear that even this small amount of testosterone strongly influences women's sexual desire. (Most anti-aging clinics now routinely prescribe small, physiologic doses of testosterone to postmenopausal women to treat sagging libido levels and improve general well-being. Even though women have less of it than men do, testosterone is vitally important to both sexes!)

We know for sure that low cholesterol is linked to low testosterone in women from studies conducted on women with a condition known as polycystic ovary syndrome (PCOS). Women with PCOS suffer from an abnormal increase in their testosterone levels, but when you lower their cholesterol their testosterone plummets, leaving little doubt about the anti-hormone effect of statin drugs.[15] The effect on men is pretty easy to document, and many studies have done just that. One study showed that Crestor, one of the most popular statin drugs, increased the risk of erectile dysfunction at least two and up to seven times![16]

If libido and sexual health were the only things disturbed by diminishing levels of testosterone, that would be reason enough to be deeply concerned. But low testosterone has a much more global influence on overall health. Low testosterone is associated with decreased life expectancy, as well as increased risk of mortality from cardiovascular disease.[17] And for those who have diminished testosterone levels, the risk is doubled! (Men: If you're over fifty, it's a good idea to have your testosterone levels assessed by a physician familiar with age-management medicine, such as the Cenegenics Medical Institute.)

The Hormone of Love

As important as it is, testosterone certainly isn't the only driver of sex and desire in either males or females. Another important hormone—known as the "hormone of love"—is oxytocin.

Oxytocin is produced in the brain, and levels are very high during childbirth and nursing because one of its functions is to help the mother bond with the child. When you cuddle after sex, you're flooded with oxytocin. (Males also make oxytocin, just a lot less of it than females do.) Researchers love to study male prairie voles because they are a rare exception to the male-female oxytocin dichotomy; male prairie voles, unlike males of most species, make a ton of the stuff. Male prairie voles are also a rare example of monogamy in the animal kingdom, and this has long been attributed to their oxytocin production, resulting in fairly permanent "pair-bondings." The bottom line is that oxytocin, which helps you feel good and bond with another person (or another prairie vole!), is an important part of human sexual desire, expression, and satisfaction.

So what does oxytocin have to do with cholesterol?

Unlike testosterone, oxytocin is not made from cholesterol. But oxytocin gets into its target organs via cell receptors, and those cell receptors are highly dependent on cholesterol-rich membranes. Critically important parts of the membranes known as lipid rafts don't work well without cholesterol, meaning that lowering cholesterol interferes with the ability of hormones such as oxytocin to reach their destination and work their magic. (As we've seen, this also happens with neurotransmitters in the brain that depend on cholesterol-rich membranes for cellular communication.)

Finally, statins also interfere with serotonin receptors in the brain.

In case you're not familiar with serotonin, it's one of the critical neurotransmitters involved in mood. The most commonly used antidepressants, including the blockbuster drugs Prozac, Zoloft, Lexapro, and the like, are known as selective serotonin reuptake inhibi-

tors (SSRIs) because they act mainly to keep sero-tonin hanging around the brain longer. Serotonin has a great deal to do with our feelings of relaxation, well-being, and satisfaction.

So how exactly do statins act on the physiology of serotonin?

Simple. Much like oxytocin (discussed above), serotonin depends on cell receptors to get into the cells. Serotonin receptors—just like oxytocin receptors—are anchored into the cholesterol-rich lipid rafts in the cell membrane. If you lower cholesterol you're going to interfere with serotonin getting into the cells. It's that simple. In fact, research has convincingly demonstrated that serotonin receptors can be rendered dysfunctional by statin drugs.[18]

The noted French researcher Michel de Lorgeril, M.D. (lead author on the Lyon Diet Heart Study), is so strongly convinced that statins are screwing up our sex lives that he devoted an entire book to the subject. His only book in English, it offers a brilliant argument supported by ninety-two references from peer-reviewed journals and textbooks. The name of the book—*A Near-Perfect Sexual Crime: Statins Against Cholesterol*—pretty much tells you what de Lorgeril thinks about statins and our sex lives.

STATINS AND ALL-CAUSE MORTALITY

Earlier, we discussed how the majority of cholesterol-lowering studies didn't show any difference in death rates between patients who took cholesterol-lowering meds and patients who didn't. In some of these cases, a slight reduction in heart disease deaths was clearly offset by a slight increase in deaths from other causes, so the overall net "gain" in terms of lives saved was a big fat zero.

But many studies show even more troubling results. For example, a study in the *Journal of Cardiac Failure* showed that low cholesterol was actually associated with a marked *increase* in mortality in heart failure cases.[19] And the Italian Longitudinal Study on Aging, published in the *Journal of the American Geriatric Society*, found that those with cholesterol levels lower than 189 were far more likely to die than those with the highest cholesterol levels. The researchers concluded, "Subjects with low total cholesterol levels are at higher risk of dying even when many related factors have been taken into account," adding that "... physicians may want to regard very low levels of cholesterol as potential warning signs of occult disease or as signals of rapidly declining health."[20]

STATINS, CANCER, AND DIABETES

There are also troubling indications that statin drugs may be associated with a higher risk for cancer and diabetes. Researchers from the Department of Medicine at Tufts Medical Center and Tufts University School of Medicine examined twenty-three statin trials looking for any connection between cholesterol levels and cancer. They concluded that "the risk of cancer is significantly associated with lower achieved LDL-cholesterol levels," adding that "the cardiovascular benefits of low achieved levels of LDL-cholesterol may in part be offset by an increased risk of cancer."[21] Statins can potentially promote cancer through a variety of mechanisms: one, through reductions in *natural killer cell cytotoxicity* (which, over time, decrease the body's immune response to tumor cells); two, through increases in *endothelial progenitor cells in the bone marrow* (which are associated with invasive breast cancer and lymphoma, and can potentially feed tumors by supporting new blood vessel growth); and three, by increasing the numbers and functionality of *regulatory T-cells* (which can impair the body's immune response against tumors and decrease the effectiveness of cancer immunotherapy).[22]

Even more disturbing, some individual statin trials have confirmed a potential cancer risk increase from statin therapy. In the Prospective Study of Pravastatin in the Elderly at Risk (PROSPER)—one of the only statin trials designed for elderly subjects—overall cancer incidence was significantly higher for participants taking pravastatin compared to a placebo. In fact, cancer rates went up so much that they cancelled out the reduction in heart disease deaths, leaving overall mortality unchanged. (For a deeper discussion of the PROSPER study see appendix A.) Likewise, in the Long-Term Intervention with Pravastatin in Ischaemic Disease (LIPID) study, the elderly subgroup (ages sixty-five to seventy-five) taking pravastatin had significantly higher cancer incidence than the placebo group. Collectively, this suggests that elderly statin users might be especially susceptible to the cancer-promoting properties of these drugs.

When it comes to diabetes, statins are also looking increasingly suspect. In a study published in *Diabetes Care* in 2014, a cohort of over 115,000 Italian residents—all freshly treated with statins during 2003 and 2004—were followed for about seven years, with researchers tracking any subsequent diabetes diagnoses or treatment they received. By the end of the study, the more consistently the participants took their statins, the greater their risk of developing diabetes: The researchers wrote, "In a real-world setting, the risk of new-onset diabetes rises as adherence with statin therapy increases."[23] In fact, compared to patients with very low adherence to the drug, those who took the drug religiously had a 32 percent greater risk of becoming diabetic.

And dose matters. Higher-potency statins were associated with an even greater risk of diabetes in one major Canadian study. Those who underwent "high-dose" statin therapy in a meta-analysis of five statin studies were found to have a significantly increased risk of diabetes.[24] In another study, researchers found that statin use increased the risk of diabetes by a whopping 46 percent. Let us point out that as recently as 2018, Dr. Jennifer Ashton went on *Good Morning America* to defend the American Heart Association's astonishing recommendation that people take whatever high dose of statins is necessary to bring their LDL down to 70 or less.[25]

Let that sink in for a minute. The American Heart Association and its apologists literally recommend that you take however high a dose you need of a drug known to cause diabetes for the sole purpose of bringing down a number ("LDL") that no longer matters. It would be funny if it weren't so sad.

Considering that statins have been shown to reduce glucose tolerance, induce hyperglycemia, induce hyperinsulinemia, and change insulin secretion patterns in the pancreas, it probably shouldn't come as a surprise that for some people, the end result is full-blown diabetes.[26] As we've noted in chapter 1, diabetes should really be considered "pre-heart disease."

Okay, so it's pretty clear that statin drug side effects are hardly uncommon. But if so many people have so many symptoms as a result of taking statin drugs, why, you might well ask, have you not heard about them? Don't doctors know about this stuff?

Okay, we've answered the first question in our inquiry—"What are the risks?" Now it's time to take a look at the second question: "What are the benefits?" Only then can we make an intelligent decision about the risk-benefit ratio and decide whether it really makes sense to take (or stay) on a statin drug.

Let's take a look at the evidence.

THE "BENEFITS" OF STATIN DRUGS: NOT EXACTLY WHAT WE'VE BEEN LED TO BELIEVE

To understand how you may have been misled about the benefits of statin drugs, it'll be useful to first understand something about how it's possible to mislead by using percentages. (Spoiler alert: If you want to make something sound better than it is—for example, the success rates for a drug—percentages are the way to go. We'll explain.)

Let's say you're on a game show and you can choose between two prizes, both of which are a big pile of money (but you don't know how much). Here's the choice: You can have 10 percent of all the money behind door number one, or you can have 90 percent of all the money behind door number two.

Which one do you choose?

It's impossible to know what's the better deal without knowing the absolute number of dollars behind each door. Sure, all things being equal, 90 percent sounds a lot better than 10 percent, but you'd have to know how much money we're talking about to know if you made the right choice. After all, I'd rather have one percent of Warren Buffet's bank account than 90 percent of the average American's.

So this is where drug companies get sleazy. Let's say a drug company advertises that their drug was shown to produce a "40 percent reduction in risk!" for a heart attack. Let's use some real numbers to show how misleading that can be, even though it sounds really good. As of this writing, Russia has the greatest rate of heart attacks of any country, 1,752 people for every 100,000. That means any given person has a 1.752 percent chance of getting a heart attack in any given year. Now let's assume you didn't know that, but you're scared to death of a heart attack because there's heart disease in your family. You're offered a drug that has a lot of potential side effects but your doctor, repeating the drug company's talking points, explains that this drug will reduce your risk of a heart attack by 25 percent. That's no small potatoes, and many of us would take a chance on side effects in order to reduce our risk of a heart attack by such a large percentage. But when you do the math and look at the actual numbers, here's what you get. Without the drug, you've got roughly a 1.75 percent chance of getting a heart attack. *With* the drug, your chance drops to . . . wait for it . . . 1.31 percent chance. Presented with the opportunity to take a drug with a lot of side effects in order to reduce your actual odds of getting a heart attack by less than a half a percent, many people might understandably say, "No thanks, doc."

The point is—you always want to know the actual numbers, whether it's the number of dollars you'll actually see at the end of the day, or the number of patients who you'll actually help. Percentages are wildly misleading.

A NEUROSCIENTIST TAKES ON THE STATIN DATA

Let's look at one of the most stunning real-life examples of how relative risk tricked us into fearing cholesterol. This one's brought to us by David Diamond, a brilliant neuroscientist whose interest in cholesterol began after he was diagnosed with *familial hypertriglyceridemia*–a genetic condition that leads to dangerously high triglyceride levels.

In his quest to get to the bottom of the heart disease and cholesterol confusion, Diamond decided to take a deeper dive into the research. He started with a highly influential study known as the MRFIT study[29] which is often used as evidence in favor of the conventional view on cholesterol and heart disease. (The MRFIT study followed a whopping near 360,000 men–at the time, the largest cohort of its kind–tracking the subjects' cholesterol levels and risk of heart attack over the years.)

The paper's claims were bold, alarming, and enough to send anyone with even *normal* cholesterol levels into a panic. The analysis seemed to show that virtually *any* increase in blood cholesterol above 150 mg/dL was associated with an incrementally greater risk of death from heart disease. For every mere 1 percent increase in blood cholesterol, in fact, heart disease risk rose by 2 percent.

In other words, it wasn't just folks with very high cholesterol that needed to worry: pretty everyone else who had a cholesterol over the "ideal" level was in trouble also!

And when the folks with the highest cholesterol were compared to the folks with the lowest? Those with levels greater than 290 mg/dL were at a *400 percent* increased relative risk of keeling over from a heart attack.

The researchers proclaimed their study proved that cholesterol "powerfully affects risk for the great majority of middle-aged American men."

If that doesn't make your doc whip out the prescription pad, we're not sure what will. Not surprisingly, the paper had a formidable impact on the nation's beliefs about cholesterol. Surely a study following *that* many people couldn't lead us astray. High cholesterol sure seemed like a bad actor. The logical conclusion from the study became "the lower, the better" where cholesterol was concerned–an assumption that still lingers today, fueling doctors' aggressive attempts to push patients' levels as far down as pharmaceutically possible (and, incidentally, making the shareholders of Big Pharma crack open the bubbly).

And that's why David Diamond wanted to see whether the study's alarmism stood on solid ground. Given how important we know cholesterol is for our body's basic survival–and, what's more, how flimsy the cholesterol hypothesis of heart disease has proven to be–something seemed fishy about such dramatic findings. So instead of trusting the *relative risk* that the researchers reported, Diamond wanted to know the *absolute* risk–how many people actually got heart attacks and died during the study.

Which is exactly what you *really* want to know.

So Diamond takes a fresh look at the MRFIT study and crunches the numbers–and the results speak for themselves. In an impressive re-analysis of the actual numbers (which he's presented in a number of recorded lectures some of which are available on YouTube), Diamond showed that in each cholesterol bracket, the number of people who *didn't* develop heart disease and the number of people who *did* was nearly identical.

Consider this: Among folks with rock-bottom cholesterol levels (150 mg/dL), the kind of numbers most conventional docs would be delighted to see, 99.7 percent didn't die of heart disease (and 0.3 percent did). Okay, sounds like really low cholesterol is a great goal. But compare those numbers to the group with really *high* cholesterol–290 mg/dL and over, the kind of numbers that would drive a conventional doctor to drink. In the super-high cholesterol group, fully 98.7 percent *didn't* die of heart disease (and a very slightly higher 1.3 percent did).

That's right. The real, absolute difference in risk between those with very low cholesterol and those with very high cholesterol was a mere 1 percent (the difference between .3 and 1.3). A lousy 1 percent difference in *absolute risk* across the entire range of cholesterol is what got everyone's knickers in a knot. Through the wizardry of statistics, the researchers were able to present those numbers as "400 percent

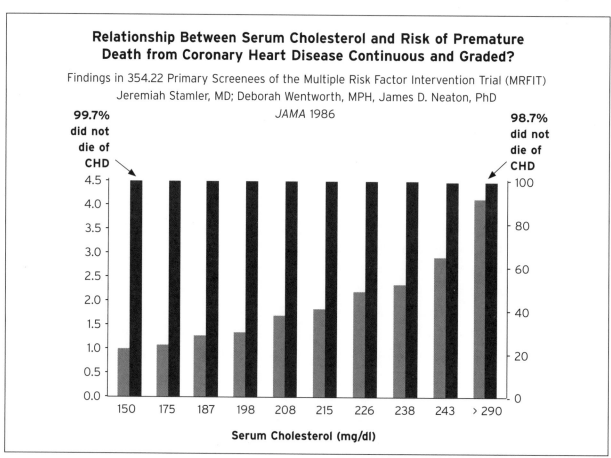

Relationship Between Serum Cholesterol and Risk of Premature Death from Coronary Heart Disease Continuous and Graded?

Findings in 354.22 Primary Screenees of the Multiple Risk Factor Intervention Trial (MRFIT)
Jeremiah Stamler, MD; Deborah Wentworth, MPH, James D. Neaton, PhD
JAMA 1986

99.7% did not die of CHD

98.7% did not die of CHD

Serum Cholesterol (mg/dl)

increased risk of death from heart disease" for people with the highest cholesterol.[30]

See why this stuff is so tricky? The original paper's relative risk wasn't *dishonest*, per se—but it certainly wasn't the kind of reporting that tells us the full story. And if it weren't for relentlessly investigative minds like Diamond's, we'd be none the wiser.

All that being said, the MRFIT paper in question was published in 1986—a great many decades ago. Has its findings, as ultimately unimpressive as they are, held up over time? Is having very low cholesterol levels really even a *tiny* boon for heart disease mortality?

The answer appears to be a resounding "no." In 2016, an even bigger analysis published in the American Heart Association's journal *Circulation*—this time following more than 1,250,00 statins-free veterans between the years 2002 and 2007—successfully called MRFIT's bluff. While folks with the highest cholesterol levels still had a higher risk for heart disease, this study found that folks with *low* cholesterol were in trouble, too: Those with cholesterol *under* 180 mg/dL had more deaths from heart disease than those with cholesterol all the way up to 240 mg/dL.

Imagine if, way back in the 1980s, we'd been told that *low* cholesterol was just as bad as high cholesterol. And that having "normal" cholesterol of, say, 175 mg/dL actually put you at a greater heart disease risk than having a "high" cholesterol of 235 mg/dL. Unfortunately, that's not what happened.

FUZZY MATH, ANYONE?

Now let's see how the drug companies use the same deceptive "relative" numbers (percentages rather than patients) to mislead you about the effects of their drugs.

The makers of Lipitor, for example, famously advertised a 36 percent reduction in heart attack risk in their magazine ads. But read the fine print. It's a relative number. Here's how they compute it.

Let's say you have a hundred randomly chosen men who are not taking medication; and let's say that out of that hundred, it's statistically likely that three of them would be expected to experience a heart attack at some point over the course of five years—in other words, 3 percent of the total number of men (one hundred) would be normally expected to have a heart attack over the course of sixty months. (The actual numbers in the study were slightly different, resulting in the "36 percent" claim, but for purposes of clarity, let's just round it out to 33 percent.)

Now, if you had put those same men on Lipitor over the course of the same five years, it turns out that instead of three men having a heart attack, only two would (2 percent of the total number of men). A reduction from three heart attacks to two heart attacks is in fact a $33\frac{1}{3}$ percent reduction in *relative* risk—"1" is obviously $\frac{1}{3}$ of the number 3—but so what?, The real, *absolute* number of heart attacks prevented is only *one*. One heart attack among a hundred men over the course of five years. The real *absolute reduction in risk* is 1 percent (the difference between the 3 percent in the no-drug group who would have had a heart attack and the 2 percent in the Lipitor group). The "33 percent reduction" figure is, again, a relative number, and because it's way more impressive than the much more truthful "1 percent" (the absolute number), researchers frequently choose to use relative risk instead of absolute risk when they report results! (Would you take a drug for five years with all the potential side effects reported above if you knew that it would reduce your chance of a heart attack by just 1 percent? Probably not, right? Which is exactly why the advertisements would tout "⅓ reduction in heart attacks" or "33 percent less risk." The drug companies may be avaricious, but they're not stupid!)

Worth noting: The fine print in that famous Lipitor ad did indeed admit that what *really* happened was heart attacks went from 3 percent to 2 percent. (You can see the original ad online—complete with fine print—by checking Google images for "Lipitor reduces heart attack risk by 36 percent.)

By the way—the aforementioned neuroscientist, Dr. David Diamond, worked his wizardry on that same Lipitor study. He created a graph to show the difference between the people treated with Lipitor and the people who got a placebo. On the graph you'll see two large bars, one in gray, one in black, that—if you squint—look like they are the exact same height.

And that's because, for all intents and purposes, they are.

The bars show the percentage of people in the study that did *not* get a heart attack. They show that in the placebo group, 97 percent of the people did not get one, while in the Lipitor group, 98.1 percent did not. When you see these bars side by side, it shows how truly minor the effect was. Lipitor basically reduced the percentage of people getting heart attacks by 1.1 percent.

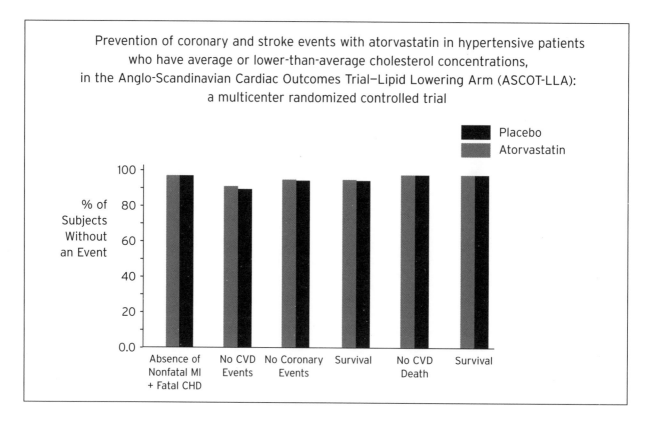

Prevention of coronary and stroke events with atorvastatin in hypertensive patients who have average or lower-than-average cholesterol concentrations, in the Anglo-Scandinavian Cardiac Outcomes Trial–Lipid Lowering Arm (ASCOT-LLA): a multicenter randomized controlled trial

Keep this in mind when you read our review of some of the studies used to promote the idea that statins save lives.

There's a second concept that would be helpful to understand before we venture into the studies themselves, and that's the distinction between *primary prevention* and *secondary prevention*. Primary prevention refers to treating people who have not had a heart attack for the purpose of preventing one. Secondary prevention refers to treating people who've already had a heart attack for the purpose of preventing another. As you'll soon see, the effect of statins on these two populations is quite different.

Before we get to that, there's something else you should know about study interpretation in general that may help you make more sense of some of the statin propaganda. Studies usually produce a mass of data that can be spun in a number of ways. Let's take one common substance we're all familiar with: alcohol. There are no shortages of studies demonstrating that moderate alcohol consumption is associated with a slightly lower risk of heart disease. So far, so good. But those same studies have also teased out a troubling connection—alcohol consumption increases the risk for breast cancer! Both facts—that alcohol helps your heart and that alcohol increases the risk for breast cancer—are absolutely true, but if you're a manufacturer of alcoholic beverages you're going to be talking up the reduction in heart disease risk and not calling attention to the association with breast cancer.

In much the same way, a drug company-sponsored study might indeed find a beneficial effect on heart disease associated with a particular drug, a beneficial effect similar to that of alcohol. But if in addition to lowering the risk for heart disease the drug increased the risk for diabetes—a finding that's shown up in a couple of statin drug studies—the connection to diabetes might easily be buried in the text where only the most determined investigators would be likely to uncover it.

At this point, in the first edition of this book, we went on a bit of a rampage, taking apart the sacred cow studies of the cholesterol establishment while bringing to light many of the studies that refute their conclusions. The "positive" studies—those showing a statistical benefit—are used by the drug companies to support the idea that statin drugs prevent heart attacks (sometimes, they claim, by as much as 36%!) and that statin drugs save lives.

In the original book we went over these studies—including the ALLHAT study, the ASCOT-LLA trial, the Japanese Lipid Intervention Trial, the PROSPER trial and the infamous JUPITER study—in great detail, exposing faulty methodology and unjustified conclusions whenever they occurred (and they occurred frequently).

But that was ten years ago, and detail that might seem mind-numbing and tedious today was needed then to expose the real flaws in the cholesterol hypothesis. We've decided to take a different approach in this edition, largely to save those who don't really care about the methodological minutiae and statistical details and would rather just get to the conclusions. We feel you.

But for those of you who *are* interested in the details of the how's and why's of misleading statistics, we've included the detailed analyses of all these studies in appendix A. Those who want to can nerd out on the numbers all they like, and the "cut-to-the-chase" crowd can break out the kazoos and keep reading, because here's the executive, "what-you-need-to-know" summary of the "case" for statin drugs.

In the ALLHAT study, there was ultimately no difference in the death rate from heart attacks between the statin-treated group and the no-statin group. Not a single life was saved by statins. The ASCOT-LLA study was the one that allowed Lipitor to claim that their drug lowered the risk of heart disease by 36 percent but for all the bragging, 100 mil was spent on the study and not a single life was saved. What's more, critics of the study pointed out a trend toward higher rates of heart failure, diabetes, and kidney impairment in the Lipitor-treated group.

The Heart Protection Study–which claimed "massive" benefits for a statin drug–actually produced a 1.8% difference in five-year survival rates between the statin and non-statin group, and that benefit was completely independent of LDL cholesterol (meaning lowering cholesterol had nothing to do with it). The PROSPER study showed a slight reduction in heart attacks and strokes, but a slight increase in cancer. And again, no change in overall mortality.

Finally, in the famous JUPITER trial that proclaimed a "50 percent reduction in risk of heart attacks," the *actual* risk went from 1.8% in the placebo group to .9 percent in the statin group and the statin group had higher rates of diabetes. (For those who want more details, please go to the appendix.) The bottom line is that the body of "evidence" for the overwhelming benefit of statins is . . . well, underwhelming at best.

THE DARKER SIDE OF

CHOLESTEROL LOWERING

Now, if you're still on the cholesterol-lowering/statin bandwagon, you might be forgiven for trying to look on the bright side. "Look," we can almost hear you saying, "maybe you guys are right. Maybe lowering cholesterol doesn't matter all that much. But clearly there are some good things statins do besides lower cholesterol, as you yourselves have pointed out. They're anti-inflammatory, they're powerful antioxidants, and they thin the blood. So what's the harm if people take them?"

Fair enough. For some people, especially middle-aged men who've already had a first heart attack, the good statins do may indeed outweigh the risks. The problem is twofold: One, statins are being prescribed left and right to people who have absolutely no business being on them, and to populations for which they have shown no real benefit. Two, the risks are significant, serious, varied, and highly underpublicized.

Before we get to our evaluation of the risks and benefits of statin drugs, let's review exactly what it is that cholesterol does in the first place. Understanding the functions of this much maligned molecule will help you understand why so many things can go wrong when we pursue lower and lower cholesterol numbers.

Cholesterol is a hormone factory. Cholesterol is actually the parent molecule for the whole family of hormones known as *steroid hormones*. These hormones include cortisol (known as the fight-or-flight hormone) and the entire family of sex steroids, including estrogens, progesterones, and testosterone. (No wonder statins produce such serious sexual

WHAT ABOUT PLAQUE?

Okay, so maybe statin drugs don't cut the risk of dying, except possibly in middle-aged men with previous histories of heart disease (and even then the effect is modest). But what about plaque? Doesn't aggressive lowering of LDL cholesterol at least reduce plaque?

Well, no.

A study published in the *American Journal of Cardiology* in 2003 used electron beam tomography to evaluate plaque in 182 patients after 1.2 years of treatment with either statins alone or statins in conjunction with niacin.[32] And yes, just like in many other studies, cholesterol did indeed go down in those patients treated with cholesterol-lowering medication. But plaque?

Sorry.

The authors wrote, "Despite the greater improvement in [cholesterol numbers] . . . there were no differences in calcified plaque progression." In fact, subjects in both groups had—on average—a 9.2 percent increase in plaque buildup. "[W]ith respect to LDL cholesterol lowering, 'lower is better' is not supported by changes in calcified plaque progression," concluded the authors.

side effects!)

Cholesterol is used by the body to synthesize bile acids. Bile acids are vitally important for the digestion of fat. The acids are synthesized from cholesterol and then secreted into the bile. Bile acids are so important to the body that the body holds on to most of them. It keeps them from being lost in the feces by causing them to be reabsorbed from the lower intestine, put into a kind of "metabolic recycling" container, and taken back to the liver. Still, even with its best efforts, the body loses some bile acids. To make up for this, the liver synthesizes approximately 1,500 to 2,000 mg of new cholesterol a day (that's about seven to ten times the amount in a large

egg). Clearly, the body thinks you need that cholesterol.

Cholesterol is an essential component of all the cell membranes in the body. It's especially important in the membranes of the brain, the nervous system, the spinal cord, and the peripheral nerves. It's incorporated into the myelin sheath, a kind of insulation or "cover" for the nerve fibers that facilitates nerve impulse transmission. And, as we've already seen, cholesterol is an integral part of the lipid raft, essentially allowing for cellular communication. (That's why there are so many cognitive problems associated with aggressive cholesterol lowering.) Cholesterol is also important for stabilizing cells against temperature changes.

Cholesterol is important for the immune system. Cholesterol has an important connection to the immune system. Research has shown that human LDL (the so-called "bad" cholesterol) is able to inactivate more than 90 percent of the worst and most toxic bacterial products.[33]

A number of studies have linked low cholesterol to a greater risk of infections. One review of nineteen large, peer-reviewed studies of more than 68,000 deaths found that low cholesterol predicted an increased risk of dying from respiratory and gastrointestinal diseases, which frequently have an infectious origin.[34] Another study that followed more than 100,000 healthy individuals in San Francisco found that those who had low cholesterol at the beginning of the fifteen-year study were far more likely to be admitted to the hospital because of an infectious disease.[35] And an interesting finding from the MRFIT study showed that sixteen years after their cholesterol was first checked, the group of men whose cholesterol level was 160 mg/dL or lower was four times more likely to die from AIDS than the group of men whose cholesterol was higher than 240 mg/dL![36]

We make vitamin D from cholesterol. It's almost impossible to overstate how important the cholesterol–vitamin D connection is. Vitamin D, which is actually a hormone, not a vitamin, is made from cholesterol in the body. If you lower cholesterol indiscriminately, it stands to reason that you may negatively affect vitamin D levels. And that's hardly insignificant.

Virtually every health practitioner worth his or her salt will tell you that massive numbers of people in the United States (and probably the world) have less than optimal vitamin D levels. According to the Centers for Disease Control and Prevention, "only" 33 percent of the U.S. population is at risk for either vitamin D "inadequacy" or vitamin D "deficiency,"[37] but the levels considered "sufficient" are still being debated, and "sufficient" is hardly "optimal."

In 2010, the Life Extension Foundation conducted a survey of its members—a self-selected sample of people who really care about these things and pay particular attention to their health, blood tests, and supplementation—and found that even in this highly health-conscious population, a whopping 85 percent had blood tests with vitamin D levels below 50 ng/mL, considered the low end of "optimal" (50 to 80 ng/mL).[38]

Why does this matter? Because there is compelling research that links less than optimal levels of vitamin D with heart disease, poor physical performance, osteoporosis, depression, cancer, difficulty in losing weight, and even all-cause mortality. Vitamin D is so important that Dr. Gregory Plotnikoff, medical director of the Penny George Institute for Health and Healing, Abbott Northwestern Hospital in Minneapolis, recently commented, "Because vitamin D is so cheap and so clearly reduces all-cause mortality, I can say this with great certainty: Vitamin D represents the single most cost-effective medical intervention in the United States."[39]

Undoubtedly, there are multiple reasons why so many people are walking around with suboptimal levels of vitamin D, not the least of which is that we are so darn sun-phobic that we now slather SPF ninety on our skin just to go to the grocery store. But is it a coincidence that vitamin D deficiencies and insufficiencies are showing up all over the place at the same time that 11 million to 30 million Americans are on statin drugs, the purpose of which is to lower the very molecule that gives "birth" to this vitally important nutrient?

AN OVERALL HEALTH BENEFIT OF ZERO

A few years ago, John Abramson, M.D., author of *Overdosed America*, analyzed eight randomized trials that compared statin drugs with placebos. His findings and conclusions were published in a column in *The Lancet*. Here's what he wrote: "Our analysis suggests that . . . statins should not be prescribed for true primary prevention in women of any age or for men older than 69 years"[40]

Dr. Abramson's conclusions echo the findings and recommendations of the researchers at Therapeutics Initiative, a kind of "consumer reports" on drug-industry studies that was started in 1994 at the University of British Columbia. Therapeutics Initiative, which is wholly independent of government and Big Pharma, evaluated five of the major statin trials (including some we talk about in the appendix) and concluded that total mortality—i.e., the number of people who actually died—was *not* impacted by statin therapy, and that "statins have *not* been shown to provide an overall health benefit in primary prevention trials"[41] (emphasis ours).

STATINS: A FINAL CAUTIONARY

NOTE

Millions of Americans will be taking statin drugs for decades, as recommended by the National Cholesterol Education Program's (NCEP) guidelines, and long-term side effects will become apparent, creating a whole host of pathologic situations.

What does all this confusion and controversy mean to practicing physicians and the patients for whom they care? Dietary factors and therapeutic life-style changes have no side effects. They should be considered the first line of defense in preventive cardiology.

Look, there's not much doubt that statin therapy can reduce the incidence of coronary morbidity and mortality for those who are at great risk of developing coronary artery disease.[42] But as research continues to implicate inflammation as the major coronary risk factor, cholesterol recommendations by groups such as the NCEP need to be modified. We're chasing the wrong villain, as you'll see in the coming chapters. Ultimately, hopefully, the attention paid to cholesterol will wind up being proportional to its importance as a causative factor in heart disease, which is to say, not much.

Rather than selecting treatment options as a technician or a computer would do and targeting cholesterol numbers alone, doctors owe it to their patients—and patients owe it to themselves!—to look further into these controversial issues before embracing potent drugs that might not truly serve the needs of the people for whom they're being prescribed.

Although the use of statins in high-risk coronary

patients—especially those with inflammatory markers—might be good medicine right now, overuse of these potent pharmacologic agents (that have both known and unknown side effects) for long-term use in otherwise healthy people is simply not justifiable.

◀ WHAT YOU NEED TO KNOW

• The benefits of statin drugs have been widely exaggerated, and any benefit of these drugs has little to do with their ability to lower cholesterol.

• Statin drugs deplete coenzyme Q_{10}, one of the most important nutrients for the heart. Depletion of CoQ_{10} can cause muscle pain, weakness, and fatigue.

• Statin drugs lead to a reduction in sex hormones, as shown by several studies. Sexual dysfunction is a common (but underreported) side effect of statin drugs.

• There are troubling indicators that statin drugs may be associated with a higher risk for cancer and diabetes.

• Statins should not be prescribed for the elderly or for the vast majority of women, and they should *never* be prescribed for children.

CHAPTER 9

THE *REAL* CAUSE OF HEART DISEASE

WE'VE ALL HEARD ABOUT THE APPARENTLY HEALTHY PERSON with no history of heart disease and no known risk factors who suddenly drops dead of a heart attack at age forty-seven while running in the park.

Everybody clucks their tongue, expresses shock and disbelief, and says some version of, "But he was so healthy!"

Well, he wasn't.

The signs and symptoms were there, probably for many years. And they were hiding in plain sight. The problem is, no one was looking for them. Because the warning signs for heart disease—the ones we *should* be paying close attention to, the ones that often show up years before an actual event—have very little to do with total cholesterol or LDL.

But they have everything to do with diabetes.

And to understand why, you first need to understand a condition that is at the root of not just diabetes, but—according to some compelling research—is at the root of *most* of the degenerative diseases of aging. It's called *insulin resistance*.

Insulin resistance is to heart disease what smoking is to lung disease.

Insulin resistance doesn't account for 100 percent of heart disease any more than smoking accounts for 100 percent of lung cancer. But it tracks with and predicts cardiovascular disease better than any other variable yet studied. We'll show you the proof a little later on—and don't worry, there's quite a bit of it. But first we have to explain exactly what insulin resistance is, and why it's so critically important to your health.

INSULIN RESISTANCE IS ESSENTIALLY AN ERROR OF METABOLISM

To understand how a *healthy* metabolism is supposed to work, imagine an eight-year-old kid back in the days before the internet and play dates. He has a healthy, undamaged metabolism. The kid comes home from third grade and eats a small snack—say an apple. His blood sugar goes up a little—it always goes up when you eat food—and so his pancreas releases a little shot of a hormone called insulin.

One of insulin's main jobs is to round up that sugar in the bloodstream and deliver it into the muscle cells where it can be "burned" for energy. This is just fine for our eight-year-old kid, because he's going to be climbing on the monkey bars, riding his bike, and playing tag. Eventually, his blood sugar goes down, and even drops a little from baseline because his muscles have eagerly used up all the sugar pro-

vided by the apple. And that's just dandy—he goes home, his blood sugar is *slightly* lower than normal because all the sugar has gone to powering his muscles. Now he's hungry, he eats a healthy dinner, and all is right with the world.

That's how insulin—and metabolism—is *supposed* to work. In theory. In fact, it does not work that way in at least 50 percent—or more—of the population. A 2015 study showed that when you combine patients with "pre-diabetes" with patients who have already been diagnosed with diabetes, and, just for good measure, throw in historically-based estimates of the large number of people who are walking around with undiagnosed diabetes, you're left with the disturbing conclusion that between 49 to 52 percent of the population has some form of diabetes.[1] And *that* figure is probably a low estimate. We'll get into all that in a moment.

Now back to our story about the kid with a healthy metabolism. Let's fast-forward thirty years or so. That same "kid"—now thirty-eight—wakes up late, stress hormones coursing through his body. Stress hormones send a message to his brain to fuel up for an anticipated emergency (read: *stock up on sugar!*). He runs out the door and stop at the local coffee emporium for a pumpkin spice latte[2] (380 calories, 49 grams of sugar) and a nice, "low-fat" blueberry muffin (350 calories, 55 grams of carbs, 29 grams of sugar).[3]

His blood sugar takes off like the Challenger.

Get to know insulin—it's more important to your health and your heart than you can imagine, and way more important than your doctor has probably told you.

The pancreas says, *"Code Red! Send out the big guns! This dude just ate the equivalent of ten packs of Ding Dongs!"* The pancreas produces a bucketful of insulin in a desperate attempt to get all that sugar out of the bloodstream and deliver it to the muscles.

Problem is the muscle cells aren't having it.

"What do we need all this sugar for?" they seem to be asking. "The only 'exercise' this guy's gonna get all day is pushing a computer mouse, and when he goes home, he's going to sit on the couch and play with the TV clicker. The last thing we need here is more fuel."

So the muscle cells begin to *resist* the effects of insulin. Like residents of New York apartments, they get so used to the "noise" that they barely notice it. They say to insulin, "Thank you but no thank you. Don't need it. Go somewhere else. We gave at the office. Buh-bye." And insulin has no choice but to take its sugar payload to another location, and guess where that is?

The fat cells. Which happily welcome the sugar in. And that's not a good thing for all sorts of reasons, starting with the fact that fat cells don't just sit there on your waist, butt, and thighs—they are actually endocrine organs, and they secrete a ton of inflammatory chemicals. And inflammation is one of the major causes and promoters of heart disease. Making your fat cells bigger only creates more inflammation.

But the fat cells get bigger anyway, whether you like it or not. Indeed, they welcome in all that excess sugar, and for a while your blood sugar levels may even be in the normal range, as the pancreas valiantly tries to pump out enough insulin to keep up with the sugar influx.

But don't be fooled. If insulin is frequently elevated beyond what it should be, that's a good clue that it's having to work awfully hard to keep sugar at manageable levels. Your blood sugar may still be hanging on in the "normal" range, but the high levels of insulin—which your doc may *not* be testing for—are a clue that the whole thing is about to come tumbling down. You can think of chronically elevated insulin as the pancreas's way of shouting *"Help!"*

Eventually, insulin will no longer be able to keep blood sugar in the "normal" range, and blood sugar will start to rise past "normal." Now your blood sugar is high—as it's got nowhere left to go! Your insulin is high, and you're *this*close to a diagnosis of full-blown diabetes.

CAUTION: HEART DISEASE AHEAD!

"Emerging evidence shows that insulin resistance is the most important predictor of cardiovascular disease and type 2 diabetes," says Robert Lustig, M.D., the pediatric endocrinologist and professor in the Department of Endocrinology at University of Southern California, San Francisco.[4]

The fact that insulin resistance is the most impor-

THE ENGINEER AND THE EMPEROR'S NEW CLOTHES: THE STRANGE CASE OF IVOR CUMMINS

Many folks–including both of us–would never have heard of Dr. Joseph R. Kraft (see page 134) had it not been for an Irish engineer named Ivor Cummins. In 2013, Ivor Cummins got some problematic blood tests back from his doctor, and wanted to figure out exactly what they meant in terms of risk. He had five kids and was a relatively young guy. What did these tests mean in terms of mortality? It was an odd assortment of out-of-range tests and Cummins wanted to know their significance.

The problem was that his doctor didn't really know. It was, after all, a strange trio of seemingly unrelated anomalies. Two doctors Cummins consulted for second and third opinions weren't much help either.

Since nothing looked particularly life threatening, many folks might have been tempted to just forget about it and see if anything weird showed up on the blood test next time around.

But Cummins wasn't–isn't–an "ordinary folks" type of guy. Cummins made his living as a master strategist, a problem-solver who led teams of other brainiac engineers in problem-solving for complex, multifactorial systems. Not content with an "I don't know" answer, he began to apply his considerable abilities in systems-analysis to metabolism and the human body.

It didn't take him long to get at what he thought was the root of his problem. In all cases, his elevated readings could be linked back to a high intake of carbohydrates.

A liver enzyme that was elevated turned out to be a marker for fatty liver, which is linked to diabetes. A high level of serum ferritin turned out to be a sixth marker for metabolic syndrome ("pre-diabetes"). What did they have in common? "They all tracked back to the metabolic syndrome and insulin resistance," says Cummins.[5]

Cummins changed his diet–not based on any diet book he read but based on the published peer-review research he carefully reviewed–and within a short time lost 30 pounds. All his weird blood tests returned to normal. Including the troublesome cholesterol numbers.

He started to research cholesterol–and fairly quickly arrived at the conclusion that the research supporting the cholesterol-causes-heart disease hypothesis, when examined rigorously from a systems biology point of view, turned out to be . . . extremely thin. (In one of his many lectures available on YouTube he said, and we're paraphrasing, "If my safety data on a product was as weak as the data on cholesterol causing heart disease, I wouldn't even be allowed to take that product to market."

He took the knowledge he had gained from his rigorous systems-analysis of metabolism and began giving seminars to other engineers.

Eventually those seminars—many of them as complex and detailed as any medical school lecture—wound up on YouTube. Where they created quite a sensation and remain wildly popular (and highly recommended: Start with "Wanna Know How To Collapse Your Heart Disease Risk? Well, then.").[5]

People started sending him their blood work and asking for advice. Doctors—notably functional medicine doctor Jeffrey Gerber, M.D.—reached out to collaborate. (Gerber and Cummins eventually wrote a terrific—and heavily referenced—book called *Eat Rich Live Long*—highly recommended.) Cummins became the director of the Irish Heart Disease Association. Andreas Eenfelt, M.D., the highly regarded low-carbohydrate advocate, posted a video interview with Cummings titled, "The engineer who knows more than your doctor."[6]

Cummins now blogs and tweets @thefatemperor. The name derives from the Hans Christian Anderson fable, and suggests an outsider telling truth to power, particularly on the subject of fat and cholesterol, and what Cummins calls "the bad science we've had on this for the last fifty years." He considers the cholesterol focus in heart disease "a farce" and—like Kraft, Reaven, and so many since—sees insulin resistance as what his engineering team would call a "root cause."[7]

Is he right? Is insulin resistance a "root cause" of chronic disease? Many researchers are coming to that conclusion. The title of one study recently published captures a growing sentiment: Hyperinsulinemia: A unifying theory of chronic disease?[8] As this book was being written, a new study was published in the journal *Aging Cell*.[9] It said that a combination drug cocktail that included a drug called Metformin had, in a small pilot study, been found to reverse biological aging by 1.5 years. Not stop aging—reverse it.

Metformin has also undergone studies at the National Institutes of Health[10] for its anti-aging effects, and was the subject of a *60 Minutes* piece.

Metformin is a drug used to fight diabetes and insulin resistance.

Let that sink in for a minute. As Bob Dylan said, many, many moons ago, "You don't have to be a weatherman to know which way the wind blows."

tant predictor of diabetes might not surprise you. But the fact that it's the single most important predictor of *cardiovascular disease* may come as a shock. Let us show you why that's true, and why *diabetic dysfunction* (aka insulin resistance syndrome) is indeed the most potent risk factor and the best predictor of heart disease on the planet.

Introducing the Insulin Assay

A good place to start is with Dr. Joseph R. Kraft, one of the most important researchers that almost no one had ever heard of, at least until fairly recently. Dr. Kraft was Chairman of the Department of Clinical Pathology and Nuclear Medicine at St. Joseph Hospital in Chicago for thirty-five years and, upon retirement, was appointed Chairman Emeritus.

Dr. Kraft invented something called the insulin assay, a then state-of-the-art test requiring glucose and insulin monitoring over anywhere from three to five hours. It goes far beyond the "fasting blood sugar" test and, by monitoring insulin levels, looks at how the body handles a given load of sugar over several hours. It was the most accurate test for insulin resistance ever devised.

In virtually every study Kraft did, very few folks with healthy insulin response got sick, while a disturbingly high percentage of those with insulin resistance did. Kraft wrote a book—still in print—summarizing all of the studies he did over the course of his career, all pointing to the same conclusion.[11]

Kraft summed up his life's work succinctly and beautifully. After rigorously testing more than 14,000 people for insulin resistance over his 30-something year career, and following them up for years to track what happened to them, this is what he concluded: *"Those with cardiovascular disease not identified (as diabetics) . . . are simply undiagnosed."*

The insulin assay is in use to this day, albeit modified a bit with modern technology. Labs like Meridian Valley now offer what they call the Kraft Prediabetes Profile, based on Kraft's seminal work.[12] In 2013, researchers found that the Kraft patterns predicted the risk of type 2 diabetes in Japanese Americans.[13] Then, in 2015, researchers led by Catherine Crofts published an important paper whose title says it all: *Hyperinsulinemia: A Unified Field Theory of Chronic Disease?*[14]

In 2017, Crofts team published another paper citing research showing that high levels of insulin (hyperinsulinemia) had been shown to be causal in hypertension, obesity, atherosclerosis, microvascular disease, neurodegenerative disorders, idiopathic peripheral neuropathy, and certain cancers.[15] They titled their paper, "Postprandial insulin assay as the earliest biomarker for diagnosing pre-diabetes, type 2 diabetes, and *increased cardiovascular risk*" (emphasis ours).

Insulin Resistance Syndrome

Kraft may have been the first to actually demonstrate the connection of insulin resistance to heart disease, but he was hardly the last. In 1988, a brilliant Stanford University medical professor and researcher named Gerald Reaven noticed that insulin resistance was almost always at the center of a cluster of conditions that, together, greatly increased the risk for cardiovascular disease: high blood pressure, abdominal obesity, low HDL cholesterol, and high triglycerides. Any of those conditions alone is a risk factor for heart disease, but together—with insulin resistance at the core—they were even more ominous.

Reaven named this dangerous collection of symptoms Syndrome X, but not long afterwards it became known as *metabolic syndrome*, and later, as *pre-diabetes*. Many researchers are now calling this syndrome—correctly in our view—*insulin resistance syndrome*. Over half of U.S. adults have it. And yes, you should be worried.

"During insulin resistance, several metabolic alterations induce the development of cardiovascular disease," said a 2018 article in the journal *Cardiovascular Diabetology*.[16] The authors point to many of the downstream by-products of insulin resistance—oxidative stress, inflammatory responses, endothelial dysfunction, hyperglycemia, and cell damage. They noted that insulin resistance leads to the well-known *lipid triad*: (1) high levels of triglycerides, (2) low levels of HDL and (3) small, dense LDL particles.

Reaven himself already knew that insulin resistance put you on the fast track to diabetes. Next, he wanted to find out if it put you on the fast track to anything else.

It did.

Reaven and his team performed sophisticated statistical tests to answer the question, *"Does insulin resistance predict bad stuff happening?"* They took 208 apparently healthy and non-obese individuals, average age sixty-one, and measured their insulin resistance and related variables. He followed them up for a period of four to eleven years, looking for incidence of hypertension, coronary heart disease, stroke, type 2 diabetes, and—just for good measure—cancer.

During follow-up, Reaven's team observed forty "clinical events" (i.e., the appearance of hypertension, coronary heart disease, stroke, cancer, and type 2 diabetes) in thirty-seven people. Several people in the study had multiple "events." Twenty-five of the thirty-seven who experienced events had scored "high" on insulin resistance syndrome. The other twelve had scored "moderate."

No one in the insulin sensitive group got sick.

To be crystal clear, the subjects with a healthy insulin response (i.e., those who had no measurable level of insulin resistance) suffered zero deaths *or* "events" of any kind over the next seven years of follow-up. And that's pretty unusual for a large sample of sixty-one-year-olds. The odds of getting those results by chance are about .00001.

It's important to know that Reaven's tests for insulin resistance were phenomenally sophisticated—far more than just measuring blood glucose, and even more accurate than fasting insulin. Reaven's results were no accident. And the fact that both Kraft's tests and Reaven's show almost the exact same thing should give us pause.

The truth is insulin resistance is a bear of a predictor. Reaven's studies demonstrated that if a person has a high degree of insulin resistance then he or she has a 40x increase in his risk for heart disease (and, frankly, other chronic diseases as well). But not just an "increase in risk" that's a doggone force multiplier. To make matters worse, insulin resistance is also linked to obesity, which, in turn, is associated with a higher risk of cardiovascular disease (CVD).[17]

Insulin resistance doesn't just put its thumb on the scale that measures your heart disease risk, it puts its whole hand on it. Researchers in the famed Insulin Resistance Atherosclerosis Study (IRAS) showed a *direct* relation between insulin resistance and atherosclerosis. And subsequent studies have consistently found insulin resistance to be an important risk factor and an excellent predictor for CVD.

A mathematical analysis of the relationship of insulin resistance (and other measures of diabetic physiology) to coronary artery disease in young non-diabetic adults concluded that preventing insulin resistance could avoid approximately 42 percent of myocardial infarctions in the next sixty years.[18]

Think about that for a minute–*over 40 percent of heart attacks could be prevented just by reversing or preventing insulin resistance!*

Here's another great example of careful research that clearly exposed the central role of insulin resistance in heart attacks. And it was research done for a very practical reason. You see, in Columbia–as in many parts of the world–heart attacks are the number one cause of mortality and disability. So Columbian researchers set out to discover what they could do to prevent second heart attacks in their people who had already had one attack, a question that probably has great relevance to more than a few people reading this book.[19]

The researchers gathered up 295 Columbians who had survived a first heart attack. The initial analysis found that there were eleven factors (including age, low income, lack of education, hypertension, and insulin over 10 IU/ml) that were initially associated with new cardiovascular events. All of those would be considered "risk factors."

But then they did what all researchers do–look at the raw data to figure out what factors were real and what factors were spurious. They did the standard multivariate analysis–which simply tells you what factors are dependent on what other factors, what factors are "noise," and what factors are "signal." (For example, sometimes "low education" shows up as a risk factor for heart disease, but it's really a stand-in for "low income," which is itself is a stand-in for a diet of cheap, processed food.) This kind of analysis teases out what factors are really responsible for the observed results.

When all the analysis was done, only one factor remained standing as a "significant predictor for new cardiovascular events"–insulin. The authors concluded that high levels of insulin were by far the most important factor related to the occurrence of new cardio-vascular disease. Insulin was a jaw-dropping 6.7x multiplier of risk. By contrast, the association between LDL and a second heart attack was non-significant, so LDL was essentially a "zero multiplier" of risk.

Now to be fair, there are studies that show a slightly higher than zero correlation between LDL and second heart attacks, but even the most touted studies don't show much better than a 1.5x correlation. And in many cases, a "bad" cholesterol test may only be a symptom of the *real* problem: insulin resistance.

One group of researchers reviewed seventy studies that had accurately documented the insulin levels of patients in the studies. The jaw-dropping results showed that out of 7seventy studies on patients with chronic disease, *sixty-seven of the studies showed that subjects in the "sick" categories had significantly elevated levels of insulin compared to subjects in the "healthy" categories.* As far as heart disease itself goes, there were a total of twelve studies included in the review, four studies on atherosclerosis, and eight more for cardiovascular disease in general. One hundred percent of the studies on people with cardiovascular disease reported significant elevation in insulin levels. That's an astonishing twelve out of twelve studies on heart disease showing *significant hyperinsulinemia in heart disease patients*.

HIDDEN DIABETES AND THE HIDDEN RISK OF HEART DISEASE

According to the data about 65 percent of U.S. adults over forty-five are pre-diabetic or diabetic—and many suspect that's an understatement. After all, those conclusions are based on *blood sugar* readings, not direct measures of insulin, nor of insulin resistance. Unfortunately, high blood sugar is a *late* sign of problems. The pancreas can be furiously producing a truckload of insulin in a gallant attempt to keep blood sugar "normal," which it may well be for a while, leading your conventional doc to say "everything's fine."

But it isn't.

Like a volcano on an island that looks peaceful to a tourist, your metabolism has hidden signs of a forthcoming eruption, and in the case of heart disease, the most important "hidden" sign is insulin resistance. And it's actually not hidden at all—you just have to know how to look for it.

And often, as we said earlier, the overwhelming importance of insulin resistance is hiding in plain sight. Take, for example, the famous EUROASPIRE study, which identified risk factors in patients with cardiovascular disease. All the patients in the study had survived a heart attack, so the study aimed to follow up with these patients for many years and to discover which risk factors were the most powerful predictors of a second event.[20]

The researchers initially separated the patient population into two groups—those with cardiovascular disease *and* diabetes, and those with cardiovascular disease *without* diabetes. One third of the initial patient population were full-blown, diagnosed diabetics. The other two thirds were classified as having "cardiovascular disease without diabetes." And here's where it got interesting—and scary.

On closer examination, a third of the "non-diabetics" in EUROASPIRE were anything but. They were actually full-blown diabetics, which when you think about it is not all that surprising, because in the U.S. alone, about one third of full-blown diabetics are walking around undiagnosed and as of 2015, more than 81 million adults in the U.S. had *pre*-diabetes.[21]

We can be pretty sure that the percentage of those "non-diabetics" that were actually diabetic would have been considerably higher if measurements of insulin were available on the patient population. Even using the imperfect measurement of blood sugar, we're still left with the conclusion that practically *three quarters* of heart disease patients studied are actually, to some important degree, diabetic.

Here's a good time to make mention of what's called *diabetes in situ*—which basically means *hidden diabetes*. Because that is exactly what these folks—and so many others reading this book—are walking around with.

See, we're all familiar with the metabolically obese unhealthy person with the collection of risk factors—including, of course, insulin resistance and hyperinsulinemia. There's nothing hidden about their health problems, whether diabetes, obesity, or heart disease. We're sad when folks like this get heart disease, but we're not really surprised. They're overweight, they have high blood pressure, they eat a bad diet, and they don't exercise. We almost *expect* they will get heart disease at some point in their lives.

But what we're always surprised by is heart disease in a person of normal weight who seems to be doing everything right. He's not overweight, he doesn't smoke, he's not downing a dozen cans of sweetened sodas . . . but yet under the hood, he's aging rapidly due, largely, to undiagnosed insulin resistance and the metabolic damage it leaves in its wake.

How Does Insulin Resistance Happen in a Person of Normal Weight?

Let's start with refined carbohydrates. Remember the gut is the largest endocrine organ in your body—it's one of the immune system organs, like your skin, that helps protect you from the outside world. This gut talks to practically everything in your body: your brain, your pancreas, your liver, your fat tissue. That's what Dr. Barry Sears means when he says, "food is information."

Carbs—most especially processed carbs—drive up insulin. And anything filled with refined carbs doesn't provide that feeling of fullness that comes with the release of satiety hormones. That's precisely why it's so easy to eat six bowls of sugared cereal while you're watching reruns of *Seinfeld*, and why it's almost impossible to eat six servings of buttered broccoli and steak. Broccoli and steak get the mes-

sage to your brain that you're full. Processed carbs do the opposite, and often create cravings for more. Never was there a truer marketing saying than, "Betcha can't eat just one!"

And this isn't just theoretical. Studies have demonstrated that Paleo-type diets constructed from protein and plenty of fibrous vegetables send satiety hormones sailing upward, while conventional "food pyramid" diets drive up the very hormones that *raise* insulin and fat storage.[22]

And remember, it's not just the food itself—it's how it's processed. Brown rice and white rice produce slightly different insulin response curves, neither of them great, but the brown rice is slightly better. Grind them up and the difference disappears. The insulin response curve for *both* forms of rice goes through the roof—the brown/white distinction goes away.[23] Processing matters!

LET'S ALL SWITCH TO VEGETABLE OIL! *NOT.*

Coming up right behind refined carbs as a culprit in this insulin resistance syndrome mess is the entire category of refined vegetable oils, or more properly, refined *seed* oils (e.g., corn, soybean, sunflower, rapeseed, safflower, and other highly processed petrochemical-extracted oils). These oils are all very high in omega-6 fats, which, while necessary for human health, are very much *pro*-inflammatory. For optimal health, they need to be consumed in balance with their *anti*-inflammatory relatives, the omega-3 fats.

But nothing of the sort is happening in the Western diet. We currently consume about sixteen

Stop worrying so much about LDL cholesterol and start looking at where you are on the insulin resistance scale.

times more omega-6 than omega-3 and some researchers think that estimate is conservative.[24] Inflammation is a key—if not *the* key—factor in the development of heart disease.

SO WHY AREN'T WE TALKING ABOUT THIS?

Conventional medicine continues to focus on LDL cholesterol—but the correlations between insulin resistance and heart disease had been known since the 1970s. What gives?

Well, for one thing, insulin resistance remains a much more complicated thing to measure properly than LDL. When LDL measurement became accepted as the gold standard of heart disease prevention, it was a very different time. And if there is one message from this book that you take home with you it should be this: Stop worrying so much about LDL cholesterol and start looking at where you are on the insulin resistance scale. And if your doctor balks at ordering an insulin resistance test, you have options.

How to Test for Insulin Resistance

The easiest option is to get yourself a fasting insulin test. These tests are now available online for as little as $28 and they don't always require an outside doctor's prescription.[25] Once you have your fasting insulin level, go to any recent blood test you've had with your doctor, and note the number next to "fasting glucose" (blood sugar).

Take those two numbers—fasting insulin and blood glucose—then go online and look for a HOMA-2 calculator, such as the Blood Code Insulin Resistance calculator. HOMA stands for *homeostatic model* of insulin resistance. HOMA-2 is a very good surrogate for insulin resistance and incredibly easy to obtain. Plug those two numbers into the calculator, just as you plug your weight and height into an online body mass index (BMI) calculator. If you have healthy insulin sensitivity, your HOMA number will be between .5 and 1.4. If it's more than 1.9, you have early insulin resistance. Over 2.9 and it's significant insulin resistance. In either case, it's time to change your diet.

If you'd like something even more accurate, and your doctor is open-minded to the information in this book, consider the LP-IR test, available through LabCorp.[26] This is the most accurate test currently available and is actually based upon data from the NMR particle test, which itself is a test we have long recommended as the gold standard for cholesterol testing. The LP-IR (the IR stands for insulin resistance) test takes the data from the NMR particle test, adds extremely sensitive inflammatory marker tests like GlycA—an excellent measure of systemic inflammation—and uses a sophisticated and validated algorithm to calculate an IR score.

Critically Important: Your Triglyceride to HDL Ratio

There are two numbers already available on just

about any blood test you've ever taken that can tell you a lot about your risk for both insulin resistance *and* heart disease: your triglycerides and your HDL. (Interestingly, these are the same two numbers that both Kraft and Reaven identified as red flags for cardiometabolic problems.) In the vast majority of cases, your triglycerides will be the larger number of the two. Divide your triglycerides by your HDL and the result is your triglycerides to HDL ratio. The ideal ratio—the one associated with the least risk for heart disease—is two or under.

Let's say, for example, that your triglycerides are 100 and your HDL is 50. You take 100 and divide by 50 giving you a ratio of 2, which is excellent. (If you are an outlier, and your HDL is *higher* than your triglycerides, you're in even better shape because your ratio will be less than 1.0!)

We can't overemphasize how important the triglyceride to HDL ratio is.

It's a good surrogate for an insulin resistance test. If your ratio is more than 2, pay attention, and if it's over 5 change your diet immediately.

It's hard to improve your ratio by raising your HDL since changing your HDL levels isn't easy., Lowering your triglycerides, however, is the easiest thing in the world to do, and will have the same effect on your ratio as bringing your HDL up. How do you lower triglycerides? Simple. With a low-carb diet. Triglycerides drop like a rock 99 percent of the time on a low-carb diet, such as the higher-fat version of the Mediterranean diet we talk about in chapter 10.

◀ WHAT YOU NEED TO KNOW

- Insulin resistance—pre-diabetes—is one of the strongest and most consistent predictors of heart disease.
- Insulin resistance happens when the body is no longer able to effectively manage your intake of sugar and starch.
- Studies going back to the 1970s show clearly that insulin resistance substantially increases the risk for many degenerative diseases and is an early warning sign for heart disease.
- You can have insulin resistance as much as a decade before the other, more "conventional" signs of heart disease show up, making it all the more important to test for insulin resistance.
- Preventing, reversing, or treating insulin resistance may be one of the most effective ways yet discovered to prevent heart disease.

PART THREE

Both of us cut our teeth in the era when something known as "functional medicine" was just beginning to gain traction among integrative medicine practitioners. (It is now a fully recognized way of practicing medicine, complete with its own conferences and certifications.) Functional medicine approaches the body as a working group of components in which every part influences the performance of the whole. It is essentially "root cause medicine." Functional medicine practitioners understand that what affects the heart affects the brain (and vice versa), what affects the adrenals affects the thyroid (ditto), and what affects the gut affects . . . well, just about everything. The motto of functional medicine might as well be "it's all connected."

In this spirit, we introduce part three of this book, the part we've affectionately referred to as our "Eat. Play. Love" section. In it we discuss three main issues: Food, Supplements, and what we might call Everything Else.

While the sections on what to eat and what supplements to take may seem pretty straightforward, the "Everything Else" section needs a few words of explanation. Maybe because each of us—at one point in our respective careers—studied psychology and psychotherapy, we are acutely aware of the impact our brain (not to mention anything more ethereal like our "soul" or "spirit") has on the health of our heart. For proof, look no further than the physiology of stress. Worry and anxiety and stress all cause the release of powerful hormones that have significant impact on everything in our body from sex drive to hunger to blood pressure to brain wave patterns to immune system function.

Stress may originate in your head, but it ends up influencing virtually every system in the human body.

There is even an entire science known as psychoneuroimmunology, which studies how what we think about affects our immune system. Thoughts are powerful. So are feelings. They can strengthen—or weaken—the heart, and as such, deserve a discussion in any book on heart health.

So in this section—in addition to learning about food and supplements—you'll also find some suggestions for self-care in general. That includes such things as deep breathing, meditation, walks in the park, and Epson salt baths. Think stuff like that doesn't affect your heart? Think again. Relaxing and relating are two of the most potent medicines in the playbook for heart disease treatment and prevention.

If either of us were presented with a choice between two prescriptions for preventing heart disease—the first for a statin drug, the second for a daily dose of laughter, cuddling, joy, healthy food, supplements, and a good night's sleep—neither of us would hesitate before choosing the second.

Not even for a second.

CHAPTER 10

BEYOND THE MEDITERRANEAN DIET: WHAT DO I EAT?

NEARLY EVERY HEALTH ORGANIZATION ON THE PLANET routinely recommends the Mediterranean Diet, as do most doctors and dietitians. But the definition of what exactly the Mediterranean Diet *is* remains far more elusive than you might think. First of all, there are twenty-one countries bordering the Mediterranean Sea—Montenegro, Spain, Albania, Greece, Turkey, Monaco, Italy, Malta, Slovenia, Cyprus, France, Croatia, Bosnia and Herzegovina, Syria, Lebanon, Israel, Egypt, Libya, Tunisia, Algeria, and Morocco. And guess what—*they don't all eat the same foods*.

Most of what we think we know about the "Mediterranean Diet" actually came from Ancel Keys's personal observations during his trips to Naples and Nicoteria in 1957,[1] based on which he launched the infamous Seven Countries Study, about which controversy has been ranging for at least a decade. What's more, there's emerging evidence that the fabled Mediterranean Diet may have included a lot more meat than is commonly believed.

Sardinia is a perfect example. Not only is it in Italy—the virtual birthplace of the concept of "Mediterranean Diet"—but it's also one of the "Blue Zones," those five areas around the world that have the greatest number of healthy centenarians and are constantly touted as having the healthiest lifestyles on the planet. So Sardinia is kind of the poster-child example of a country with a much-envied diet. And that diet is hardly meat-free.

On the "Sardinia Unlimited" website, the third most popular traditional Sardinian dish is roast suckling pig.[2] And a look at the Italian cookbooks of famed food writer Elizabeth David[3] or at the menu of any fine Sardinian restaurant will reveal—along with the vegetables—plenty of bacon, pork, chops, veal, and ribs.[4] So rather than echoing the standard fare about following the ill-defined "Mediterranean Diet" we'd rather talk about the best things in the Mediterranean pattern of eating and about the best things in the Mediterranean pattern of *living*.

Great foods that are part of a "Mediterranean Diet"—such as walnuts and olive oil and fish—can be beneficial to anyone, following any eating plan. Many of the things we like about the Mediterranean diet can actually be compatible with any number of healthy diets. (You could even do a keto diet using primarily extra-virgin olive oil as your fat, or a low-carb diet using traditional Mediterranean foods without the grains. And even keto diets can incorporate nuts and green vegetables!)

Researchers writing in the *American Journal of Clinical Nutrition* recently tested a "Mediterranean-type" diet supplemented with unprocessed red meat on overweight or obese adults. They found significant benefits to the meat-supplemented diet when compared to the "traditional" Mediterranean diet.[5]

The point, we feel, is not to be slavish to a diet, but rather to be conscious about what foods you eat *in general*. Which is what this section is about.

BEYOND DIET—*WAY* BEYOND

But food is not the only thing experts mean when they say "Mediterranean Diet." With that diet—however ill-defined it is—goes an entire lifestyle that is, frankly, quite different than ours, in ways it would benefit us to understand.

Men share their emotional lives much more freely there than they do here. There is much activity in the public square. People take naps. They have their big meal during the day. They spend time in the sun. If we should be talking about anything Mediterranean, it should be the Mediterranean *Lifestyle*—at least as much as the food itself.

But now it's time to focus on food. The rest of this section is divided into two parts—what to eat and what *not* to eat for optimal heart health. Fortunately, the list of what *not* to eat is fairly short, so let's get that one out of the way first. We call it the "Dump It!" list and provide you with specific "fast action plans" to help you remove these nutritionally empty, heart-unfriendly foods from your diet. The second part of this section is called "Eat This!" and reveals some of the healthiest foods on the planet.

Dump It: Sugar

As we've said throughout this book (see chapter 6), sugar is a far worse threat to your heart than fat ever was. The 2010 Dietary Guidelines for Americans suggest that no more than 25 percent of your calories should come from added sugars, but we think that's a ridiculously high amount. (The American Heart Association recommends no more than 5 percent.) Research by Kimber Stanhope, Ph.D., at the University of California, Davis, has shown that when people consume 25 percent of their calories from fructose or high-fructose corn syrup, several factors associated with an increased risk for heart disease—including triglycerides and a nasty little substance called *apolipoprotein-B*—escalate.[6]

Remember, it's the fructose in sugar that's the problem. High-fructose corn syrup is 55 percent fructose, and regular sugar is 50 percent fructose, so for all intents and purposes, they have the same bad effect on your heart and your health.

Fast Action Plan: Cut out soda. Soda is probably the worst offender in this category, but not by much. Fruit juices are loaded with sugar and only marginally better than soda. "Energy drinks" aren't any better. Most are loaded with sugar, and the sugar-free versions are loaded with chemicals. Many processed carbs (see below) are also full of sugar, and virtually all cakes, candies, pastries, doughnuts, and other sources of empty calories are also sugar heavyweights.

Dump It: Processed Carbohydrates

Processed carbs include almost any carbohydrate food that comes in a package: cereals, pasta, bread, minute rice, you name it. These foods are almost always high-glycemic, meaning they quickly and dramatically raise your blood sugar, which is exactly what you do not want. A study in the *Archives of*

Internal Medicine demonstrated that women who ate the highest amount of carbohydrates had a significantly greater risk of coronary heart disease than those who ate the lowest amount, and that carbohydrates from high-glycemic carbs were particularly associated with significantly greater risk for heart disease.[7] (This association was not confirmed for men in this particular study, but we suspect that future studies will discover that it's true for both sexes.)

There's no two ways about it—high-glycemic carbohydrates are inflammatory. As researchers from Harvard Medical School and the Harvard School of Public Health noted, quickly digested and absorbed carbs (i.e., those with a high glycemic load) are associated with an increased risk of heart disease.[8]

Full disclosure: We don't much buy into the argument that "whole grains" eliminate all the problems associated with processed carbs, and here's why: Number one, most commercial products that are made with whole grains don't contain all that much of them. Number two, whole grains raise blood sugar almost as much as processed grains do. Number three, whole grains still contain gluten, which can be very inflammatory for people who are gluten-sensitive. That said, real whole-grain products (Ezekiel 4:9 breads, for example) are way better than their processed counterparts. But be a careful consumer—just because a label says "wheat" instead of "white," don't assume it's good for you.

Fast Action Plan: Reduce (or eliminate) consumption of processed carbohydrates. At the same time, increase non-processed carbohydrates such as vegetables and low-sugar fruits. Replace your bagel

CORNFLAKES A GREAT BREAKFAST? THINK AGAIN!

If any of you out there still think cornflakes are a great, wholesome breakfast, read on. A landmark research study conducted by Michael Shechter, M.D., of Tel Aviv University's Sackler School of Medicine and the Heart Institute of Sheba Medical Center, with collaboration from the Endocrinology Institute, shows exactly how high-carbohydrate foods increase the risk for heart problems.[9]

Researchers looked at four groups of volunteers who were given different breakfasts. The first group was given a cornflake mush mixed with milk, not unlike the typical American breakfast. The second group was given a pure sugar mixture. The third group was given bran flakes. And the fourth group was given a placebo (water).

Over four weeks, Shechter applied a test that allows researchers to visualize how the arteries are functioning. It's called *brachial reactive testing*, and it uses a cuff on the arm (similar to those used for measuring blood pressure) that can visualize arterial function in real time.

The results were dramatic. Before any of the patients ate, their arterial function was basically the same. After eating, all had reduced functioning except for the patients in the water-drinking placebo group. Enormous peaks indicating arterial stress were found in the high GI groups: the cornflakes and sugar groups.

"We knew high glycemic foods were bad for the heart. Now we have a mechanism that shows how," Shechter wrote. "Foods like cornflakes, white bread, French fries, and sweetened soda all put undue stress on our arteries. We've explained for the first time how high-glycemic carbs can affect the progression of heart disease." During the consumption of foods high in sugar, there appears to be a temporary and sudden dysfunction in the endothelial walls of the arteries. Endothelial health can be traced back to almost every disorder and disease in the body. According to Shechter, it is the "riskiest of the risk factors."

Shechter recommended sticking to foods such as oatmeal, fruits and vegetables, and legumes and nuts, which all have a low glycemic index. Exercising every day for at least thirty minutes, he added, is an extra heart-smart action to take.

These same researchers examined the diets of 244 apparently healthy women to evaluate the association between glycemic load and blood levels of CRP (C-reactive protein, the systemic measure of inflammation discussed earlier in this chapter). They found "a strong and statistically significant positive association between dietary glycemic load and [blood levels of] CRP."[10] And that's putting it mildly.

Women whose diets were highest in glycemic load had almost twice the amount of CRP in their blood as women whose diets were lowest in glycemic load (3.7 for high-glycemic load ladies, 1.9 for low-glycemic load ladies). The difference in inflammation levels was even more pronounced for overweight women. Among women with a body mass index (BMI) greater than 25, those whose diets were lowest in glycemic load, had an average CRP reading of 1.6, but those whose diets were highest in glycemic load had a CRP reading more than three times that amount (average measurement: 5.0 mg/L).[11]

and orange juice with some eggs, veggies, and a slice of avocado. Have berries for dessert. When eating out, say "no" to the breadbasket.

Dump It: Trans Fats

According to findings presented at the annual meeting of the American Heart Association in 2006, women who ate the most trans fats were more than three times as likely to develop heart disease as women who ate the least.[12] Harvard researcher Charlene Hu examined data from the long-running Nurses' Health Study, which has followed 120,000 female nurses for more than thirty years. His research shows that for each 2 percent increase in trans fat calories consumed, the risk for coronary heart disease roughly doubles![13] Trans fats raise LDL cholesterol levels, which doesn't mean very much by itself, but at high intakes they also reduce HDL levels, which definitely isn't good.[14]

The worst offenders include nondairy "creamers," most margarines, cake mixes, ramen noodles, soup cups, virtually all packaged baked goods (e.g., Twinkies, chips, and crackers), doughnuts, many breakfast cereals, "energy" bars, cookies, and definitely fast food. (Just for example, a medium order of fries contains an incredible 14.5 g of trans fat, and a Kentucky Fried Chicken Original Recipe chicken dinner has 7 g. The ideal intake for humans is 0 g.)

Worth knowing: There is one exception to the don't-eat-trans-fats rule, and that's something called *conjugated linoleic acid*, or CLA. CLA is a trans fat that's not man-made; rather, it's made naturally in the bodies of ruminants (cows). Factory-farmed meat doesn't have any, but grass-fed meat—and products that come from pasture-raised animals—do. CLA has both anticancer and antiobesity properties. CLA is good for you, unlike man-made trans fats —which are definitely *not* good for you.

Fast Action Plan: Stop eating fast food. On all packaged foods from the supermarket, check the ingredients list for "partially hydrogenated" oils. If you see it in the ingredients list, don't eat it. Look in

THE "NO TRANS-FATS!" SCAM

When the government mandated that trans fats be listed on the nutrition facts label of food, big food lobbyists sprang into action. They somehow created a loophole that lets manufacturers use trans fats while legally claiming "no trans fats!" on their packaging. Here's how:

Manufacturers can claim "no trans fats" as long as there is less than half a gram of the stuff per serving. Sounds reasonable, until you remember how clever and ruthless Big Food can be. By making "serving sizes" ridiculously small, and by keeping trans fats to just under half a gram per "serving," they were able to technically comply with the rules. But the end result is that if each artificially small "serving" contains, say 0.4 g of trans fats, you could quite easily consume a gram or two of the stuff just by eating what most people would consider a "normal" serving size. Do that a few times a day and before you know it you've raised your heart disease risk by quite a few percentage points.

What to do? Simple. Ignore the "no trans fats!" legend on the front of the package and read the ingredients list instead. No matter what the label says, if the list of ingredients contains partially hydrogenated oil or hydrogenated oil, the product has trans fats. Period. (Typically, you'll see partially hydrogenated soybean oil in the ingredients list, but it could be any type of oil at all. What you're looking for are the keywords *hydrogenated* and *partially hydrogenated*.)

particular at margarines, cookies, cakes, pastries, doughnuts, and, as mentioned, fast food.

Dump It: Processed Meats

Processed meats contribute to both inflammation in general and heart disease specifically. Harvard researchers investigated the effect of eating processed meat versus unprocessed meat. Processed meat was defined as any meat preserved by curing, salting, smoking, or with the addition of chemical preservatives, such as those found in salami, sausages, hot dogs, luncheon meats, and bacon.

(Previous studies had rarely separated processed meat from unprocessed meat when investigating the relationship between disease and meat eating.) The researchers analyzed twenty studies that included a total of 1,218,380 people from ten countries on four continents (North America, Europe, Asia, and Australia). They found that each 1.8-ounce daily serving of processed meat (about one hot dog or a couple slices of deli meat) was associated with a 42 percent higher risk of developing heart disease. (In contrast, no relationship was found between heart disease and nonprocessed red meat.)[15]

Although the study didn't identify which specific ingredients in processed meat could be responsible for the association, many health professionals believe that the high levels of sodium and nitrates might be responsible. "When we looked at average nutrients in unprocessed red and processed meats eaten in the United States, we found that they contained similar average amounts of saturated fat and cholesterol. In contrast, processed meats contained, on average, four times more sodium and 50 percent more nitrate preservatives," said Renata Micha, a research fellow in the department of epidemiology at the Harvard School of Public Health and lead author of the study. "This suggests that differences in salt and preservatives, rather than fats, might explain the higher risk of heart disease and diabetes seen with processed meats, but not with unprocessed red meats."[16]

Fast Action Plan: Cut out processed (e.g., deli) meats.

Dump It: Excessive Omega-6 Fats

Vegetable oils (corn, canola, and soybean) are mostly made up of pro-inflammatory omega-6 fats, and you should reduce (not necessarily eliminate) your consumption of them while increasing your consumption of anti-inflammatory omega-3 fats.

This is the one recommendation that comes with an asterisk. Omega-6 fats, the ones that are most prevalent in vegetable oils, are not in and of themselves "bad." But they *are* pro-inflammatory, and they need to be balanced by an equal (or near-equal) intake of anti-inflammatory omega-3s. (You can review this information in chapter 7.) The optimal ratio of omega-6 to omega-3 in the human diet is no

higher than 4:1, and many believe the ideal ratio is 1:1. In the average Westernized diet, the ratio is anywhere between 15:1 and 25:1, which creates a highly inflammatory state in the body. Because heart disease is primarily a disease of inflammation, such a state should be avoided as much as humanly possible.

And by the way, it's not just the oils you use for cooking that tip the scales into inflammation land. Omega-6 fats are everywhere in the food supply—you can't swing a rope without hitting a food product loaded with omega-6s. Nearly all processed foods contain them. They're used almost exclusively in restaurants, for frying, sautéing, and baking, so virtually anything you order from the menu has got a ton of omega-6 fats.

So choose your omega-6 fats carefully and use them sparingly. (The best choices are cold-pressed, unrefined oils—sesame oil is a particularly good choice.) Use highly processed supermarket oils (such as corn oil) infrequently or not at all. When you sauté food, try substituting monounsaturated fats such as olive oil and macadamia nut oil for high omega-6 oils such as canola or soybean. And, above all, increase your intake of omega-3 fats to help balance your intake of omega-6s (see the "Eat This!" section on page 150).

Fast Action Plan: Never use generic processed oils such as Wesson or Crisco. Cut down on corn oil, safflower oil, soybean oil, and canola oil (see Dr. Sinatra's personal story on canola oil in chapter 7). Whenever possible, use olive oil, sesame oil, or macadamia oil. And pay attention to the "Eat This!" section in this chapter on omega-3s.

THE "EAT THIS!" LIST

Both of us are frequently interviewed about the best foods for health. Virtually every reporter either of us has ever spoken with winds up asking, "How much of this food do you need to eat to get its benefits?" It's a reasonable question, but there's almost never a perfect answer. We know of no study, for example, that has systematically tested the effects of eating five portions of blueberries a week as opposed to three, or compared eating two portions of salmon per week with eating it daily. Our recommendation is to put these foods in heavy rotation in your diet, enjoying them as frequently as you like.

Here are the foods you want to include in your diet on a regular basis.

Eat This: Wild Alaskan Salmon

Salmon is one of the best sources of anti-inflammatory omega-3s. But not all salmon is created equal. Wild Alaskan salmon is far superior to the farm-raised variety. (According to independent lab tests by the Environmental Working Group, seven out of ten farmed salmon purchased at grocery stores were contaminated with polychlorinated biphenyls [PCBs] at levels high enough to raise health concerns.) Wild salmon is far cleaner, and it has the added benefit of containing one of the most powerful antioxidants on the planet, *astaxanthin*. A 4-ounce serving also contains 462 mg of heart-healthy potassium, the same amount in a medium banana.[17]

Both of us have been buying our salmon from a wonderful company called Vital Choice for many years. Vital Choice is run by third-generation Alaskan fishermen who are scrupulous about using sustain-able fishing and equally scrupulous about testing their fish thoroughly for contaminants and metals. They ship in dry ice, and they have the best fish we've ever tasted.

Fast Action Plan: Eat wild salmon twice a week.

Eat This: Berries

All berries are loaded with natural anti-inflammatory properties and natural antioxidants. They're also very low in sugar. Blueberries contain a beneficial compound called *pterostilbene*, which helps prevent the deposit of plaque in the arteries and also helps prevent some of the damage caused by oxidized cholesterol.[18] Raspberries and strawberries contain another substance, *ellagic acid*, which offers similar protection against oxidized LDL.[19] And all berries—blueberries, raspberries, strawberries, and others—contain anthocyanins, plant compounds that help lower inflammation (see "Cherries" below).

Fast Action Plan: Eat berries three (or more) times a week.

Eat This: Cherries

Cherries and cherry juice have long been known to be effective against the pain of gout, and scientists believe that the compounds in cherries responsible for this are *anthocyanins*. Anthocyanins act like natural COX-2 inhibitors. "COX" stands for *cyclooxygenase*, which is produced in the body in two forms called COX-1 and COX-2. COX-2 is used for signaling pain and inflammation.

The popularity of arthritis drugs such as Vioxx and Celebrex was based on their unique ability to block the pain and inflammation messages of COX-2 while leaving the non-inflammatory COX-1 alone. Unfortunately, there were some really unpleasant side effects associated with Vioxx, and it was taken off the market. But anthocyanins produce a similar effect with none of the problems of such drugs. Cherries (along with raspberries) have the highest yields of pure anthocyanins. In one study, the COX inhibitory activity of anthocyanins from cherries was comparable to that of ibuprofen and naproxen. Researchers feel that in addition to helping with pain and inflammation, consuming anthocyanins on a regular basis may help lower heart attack and stroke risk.

Fast Action Plan: Eat cherries two (or more) times a week.

Eat This: Grass-Fed Beef

We're not anti-meat guys, but we are very much against factory-farmed meat. The majority of the meat we consume, unfortunately, is feedlot-raised meat from factory farms. It's loaded with antibiotics, steroids, and hormones; it's very high in inflammatory omega-6 fats; and it contains virtually no anti-inflammatory omega-3s.

Grass-fed meat is a whole different "animal." (Okay, bad pun, sorry, we couldn't resist.) Raised on pasture, it contains less omega-6s plus a fair amount of omega-3s, resulting in a much better omega-6:omega-3 ratio. Grass-fed meat is almost always raised organically, and, in any case, it never has hormones, steroids, or antibiotics. If you eat meat, grass-fed is the only way to go.

Fast Action Plan: Eat only grass-fed meat when you eat meat.

Eat This: Vegetables (and Some Fruit)

No matter what kind of diet you're on—from vegan to Atkins—you can probably benefit from eating more vegetables than you already do. The entire vegetable kingdom is loaded with natural anti-inflammatories, antioxidants, and other plant compounds, such as flavonoids, that are good for your heart.

In two long-running Harvard-based research projects, the Nurses' Health Study and the Health Professionals Follow-up Study, the higher the average daily consumption of vegetables and fruits, the lower the chances of developing cardiovascular disease. Compared with those in the lowest category of fruit and vegetable intake (fewer than one and a half servings daily), those averaging eight or more servings per day were a whopping 30 percent less likely to have had a heart attack or stroke.[20]

Although all vegetables and fruits probably contributed to this stunning effect, the researchers felt that the most outstanding contributors were the green, leafy veggies (such as spinach and Swiss chard) and the cruciferous ones (broccoli, Brussels sprouts, kale, cabbage, and cauliflower). (In the fruit department, citrus fruits such as oranges, lemons, limes, and grapefruit were particularly protective.[21])

When researchers took the Harvard studies mentioned above and combined them with several other long-term studies both in Europe and the United States, they found a similar protective effect. Individuals who ate more than five servings a day of vegetables and fruits had a roughly 20 percent lower risk of coronary heart disease,[22] and a similar reduction in the risk of stroke.[23]

FIGHT HEART DISEASE WITH FOOD

In a fascinating and much-discussed article that appeared in the December 16, 2004, issue of the *British Medical Journal*, researchers put forth an idea called the *polymeal*. They examined all of the research on foods and health to see whether they could put together the ideal meal (the polymeal) that, if you ate it every day, would significantly reduce your risk for cardiovascular disease. They came up with a theoretical meal that, eaten daily, would reduce cardiovascular risk by a staggering 75 percent (there's not a pill in the world that can do that!).

The ingredients of the polymeal? Wine, fish, almonds, garlic, fruits, vegetables, and dark chocolate.

One of the many reasons for the protective effect of nuts may be an amino acid named *arginine*. Remember our earlier discussion about the endothelium (the inner lining of the arterial walls)? Arginine has a role in protecting this inner lining, making the arterial walls more pliable and less susceptible to atherogenesis. Arginine is needed to make an important molecule called *nitric oxide*, which helps relax constricted blood vessels and ease blood flow.[25]

The reason we're not as over-the-top enthusiastic about fruit is that despite its terrific benefits, it still contains sugar, which can be a problem for many folks. For the large number of people whose blood sugar rises when they merely look at a candy bar, unlimited fruit is a bad idea. Low-sugar fruits (such as apples, grapefruit, cherries, berries, and oranges) are fine in moderation. Vegetables, on the other hand, can be virtually unlimited.

Fast Action Plan: Eat five to nine half-cup servings of vegetables and fruit a day.

Eat This: Nuts

Although an apple a day may indeed keep the doctor away, the same can also be said of a handful of nuts. People who eat nuts regularly are less likely to have heart attacks or die from heart disease than those who don't. Five large studies—the Adventist Health Study, the Iowa Women's Health Study, the Nurses' Health Study, the Physicians' Health Study, and the CARE Study—have all found a consistent 30 to 50 percent lower risk of heart attacks or heart disease associated with eating nuts several times a week.[24]

In addition, nuts are a great source of numerous *phytonutrients*—bioactive chemicals found in plants. These compounds have powerful health benefits, not the least of which is their antioxidant activity, which is linked to the prevention of coronary heart disease. And if you're worried about calories, consider this: In the Nurses' Health Study out of Harvard, nut consumption was inversely related to weight gain.[26] Several large studies, including the Physicians' Health

Study (22,000 men) and the Adventist Health Study (more than 40,000 people), have demonstrated a link between nut eating and a reduction in heart disease.[27] Just keep portions reasonable—an ounce or so a day is great.

Fast Action Plan: Eat 1 ounce of nuts five times a week.

Eat This: Beans

Fact number one: Fiber is good. (High-fiber diets have been associated with lower rates of a host of diseases, including heart disease.) Fact number two: We don't get enough of it. (Most health organizations recommend a daily intake of 25 to 38 g daily; the average American gets 11 g.) Fact number three: Beans are a fiber heavyweight. Case closed.

Regarding heart disease, the big selling point of beans used to be that they lowered cholesterol.[28] That's definitely true, but, as you've learned, it's not nearly as important as whether they actually lower *heart disease*. And they do. One study found that one serving of beans on a daily basis lowered the risk of a heart attack by an eyebrow-raising 38 percent![29] Another study found that individuals eating beans and legumes at least four times a week had a 22 percent lower risk of heart disease than individuals consuming beans/legumes less than once a week.[30]

One study found that one serving of beans on a daily basis lowered the risk of a heart attack by 38 percent.

Their high fiber content alone would make beans a top food for the heart, but beans offer a lot more than fiber. The U.S. Department of Agriculture ranking of foods by antioxidant capacity lists small red dried beans as having the highest antioxidant capacity per serving size of any food tested. In fact, of the four top-scoring foods, three were beans (red beans, red kidney beans, and pinto beans). Many bean varieties have a lot of folic acid (especially adzuki beans, lentils, black-eyed peas, and pinto beans). Folic acid is one of the key players in bringing down the inflammatory compound *homocysteine*, itself a risk factor for heart disease.

Fast Action Plan: Eat a serving of beans or lentils at least four times a week. (One serving is 1/2 cup to 1 cup cooked beans.)

Eat This: Dark Chocolate

Study after study is confirming that plant chemicals in cocoa-rich dark chocolate called *flavanols* can lower blood pressure and reduce inflammation. A 2011 study in the *British Medical Journal* found that high levels of chocolate consumption are associated with a one-third reduction in the risk of developing heart disease. The highest levels of chocolate consumption were associated with a 37 percent reduction in cardiovascular disease and a 29 percent reduction in stroke when compared to the lowest levels.[31]

Flavanol-rich cocoa lowers blood pressure.[32] And the Zutphen Elderly Study of 470 elderly men found that those who ate the most cocoa had literally half the risk of dying from heart disease than men who ate the least.[33]

Now the thing about chocolate is that all the good stuff is found in the cocoa that it's made from, so you really want high-cocoa chocolate. We're not talking about the candy bars you get at the 7-Eleven here; we're talking about a cocoa-rich chocolate that contains all the flavanols that have been found to be so healthy. White chocolate and milk chocolate have hardly any flavanols to speak of, so it's got to be dark. Many dark chocolate bars will now tell you their cocoa content in percentage form—look for at least 60 percent cocoa. (The higher the cocoa content, the less sweet the bar.)

You'll also find that this kind of chocolate is easy to eat in small quantities—it's not so sweet that it causes you to crave more and more of it, and it's easy to be satisfied with just a square or two, which is all you need for the health benefits.

Fast Action Plan: Eat one to two squares of dark chocolate four to six days a week.

Eat This: Turmeric

Turmeric is the spice that makes curries yellow. It occupies a place of distinction in both Ayurvedic and Chinese medicine, largely because of its phenomenal anti-inflammatory properties. (It also has anticancer activity and is very helpful for the liver.) The active ingredients in turmeric are a group of plant compounds called *curcuminoids* (collectively known as curcumin). In addition to being anti-inflammatory, curcumin is a powerful antioxidant. Because oxidized LDL is a big player in the cascade that leads to inflammation and heart disease, turmeric's antioxidant properties are a big benefit.

Fast Action Plan: Put turmeric at the front of your spice cabinet and use it often. It goes well on veggies, eggs, sautéed dishes, meats, fish, and poultry.

Eat This: Pomegranate Juice

Pomegranate juice is one of the few "trendy" health foods that actually lives up to its hype. Researchers at the Technion-Israel Institute of Technology in Haifa suggest that long-term consumption of pomegranate juice may help slow aging and protect against heart disease.

In a study published in the *American Journal of Cardiology*, forty-five patients with heart disease drank either 8 ounces of pomegranate juice or 8 ounces of a placebo drink for three months. The pomegranate juice drinkers had significantly less oxygen deficiency to the heart during exercise, suggesting that they had increased blood flow to the heart.

Pomegranate juice has the ability to inhibit the oxidation of LDL cholesterol.[34] (Remember that LDL cholesterol is only a problem when it's oxidized!) And an impressive number of studies have demonstrated a beneficial effect of pomegranate juice on cardiovascular health, including one that showed 30 percent reduced arterial plaque.[35] Pomegranate juice also enhances the activity of nitric oxide, a molecule essential for cardiovascular health.[36]

One caution: Avoid "juice blends" and "juice cocktails," because these have much less pomegranate juice in them and much more sugar. We like pure pomegranate juices such as Just Pomegranate, which are admittedly expensive but contain absolutely nothing but pure pomegranate juice. Another popular brand we like a lot is Pom Wonderful.

Fast Action Plan: Put pomegranate juice in "heavy rotation" on your menu: 4 to 8 ounces a day, or as often as you like.

Eat This: Red Wine

For years, it was believed that the reason the French could "get away" with eating high-fat foods—while still having remarkably lower rates of heart disease than Americans—was because of their regular consumption of red wine, which contains numerous compounds that protect the heart. Chief among these is *resveratrol*, a polyphenol (plant compound) that's found in the skins of dark grapes and is highly concentrated in red wine. Resveratrol is a potent antioxidant that can prevent harmful elements in the body from attacking healthy cells. Red wine has been shown to be cardio-protective in quite a number of studies.[37]

And resveratrol isn't the only reason. Other compounds in red wine such as flavonoids inhibit the oxidation of LDL cholesterol, which is pretty darn important because oxidized LDL cholesterol initiates and intensifies the inflammatory process.[38] Red wine also limits the tendency of compounds in the blood to clot and increases HDL cholesterol to boot.[39] Interestingly, in one study, moderate consumption of red wine was associated with lower levels of three markers we told you about earlier: CRP, fibrinogen, and interleukin-6.50 It's hard to think of a more heart-healthy drink.

Worth noting: The dark side of alcohol is well known, and we don't have to recount it here. If you're not a drinker, please don't start because of the benefits of red wine. Not everyone can handle alcohol, and if you suspect you're someone who doesn't do well with it, for goodness' sake, don't drink it! (With all the talk about how the wine-drinking French have the lowest rates of heart disease in Western Europe, it's fre-quently forgotten that they also have the highest rates of liver cirrhosis!) The key to enjoying wine's beneficial effects is moderate consumption, defined as about two glasses a day for men and about one a day for women, about three to four times a week. Also worth mentioning is that alcohol increases the risk for breast cancer in women who aren't consuming enough folic acid, so make sure you're getting at least 400 mg of folic acid a day through food or supplementation.

Fast Action Plan: If you are a drinker, have a glass of red wine with dinner. (If you're not, don't start!)

Eat This: Green Tea

Apart from water, tea is probably the most consumed beverage in the world, and it's also one of the healthiest. That's because it's absolutely loaded with protective plant-based chemicals known as polyphenols. Green tea in particular has gotten a ton of attention in the media, largely for the anticancer action of one of its compounds, *epigallocatechin gallate (EGCG)*.

But green tea also contributes to cardiovascular health. Although much has been written about its cholesterol-lowering effect, we find it much more interesting that green tea lowers fibrinogen, a substance in the body that can cause clots and strokes. In an article in the journal *Circulation* titled "Effects of Green Tea Intake on the Development of Coronary Artery Disease," researchers from the department of medicine at Chiba Hokusoh Hospital, Nippon Medical School, Chiba, Japan, concluded that "the more green tea patients consume, the less likely they are to have coronary artery disease."[40]

Worth knowing: Just because green tea gets the lion's share of attention from health writers doesn't mean there's not great stuff in other teas, such as black, oolong, white, and yerba matte. At Boston University's School of Medicine, Joseph Vita, M.D., conducted a study in which sixty-six men either drank four cups of black tea a day or took a placebo. The researchers showed that drinking black tea can help reverse an abnormal functioning of blood vessels that can contribute to stroke or heart attack. Best of all, improvement in the functioning of the blood vessels was visible within two hours of drinking just one cup of black tea![41]

"What we found was that if you take a group of people with heart disease who have abnormal blood vessel function to begin with and asked them to drink tea, their blood vessels improved," said Vita.[42]

Fast Action Plan: Remember, any form of tea contains caffeine, so drink in moderation. Make a big pitcher of green tea and keep it in the fridge. Drink it in the earlier part of the day, up to two glasses.

Eat This: Olive Oil

Olive oil is the primary fat used in the Mediterranean area and the one most associated with what's been called the Mediterranean Diet. (As we said earlier, there's no single "Mediterranean Diet," but all variations of it contain high amounts of fish, fruits, vegetables, nuts, wine, and olive oil.) There are countless studies on the Mediterranean Diet and heart health and virtually all of them show enormous benefits for the heart and the brain. These studies have left olive oil with an unimpeachable reputation as one of the healthiest fats for the heart.

Research in the *Archives of Internal Medicine* concluded that greater adherence to the traditional Mediterranean Diet (including plenty of olive oil and other monounsaturated fats such as nuts and avocados) was associated with significant reduction in mortality among people who had been diagnosed with heart disease.[43]

Another study in the same journal compared two groups of people with high blood pressure.[44] One group was given sunflower oil, a typical high omega-6 oil used in Western diets, and one group was given the good stuff: extra-virgin olive oil. The olive oil decreased the second group's blood pressure by a significant amount; it also decreased their need for blood pressure meds by a whopping 48 percent. As the English might say, "Not too shabby."

Like red wine and green tea, olive oil contains polyphenols that are anti-inflammatory and act as powerful antioxidants. (Researchers have isolated one in particular, *oleocanthal*, which acts similarly to ibuprofen.[45]) Because so many of these polyphenols have significant health benefits, some people believe that the fat in olive oil may not be the only reason olive oil is so darn healthy. They think that the main health benefits of olive oil come from the fact that it is a delivery system for these powerful polyphenols. Either way, the stuff is great, and you should make it a part of your heart-healthy diet.

Worth knowing: All olive oil is not created equal. Unfortunately, commercial manufacturers, trying to ride the health hype on olive oil, have rushed to market all kinds of imitation and inferior products that say "olive oil" on them but are highly processed and refined and have questionable benefits. That's why you want "extra-virgin" olive oil, which is the least processed, the most like what you'd get if you walked around barefoot in barrels of olives. It's made without the use of heat, hot water, or solvents, and it is left unfiltered. The first pressing produces the best stuff, known as "extra-virgin," but virgin isn't bad either.

Once you begin machine harvesting and processing with very high heat, you start damaging the delicate compounds in olive oil responsible for all those great health benefits. The antioxidant and anti-inflammatory polyphenols are water soluble and can be washed away with factory processing. That's one reason that factory-produced olive oil has a shorter shelf life—no antioxidants to protect it. Real olive oil—the extra-virgin kind, made with care and love and the absence of high heat and harsh chemicals—lasts for years. Dr. Sinatra feels so strongly about the healing powers of olive oil that he invested in a company that makes superb, authentic (and delicious) extra-virgin olive oil. It's called Vervana. Vervana is true extra-virgin olive oil—not a blend, like many imposters—and is one of the finest (and best-tasting) olive oils either of us has ever had! You can find links to the company on both our websites. And it's reasonably priced to boot!

Fast Action Plan: Switch to extra-virgin olive oil. Use it for salad dressing, low-heat stir-fries, and sautées.

Eat This: Garlic

Garlic is a global remedy. More than 1,200 (and counting) pharmacological studies have been done on garlic, and the findings are pretty impressive. In addition to lowering lipids and preventing blood coagulation, it has antihypertensive, antioxidant, antimicrobial, and antiviral properties. Garlic has been shown to lower triglyceride levels. It can also reduce plaque, making it a powerful agent for cardiovascular health.

In one study, subjects receiving 900 mg of garlic powder for four years in a randomized, double-blinded, placebo-controlled study had a regression in their plaque volume of 2.6 percent; meanwhile, a matched group of subjects given a placebo (an inert substance) saw their plaque increase over the same time period by 15.6 percent![46]

One of the active ingredients in garlic—allicin—also has significant antiplatelet activity. That means it helps prevent platelets in the blood from sticking together. To understand just how important that is, consider that many heart attacks and strokes are caused by spontaneous clots in the blood vessels. The anticoagulant effect of garlic is an important health benefit.

Worth knowing: The preparation of garlic is critical for it to release its health-providing benefits. If for any reason you had the impulse to swallow a garlic clove whole, not much would happen. The garlic clove has to be crushed or chopped—the more finely the better—for the compounds in it to mix together to create allicin, the active ingredient responsible for the health benefits. Allicin starts degrading immediately after it's produced, so the fresher it is when you use it, the better. (Microwaving destroys it completely.) Garlic experts advise crushing a little raw garlic and combining it with cooked food. If you add it to food you're sautéing, do it toward the end so the allicin is freshest.

Fast Action Plan: Start cooking with garlic.

◀ WHAT YOU NEED TO KNOW

Eat Less of These

- Sugar
- Soda
- Processed carbs
- Trans fats
- Processed meats
- Excess vegetable oils

Eat More of These

- Wild salmon
- Berries and cherries
- Grass-fed meat
- Vegetables
- Nuts
- Beans
- Dark chocolate
- Garlic and turmeric
- Pomegranate juice, green tea, and red wine
- Extra-virgin olive oil

CHAPTER 11

HELP YOUR HEART WITH THESE SUPPLEMENTS

ASK YOUR TYPICAL DOCTOR ABOUT NUTRITIONAL SUPPLEMENTS and the first thing you're likely to hear is this: *"There's no good research showing they work."* Both of us have heard this refrain time and time again when we discuss nutritional medicine with our more conservative colleagues.

It's not true.

You or your doctor can go online to the National Institute of Medicine's library (www.pubmed.com), enter into the search box the name of virtually any vitamin or herb you can think of, and, depending on what you choose, hundreds to thousands of citations will pop up. So the problem isn't an absence of research.

The problem is twofold. One, the conventional training of medical doctors in this country is highly biased toward pharmaceuticals. From the time they enter med school, doctors are courted by the pharmaceutical companies in myriad ways, some subtle, some not so subtle. Free lunches, symposiums, honorariums, consulting and lecturing contracts, vacations, perky pharmaceutical reps showing up at offices with the latest studies that show their products in a favorable light, free samples, and pens and prescription pads bearing the company's name—all create a culture in which pharmaceuticals are the first choice in any treatment plan. (Most docs will tell you these practices have no influence on them or what they choose to prescribe, but the research tells a very different story.)

The second part of the problem is that much of the research on vitamins flies beneath the radar. Your overworked doctor barely has time to scan the abstracts of the *New England Journal of Medicine* every month, let alone dig deeply into the hundreds of studies that are published every year on vitamins and nutrients in journals like the *American Journal of Clinical Nutrition*. The vast majority of doctors in this country get no training whatsoever in nutrition, and those who do receive only the most rudimentary and superficial introduction to the subject. Put this together with the built-in medical school bias in favor of patent medicines, and it's easy to see why doctors often fail to think of natural substances as legitimate tools that can help keep people healthy.

The third part of the problem is that the protocols that are suitable for testing pharmaceuticals are not always suited for vitamins and nutraceuticals. Many compounds—like flavonoids in apples—work synergistically and support and augment the impact of the vitamins found in that food (like vitamin C in the apple). An isolated nutrient rarely shows up in the natural world, so testing isolated nutrients—separated from the nutrients they are normally found with in nature—may not reveal what these nutrients actually can accomplish.

And the fourth problem is that medical researchers are often so removed from the world of nutrition, or so biased against it, that they test nutrients in doses that no nutritionist would expect to "work." In the period between editions of this book, a highly publicized randomized placebo-control trial was published in a reputable medical journal that purportedly "tested" the effect of omega-3s on heart disease.[2]

The study concluded that they did not. The study was widely reported, and the notion that omega-3s were helpful for heart disease even wound up on the *New York Times* list of "medical myths."[3]

But the study tested extremely sick people with multiple risk factors for heart disease, and they used a dose of omega-3 that no functional medicine doctor on earth would expect to do a damn thing for any but the healthiest people in the world. They used 1000 mg of "fish oil" and didn't specify how *much* of that oil was EPA and DHA, the two omega-3s that you take fish oil for in the first place. So the subjects likely got less than a gram of combined EPA and DHA, which is about $1/3$–$1/2$ the recommended dose. *And* the "placebo" was olive oil, which has anti-inflammatory properties of its own and is hardly an inert substance—just ask the PREDIMED investigators who reported that olive oil had remarkable medicinal and therapeutic effects. (To our way of thinking, olive oil is the secret sauce in Mediterranean-type diets—it's anything but a "placebo.")

Let's be clear. Conventional medicine is simply terrific at keeping people alive in emergencies. Both of us know that if we were to be in a car accident, we wouldn't want the ambulance rushing us to the nearest herbalist's office. We'd want to go to the emergency room of the best hospital we could find. But as good as conventional medicine is at treating people in acute situations, it's astonishingly bad at overall preventive care. It's great at keeping your heart beating if you've just had a heart attack. It's not nearly as good at keeping your heart healthy for the long run and keeping you, the heart's owner, out of the hospital in the first place.

The supplements listed in this chapter are some of the superstars for heart health that Dr. Sinatra uses in his practice (as he has for decades) and that Dr. Jonny has recommended to clients and written about extensively in his books and columns. Neither of us is saying you should just throw out your prescriptions and start randomly taking vitamins. But we *are* saying that natural substances such as vitamins, antioxidants, omega-3 fats, and many of the thousands of compounds found in foods may affect the health of the heart in an even more profound way than many of the medicines routinely prescribed as the first order of business.

Even if you're already on medication, nutritional supplements can still improve your health. In the case of coenzyme Q_{10} (CoQ$_{10}$), for example, supplementation is an absolute must if you're on a statin drug (more on that in a moment). Magnesium is often used in conjunction with blood sugar drugs such as Metformin (Glucophage) or blood pressure medications such as beta blockers. And virtually everyone needs a little help in reducing oxidation and inflammation, two of the most important drivers in the development of heart disease. Omega-3 fatty acids, for example, can be used by just about anyone, whether he or she is on medication or not (check with your doctor for any possible contraindications, such as right before going into surgery).

The following list is far from exhaustive, but it will give you a good idea of how you can use supplements to keep your heart healthy, either alone or, in some cases, as an adjunct to conventional therapy.

COENZYME Q$_{10}$: THE SPARK OF LIFE

Coenzyme Q_{10} is a vitamin-like substance found throughout the body and made in every cell. Among the many important things it does, CoQ$_{10}$ helps create energy from fuel (food) in the human body, just as a spark plug creates energy from fuel (gasoline) in a car.

A CoQ$_{10}$ deficiency affects your heart as profoundly as a calcium deficiency would affect your bones. We create less of it as we age, making it all the more important to supplement with CoQ$_{10}$ as we grow older.

Here's how it works: Your body uses a molecule called *adenosine triphosphate*, or ATP, as a source of energy (which is why ATP is nicknamed "the energy molecule"). Much like gasoline is the fuel that allows you to actually drive a car to any of a million destinations, ATP is the fuel that allows your body to perform any of a million activities, ranging from cellular metabolism to doing bench presses to dancing the tango. The body makes ATP by stripping electrons—tiny subatomic particles that carry a negative electrical charge—from food and then delivering those electrons to oxygen, which is an *electron receptor*. CoQ$_{10}$ is one of the carriers of these electrons, so it essentially helps the cells use oxygen and create more energy. Bottom line: CoQ$_{10}$ has the ability to increase the body's production of the energy molecule ATP, and this is a very good thing indeed.

Just as a gasoline engine can't work without spark plugs, the human body can't work without CoQ$_{10}$. It's an essential component of the *mitochondria*, which is command central for the production of cellular energy (ATP). Not coincidentally, the heart is one of the major organs where the most CoQ$_{10}$ is concentrated (the others, being the liver and kidney). The heart never sleeps, and it never takes a vacation. It beats more than one hundred thousand times a day, making it one of the most metabolically active tissues in the body, so it's very dependent on the energy-generating power of CoQ_{10}.

A CoQ_{10} deficiency affects your heart as profoundly as a calcium deficiency would affect your bones. We create less of it as we age, making it all the more important to supplement with CoQ_{10} as we grow older. Although it's present in food, the only foods that have any CoQ_{10} to speak of are organ meats such as heart and liver. Beef has some carnitine but—other than organ meats—the best source of carnitine in the entire animal kingdom is young lamb. Note: CoQ_{10} is easily destroyed by too much heat or overcooking.

As we've said, one of the biggest problems with statin drugs is that they significantly deplete CoQ_{10} levels. You may recall from the previous chapter on statins that the same pathway that produces cholesterol (the mevalonate pathway) also produces CoQ_{10}, so when you block that pathway at its virtual starting gate (as statin drugs do), you not only reduce the body's ability to make cholesterol but you also interfere with its ability to make CoQ_{10}.

We've said this before, but in case you missed it the first time, it's important enough to repeat: If you are on a statin drug you must, repeat *must*, supplement with CoQ_{10}. We recommend at least 100 mg twice a day.

But CoQ_{10} isn't just essential for those on statin drugs. We believe it's essential for everyone else as well, and *especially* for anyone at risk for heart disease.

CoQ_{10} has been approved in Japan as a prescription drug for congestive heart failure since 1974. And even in the United States, the benefits of CoQ_{10} for the heart have been well known since at least the mid-1980s. A study published in the *Proceedings of the National Academy of Sciences of the United States of America* in 1985 gave either CoQ_{10} or a placebo to two groups of patients having class III or class IV cardiomyopathy according to the definitions put forth by the New York Heart Association (NYHA).[4] These are seriously ill folks. Class III patients have marked limitation in activity because of symptoms and can basically only be comfortable at rest or with minimal activity; class IV patients have severe limitations and experience symptoms even while resting. (Most class IV patients are bedbound.)

So what happened when these very sick patients were given CoQ_{10}? Here's how the researchers themselves summarized the results: "These patients, steadily worsening and expected to die within two years under conventional therapy, generally showed an extraordinary clinical improvement, indicating that CoQ_{10} therapy might extend the lives of such patients. This improvement could be due to correction of a myocardial deficiency of CoQ_{10} and to enhanced synthesis of CoQ_{10}-requiring enzymes."[5]

Another study that lasted six years and was published in 1990 looked at 143 patients, 98 percent of whom were in the same two classes as the patients in the 1985 study.[6] The participants were given 100 mg of CoQ_{10} (orally), in addition to being treated in their conventional medical program. Eighty-five percent of the patients improved by one or two NYHA classes, and there was no positive evidence of toxicity or intolerance. "CoQ$_{10}$ is safe and effective long-term therapy for cardiomyopathy," the study authors concluded.

CoQ$_{10}$ also has the ability to reduce blood pressure. A recent meta-analysis of CoQ$_{10}$ in the treatment of high blood pressure reviewed twelve different clinical trials and found that across the board, patients who received CoQ$_{10}$ supplementation had significant reductions in blood pressure compared to control subjects who didn't receive supplemention.[7] It's no wonder that several studies have demonstrated a strong correlation between severity of heart disease and severity of CoQ$_{10}$ deficiency.[8]

Since the publication of the first edition of this book, there has been an explosion in the medical literature on the cardiovascular merits of CoQ$_{10}$. We now know that CoQ$_{10}$ reduces Lp(a) (see page 170), improves endothelial function, decreases cholesterol/triglyceride levels, increases HDL, decreases fasting blood sugar, decreases Hba1c, and—just for good measure—reduces LDL oxidation.

You might recall that oxidative damage (oxidation) is one of the four major culprits in heart disease, and you might also remember that cholesterol in the body is never a problem until it becomes oxidized. It's only this oxidized cholesterol—specifically, pattern B LDL cholesterol—that is a problem, because pattern B LDL molecules are the ones that adhere to the cell walls and initiate or accelerate the process of inflammation.

Why do we mention that here? Simple. CoQ$_{10}$ is a powerful antioxidant, inhibiting oxidative damage to LDL cholesterol and thus helping to prevent cholesterol from becoming a "problem" in the first place. It's far smarter to prevent LDL from getting oxidized and

thus damaged and sticky in the first place than to use a sledgehammer pharmaceutical to reduce LDL as much as possible!

Coenzyme Q$_{10}$ and vitamin E have a strange, almost symbiotic relationship. In rats given supplemental vitamin E, increases in blood levels of CoQ$_{10}$ were observed; in baboons given supplemental CoQ$_{10}$, the anti-inflammatory effects of vitamin E were increased; and in one study, CoQ$_{10}$ plus vitamin E actually lowered C-reactive protein (CRP), a systemic measure of inflammation. We think it's wise to make sure you're getting about 100 to 200 IUs or so of vitamin E a day (from mixed tocopherols) in addition to your CoQ$_{10}$ supplement. (But read the section on vitamin E, "The Good, the Bad, and the Ugly," on page 171 first!)

D-RIBOSE: THE MISSING LINK

D-ribose, a five-carbon sugar, is one of the components of ATP, the energy molecule the body uses to power all activities. Without D-ribose, there would be no ATP; without ATP, there would be no energy.

Both CoQ$_{10}$ and the nutritional supplement L-carnitine help facilitate the process by which the body manufactures ATP. Metaphorically speaking, they act like little elves, shuttling the material needed to make ATP to the factories where it's made, resulting in more efficient production of this important energy molecule. CoQ$_{10}$ and L-carnitine can be said to function like very efficient trucks transporting building materials to the factories where stuff actually gets built, but D-ribose is one of the actual building *materials*. A shortage of D-ribose means a shortage of ATP, and a shortage of ATP, especially in the heart, is bad news indeed.

D-ribose is synthesized in every cell in the body, but only slowly and to varying degrees depending on the tissue. Tissues such as the liver, adrenal cortex, and adipose tissue make plenty of D-ribose because they produce chemical compounds used to synthesize fatty acids and steroids, which are in turn used to make hormones.

But molecules of D-ribose made by these tissues have to be used right then and there and can't be "transferred" to other tissues that might need them, such as the heart. The heart, as well as the skeletal muscles and brain, can only make enough ribose for their day-to-day needs. They have no D-ribose saving account. When the cells of the heart, for example, encounter a stressor such as oxygen deprivation, they lack the metabolic machinery needed to quickly whip up some badly needed D-ribose. Tissues that are stressed because they don't get enough blood flow or oxygen can't make enough D-ribose to replace lost energy quickly. And when oxygen or blood flow deficits are chronic—as in heart disease—tissues can never make enough D-ribose, and cellular energy levels are constantly depleted.

The D-ribose connection to cardiac function was first discovered by the physiologist Heinz-Gerd Zimmer at the University of Munich. Zimmer's research found that D-ribose plays an enormous part in both energy restoration and the return of normal diastolic cardiac function. (Diastolic *dys*function is basically a kind of heart failure.) One 1992 clinical study from Zimmer's group showed that administering D-ribose to patients with severe but stable coronary artery disease increased their ability to do exercise and delayed the onset of moderate angina (chest pain). Since then, the benefits of D-ribose have been reported for heart failure, cardiac surgery recovery, restoration of energy to stressed skeletal muscles, and control of free radical formation in tissues that have been deprived of oxygen.

Here's one dramatic story from Dr. Sinatra's practice that illustrates the almost miraculous power of D-ribose supplementation to improve the quality of life of cardiac patients:

Dr. Sinatra: The Case of Louis and D-Ribose

Louis came to my office suffering from severe coronary artery disease. He had been previously treated by having a stent placed in a major coronary artery, but he still had severe blockage in a small arterial branch that was difficult to dilate with a stent and next to impossible to bypass with surgery. He had what's called refractory angina, which means he experienced chest pain even with normal activities such as walking across a room. He'd also feel chest pain anytime he had even mild emotional stress. Louis had visited a number of cardiologists for his heart problem and had been placed on a number of common heart drugs, but his problems persisted.

When Louis came to my office I noticed high levels of uric acid in his blood, indicating faulty ATP metabolism. At the time, he was already taking L-carnitine and CoQ$_{10}$ at "maintenance doses." Realizing that it would help him enormously if he could build up his ATP stores, I immediately recommended D-ribose as well as increased doses of

L-carnitine and CoQ_{10}. In just a few short days, Louis showed remarkable improvement. His son-in-law, a dentist, called me a few days later and reported, "You fixed Louis!"

An adequate dose of D-ribose usually results in symptom improvement very quickly, sometimes within days, as in Louis's case. If initial response is poor, the dose should be increased to 5 g (1 teaspoon) three times a day. Logically, those who are the sickest and the most energy depleted will notice the most improvement in the quickest time.

Despite accumulating scientific evidence of the benefit of D-ribose, very few physicians in the United States have even heard of it outside of their first-year med school biochemistry class. Fewer still recommend it to their patients. Those who are familiar with it have the wonderful gratification of seeing it help patients on a regular basis.

Although the optimal level of D-ribose supplementation will differ depending on the person and the particular condition, here are some good recommended starting points for supplementation:

- 5 g daily for cardiovascular prevention, for athletes on maintenance, and for healthy people who engage in strenuous activities or hard-core workouts
- 10 to 15 g daily for most patients with heart failure, ischemic cardiovascular disease, or peripheral vascular disease; for individuals recovering from heart attacks or heart surgery; for treatment of stable angina; and for athletes who engage in chronic bouts of high-intensity exercise
- 15 to 20 g daily for patients with advanced heart failure, dilated cardiomyopathy, or frequent angina; for individuals awaiting heart transplant; and for individuals with severe fibromyalgia, muscle cramps, or neuromuscular disease

Reported side effects are minimal and infrequent, and there are no known adverse drug or nutritional interactions associated with D-ribose use. The toxicology and safety of D-ribose have been exhaustively studied, and the supplement is 100 percent safe when taken as directed. (Thousands of patients have taken D-ribose with minimal, if any, side effects.)

However, even though there are no known contraindications for supplementation with D-ribose, we recommend that pregnant women, nursing mothers, and very young children refrain from taking D-ribose in the absence of congestive heart failure simply because there is not enough research in these populations.

L-CARNITINE: THE SHUTTLE BUS FOR FATTY ACIDS

As previously stated, the best way to conceptualize L-carnitine is to think of it as a transportation system. It acts as a kind of shuttle bus, loading up fatty acids and transporting them into tiny structures within each cell called *mitochondria*, where they can be burned for energy. Because the heart gets 60 percent of its energy from fat, it's very important that the body has enough L-carnitine to shuttle the fatty acids into the heart's muscle cells.

Studies of patients being treated for various forms of cardiovascular disease provide the strongest evidence for the benefit of L-carnitine supplementation. One study showed that people who took L-carnitine supplements after suffering heart attacks had significantly lower mortality rates compared to those of a control group (1.2 percent of the L-carnitine takers died versus 12.5 percent of the subjects in the control group).[9] One randomized, placebo-controlled study divided eighty heart failure patients into two groups. One group received 2 g of L-carnitine a day, and the other group received a placebo. There was a significantly higher three-year survival rate in the group receiving L-carnitine.[10]

L-carnitine improves the ability of those with angina to exercise without chest pain.[11] In one study, the walking capacity of patients with intermittent claudication—a painful cramping sensation in the muscles of the legs because of a decreased oxygen supply—improved significantly when they were given oral L-carnitine. In another study, patients with peripheral arterial disease of the legs were able to increase their walking distance by 98 meters when they supplemented with L-carnitine; they were able to walk almost twice as far as those who were given a placebo. Further, congestive heart failure patients have experienced an increase in exercise endurance on only 900 mg of L-carnitine a day.

And if that were not enough to establish L-carnitine's bona fides, it has been shown to be a powerful cardio-protective antioxidant. One paper published in the *International Journal of Cardiology* found that L-carnitine had a direct stimulatory effect on two important oxidative stress-related compounds (HO-1 and ecNOS). Both of these markers have antioxidant, antiproliferative (meaning they have an inhibitory effect on tumor cells), and anti-inflammatory properties, so ratcheting up their activity a notch is a very good thing indeed. The researchers concluded that this action of L-carnitine "would be expected to protect from oxidative stress related to cardiovascular and myocardial damage."[12]

Dr. Sinatra: L-Carnitine and CoQ10

Eighty-five percent of my patients with congestive heart failure have improved significantly on CoQ_{10}. But I was concerned about the 15 percent who, despite supplementation with CoQ_{10}, still had symptoms that severely compromised their quality of life.

These folks were supplementing with CoQ_{10} and had excellent blood levels to show for it, typically 3.5 ug/mL or higher (the normal level of CoQ_{10} is 0.5 to 1.5 ug/mL.) Nonetheless, these folks seemed to be unable to utilize what was in their own bodies.

As I read more about L-carnitine, I came to see that it might work in synergy with coenzyme Q_{10}, stoking the fire in the ATP production phase of the Krebs cycle (a sequence of reactions by which living cells generate energy). I finally got comfortable enough to recommend to some of my worrisome patients that they give it a try in combination with CoQ_{10}, and wow, what a difference!

These treatment-resistant folks came in with better color, breathed easier, and walked around the office with minimal difficulty. I was genuinely amazed. It was as if the L-carnitine provided a battery, working perfectly with the coenzyme Q_{10}. The medical literature is also a testimony on carnitine's benefits. In the Mayo Clinic Proceedings, a meta-analysis of thirteen clinical studies on L-carnitine was published in 2013. In a review of 3,629 patients with heart attack, the survival benefits of those taking L-carnitine were realized. There were improvements in cellular energy metabolism and stabilization of heart cell membranes, which resulted in not only the reduction of ventricular arrhythmias and angina symptoms but a significant reduction in death as well.

The bottom line is that the heart is the most metabolically active tissue in the body, and thus it requires a huge and constant amount of energy molecules, or ATPs.

Remember, the heart has to pump sixty to one hundred times a minute, twenty-four hours a day, for years and years with no time off for good behavior! Cardiac muscle cells burn fats for fuel, so the heart is especially vulnerable to even subtle deficiencies in the factors contributing to ATP supply: coenzyme Q_{10}, D-ribose, and L-carnitine.

These nutrients make up three of what I call the "Awesome Foursome" in metabolic cardiology. Now let's introduce the fourth.

MAGNESIUM: THE GREAT RELAXER

Dr. Robert Atkins once referred to magnesium as a "natural calcium channel blocker," and he was 100 percent correct. A few paragraphs from now, you'll understand just why magnesium's ability to block the channels by which calcium gets into the cells is so important for the health of your heart.

Recent research strongly suggests that calcium in the heart can be a huge problem. One meta-analysis examined fifteen eligible trials with the objective of investigating the relationship between calcium supplements and cardiovascular disease. The researchers concluded that calcium supplements (administered without vitamin D) were associated with a modest but

significant *increase* in the risk of cardiovascular disease—an increase, they noted, that might well translate into "a large burden of disease in the population." The authors called for a reassessment of the role of calcium supplements in the management of osteoporosis.[13]

A second study had a different purpose, one particularly relevant to our story.[14] The researchers began with the premise that statins reduce cardiovascular risk and slow the progression of coronary artery calcium. The purpose of the study, then, was to determine whether lowering LDL cholesterol (as statins do) is in some way complementary to slowing the progression of coronary artery calcium. The researchers basically wanted to illuminate the relationship of these two phenomena as they relate to heart disease.

Here's what they did. They measured the change in coronary artery calcium in 495 patients who were basically symptom-free at the beginning of the study. They did this by using a method known as electron beam tomography scanning. Right after their first scan, the patients were started on statin drugs, and they were followed for an average of 3.2 years, during which time their cholesterol was checked and they were scanned on a regular basis. Over the course of the 3.2-year follow-up period, forty-one of the patients had heart attacks.

On average, the 454 patients who did *not* suffer heart attacks saw their arterial calcium go up by approximately 17 percent every year. But the forty-one patients who *did* experience heart attacks saw a whopping 42 percent increase per year in their arterial calcium. According to the researchers, having a faster progression of coronary artery calcium gives you an astonishing 17.2-fold increase in your heart attack risk.[15]

And get this: LDL cholesterol did *not* differ between the two groups. Ironically, the LDL levels of the folks who did *not* suffer heart attacks were slightly *higher* (though not significantly so) than the average LDL levels of the folks who *did* suffer heart attacks.

So let's summarize the results. Both groups—the forty-one folks who *had* heart attacks and the 454 folks who didn't—essentially had the *same* LDL levels. (So if you were using patients' LDL levels to predict heart attacks, you'd get no better accuracy than you would by reading their horoscopes!) But if instead of LDL levels you looked at the levels of calcium in the arteries, it would be a whole different story. Those who suffered myocardial infarctions were the *most* likely to have higher calcium levels in their arteries, especially when the arteries became totally blocked.

Coronary artery calcification has long been recognized as a big risk factor for heart disease, but for some reason we continue to obsessively focus on cholesterol, while few people have heard much about the calcium connection.

Arthur Agatston, M.D., a Florida cardiologist best known as the author of *The South Beach Diet*, actually invented a scoring method to determine the severity of calcification in the arteries—it's known as the Agatston score. (Research shows that people with Agatston scores higher than 400 are at a significantly increased risk for coronary "events"—myocardial infarctions—as well as for most coronary artery procedures [bypasses, angioplasty, etc.].[16])

Calcium in the bones? Very good. Calcium in the arteries? Not so good.

Enter magnesium.

Magnesium and calcium have an interesting, symbiotic relationship. When magnesium is depleted, intracellular calcium rises. Magnesium also inhibits platelet aggregation, an important step in the development of clots. Calcium channel blockers widen and relax the blood vessels by affecting the muscle cells found in the arterial walls, which is exactly what magnesium does—splendidly, we might add. Magnesium dilates the arteries, thus reducing blood pressure and making it far easier for the heart to pump blood and for the blood to flow freely.

In most of the epidemiologic and clinical trials, a high dietary intake of magnesium (at least 500 to 1,000 mg a day) resulted in reduced blood pressure.[17] These studies showed an inverse relationship between magnesium intake and blood pressure; people who consumed *more* magnesium had *lower* blood pressure. One study of sixty hypertensive subjects who were given magnesium supplementation showed a significant reduction in blood pressure over an eight-week period.[18]

So basically, you can think of magnesium as a "relaxer." One of the most relaxing things you can do is to bathe in Epsom salts, which is basically a compound of magnesium with a little bit of sulfur and oxygen. If you've ever worked with an integrative medicine practitioner who happens to use vitamin drips, you might have found that the most amazing and restful sleep you've ever had occurred after getting a magnesium-heavy vitamin push.* Just as magnesium has a relaxing effect on your body, it also

* A form of vitamin injection administered slowly over the course of ten to fifteen minutes.

has a relaxing effect on your arteries. And that's a very good thing from the perspective of the heart, which instead of having to push blood through a narrow or constricted vessel (dangerously raising blood pressure) now has the much easier task of pumping it through a relaxed, widened vessel that doesn't put up so much resistance. Your heart doesn't have to work as hard, your blood pressure goes down, and all is well with the world.

There's another interesting connection between magnesium and the heart, and if you've followed our argument so far, you'll love the elegance of how it all comes full circle. The connection? Sugar.

You'll recall from chapter 6 that sugar is one of the worst things you can eat if you want to have a healthy heart. Here's why: Sugar is highly inflammatory. It also creates dangerous compounds known as advanced glycation end products, or AGEs, which play a pivotal role in atherosclerosis.[19] AGEs play a role of particular importance in type 2 diabetes, which, as you know, is a condition in which blood sugar and insulin are essentially at unhealthy levels and have to be brought under control. And diabetes is one way to fast-track your path to heart disease.

One of the very best things magnesium does is help manage blood sugar. In several studies of diabetic patients, magnesium supplements of 400 to 1,000 mg per day, given for anywhere from three weeks to three months, improved a number of measures of glycemic (blood sugar) control, including the requirement for insulin.[20] One study measured serum concentrations of magnesium in 192 people with insulin resistance and found that the prevalence of a low magnesium level was about 65 percent among those with insulin resistance, as opposed to only 5 percent of those in a control group[21]

Clearly, there's a strong association between magnesium deficiency and insulin resistance. You'll recall that people with insulin resistance are at great risk for diabetes, which in turn puts them at great risk for heart disease. Helping to control blood sugar and insulin is just one more important way in which magnesium is critical for heart health.

Magnesium is necessary for more than three hundred biochemical reactions in the body, and many of these are enzymatic reactions, essential for heart health (or what scientists call *myocardial metabolism*).[22] Even borderline deficiencies of magnesium can negatively affect the heart, and not surprisingly, there is a considerable amount of evidence associating low levels of magnesium with cardiovascular disease.[23]

Bottom line: Magnesium supplements are a must for those who want to protect their hearts. Magnesium lowers blood pressure, helps control blood sugar, and relaxes the lining of the blood vessels. And almost all dietary surveys show that Americans aren't getting nearly enough.[24] We recommend supplementing with at least 400 mg per day.

NOTE: Magnesium supplementation is *not* recommended for anyone with renal insufficiency (kidney disease).

NIACIN AND ITS EFFECT ON CHOLESTEROL

Even if your doctor hasn't studied nutrition and is skeptical (or worse) when it comes to supplements, chances are he or she will be familiar with the benefits of niacin. It's been known since 1955 that cholesterol can be effectively lowered with doses of 1,000 to 4,000 mg of niacin daily.[25] Subsequent studies have shown that niacin will lower triglycerides by 20 to 50 percent and LDL cholesterol by 10 to 25 percent.[26]

Niacin is one of two major forms of vitamin B_3—the other is nicotinamide. Although both forms can be used for different things in the body, only the niacin form has an effect on your cholesterol, triglycerides, and related compounds. And the effect is not just on overall cholesterol. Studies have shown that when LDL cholesterol is reduced with niacin, there is a preferential reduction of the really nasty LDL molecules, the hard, small, BB gun pellet-type particles that stick to the artery walls, get oxidized, and cause damage.

Niacin also reduces lipoprotein(a), or Lp(a). Lipoprotein(a) is basically a special kind of LDL, and it's a really bad one. This, folks, is the *real* cholesterol story! Lp(a) is an independent risk factor for heart disease and for heart attacks, yet it doesn't get as much attention as cholesterol does because there aren't effective drug treatments for lowering it, and no one really knows what to do about it. Niacin lowers Lp(a) levels by a remarkable 10 to 30 percent.[27]

Equally terrific, if not more so, is the fact that niacin *raises* HDL cholesterol. That alone would be worth shouting from the rooftops, because we consider HDL cholesterol to be a much undervalued player in the heart disease story. (We'll delve into this topic later on in the book.) Niacin raises HDL levels by 10 to 30 percent.[28] But even better is the fact that it *preferentially* increases HDL-2, which is the most beneficial of the HDL subclasses.[29] (HDL-3 is actually pro-inflammatory, even though it's a member of the so-called "good" cholesterol family—HDL—once again demonstrating how obsolete and ridiculous the classification of cholesterol into just "good" and "bad" really is!)

The most clinically important side effect of too much niacin is that it can be very taxing on the liver (a condition known as hepatotoxicity), although as Dr. Alan Gaby points out in his exhaustive review of nutritional supplements and disease, this is almost never seen in patients taking 3 g or less per day.[30]

Abram Hoffer, M.D., the great pioneer of nutritional and integrative medicine, stated that his thirty years of experience with niacin therapy (usually 3 g a day or more) showed that one out of every two thousand patients will develop hepatitis from large doses of this vitamin. However, Hoffer also pointed out that in all of his patients who developed hepatotoxicity, liver function returned to normal after treatment was discontinued.[31]

Sustained-release niacin is actually more hepatotoxic than regular niacin, and liver problems may occur at lower doses.[32] Nausea may be an early warning sign of niacin-induced hepatotoxicity; if nausea occurs, the dose should be reduced, or treatment should be stopped.[33] For folks taking therapeutic doses of niacin, it's a good idea to have your doctor check your liver enzymes periodically using a standard liver function test.

Dr. Jonny: Niacin Flush

The first time I experienced the "niacin flush" I was working as a personal trainer. It was five o'clock in the morning, and I was getting ready for my 6 a.m. client. I remember drinking my protein shake, swallowing my vitamins, and then, a very short time later while getting dressed, having the distinct feeling that I was going to die. My skin was flushed, warm to the touch, and my cheeks (and arms) were pinkish red. It wasn't painful, but it was deeply unpleasant.

My 6 a.m. client happened to be the president of a high-end makeup company whose husband was an equally well-known Manhattan dermatologist (as well as the only doctor I knew who was likely to be awake at this ungodly hour). I called my client, and she immediately put her husband on the line. I described my symptoms, and he asked me if I'd taken or eaten anything unusual. "Just my vitamins," I said, to which he replied without hesitation, "Oh, it's just the niacin. Nothing to worry about, it'll pass in a few. I'm going back to bed now."

So that was my first encounter with the infamous "niacin flush." It's basically a temporary flushing of the skin, not at all dangerous (especially if you know it's coming!), and it's actually a result of the dilation of the blood vessels in the skin (which is why my skin turned pink). Some people experience itching as well or even a mild burning sensation. It typically goes away within a couple of weeks and can usually be counteracted with a baby aspirin taken beforehand.

NOTE: If you are diabetic or have a liver ailment, be sure to check with your doctor before supplementing with niacin.

Dr. Sinatra's Niacin Know-How

- Look for straight, non-time-release niacin (also known as nicotinic acid). Take after meals at dosages of 500 mg to 3 g daily.
- Start slowly at 100 mg. Work your way up gradu-

ally to a higher level, in divided doses.

- If the flush is too uncomfortable, take a baby aspirin before the first meal of the day and then take the niacin after the meal. Use the aspirin only as long as you experience the flush and whenever you increase your niacin dosage, which will trigger a flush.
- You can also try taking an apple pectin supplement with the niacin to reduce a flush.
- Niacin may increase the enzyme levels in liver function tests. This does not necessarily mean that niacin is causing a liver problem, but have your doctor keep an eye on it. He or she may suggest stopping the niacin for five days before your next liver test to avoid possible confusion. Be aware, though, that when you resume the niacin you will develop a flush.

VITAMIN E: THE GOOD, THE BAD, AND THE UGLY

For decades, the nutritional world revered vitamin E as something of a heart savior, a major antioxidant that defended against lipid peroxidation, which was thought to be the cause of cardiovascular disease. (*Lipid* simply means fat, and *peroxidation* is a fancy way of saying oxidative damage from free radicals.) During the 1990s the adulation for vitamin E even extended to mainstream medicine, going as far as the American Heart Association. In 1996, for instance, vitamin E was celebrated in a well-publicized study for significantly reducing cardiovascular events over the course of one year among some 2,000 patients with documented heart disease.

The successes and reputation of vitamin E

prompted many to believe that if a little vitamin E was good, then more would be even better! Critical studies that followed, however, began demonstrating that daily doses of vitamin E at 400 IUs and above didn't necessarily generate beneficial results, and, in fact, might be detrimental to health. (As early as 2003, Dr. Sinatra wrote in his newsletter about his own reluctance to back high-dose vitamin E because the emerging research indicated possible pro-oxidant effects.)

That said, both of us found ourselves puzzled by the negative study results that have popped up since then. Sure, problems could come from using the synthetic form of vitamin E (designated *dl-alpha-tocopherol*) instead of the "natural" form (designated *d-alpha-tocopherol*). But a *pro*-oxidant effect from natural vitamin E, considered one of the powerhouses in the antioxidant armamentarium? How could that be?

Sharp-eyed readers may have noticed that we put quotation marks around the word *natural* when referring to natural vitamin E in the above paragraph. That's because d-alpha-tocopherol by itself is only one *part* of natural vitamin E. Vitamin E is actually a collection of eight related compounds that are divided into two classes: *tocopherols* and *tocotrienols.* The tocopherols come in four forms: *alpha, delta, beta,* and *gamma.* Of these four forms, the best known is alpha. When you purchase a "natural" vitamin E supplement, most of the time it is 100 percent *alpha*-tocopherol.

And therein lies the problem.

Gamma-tocopherol is turning out to be the most potent of the four tocopherols, and the one most responsible for vitamin E's positive effects as an antioxidant. Thus, people taking high-dose alpha-tocoph-

erol alone and not getting enough gamma-tocopherol in their diets, or in their supplements, could run the risk of experiencing a pro-oxidant effect from vitamin E. Moreover, large doses of alpha-tocopherol could also deplete the body's existing gamma-tocopherol stores.

A 2011 study provided an even sharper image of the two faces of vitamin E. In laboratory experiments, researchers in Belfast found that vitamin E (alpha- and gamma-tocopherol) protects very low-density lipoprotein (VLDL) and LDL cholesterol against oxidation. That's a good thing! Yet they found a "surprising" pro-oxidant effect on HDL (high-density lipoprotein), the cholesterol particle that acts like a garbage truck, picking up harmful oxidized LDL and transporting it back to the liver for removal. Anything that can hinder HDL is of real concern.

Worth noting is that the researchers referenced a previous study in which taking a small amount of vitamin C along with your alpha-tocopherol helped *prevent* the negative, pro-oxidant effect of vitamin E on HDL. That wouldn't be the first time one nutrient helped another one out. We already know that CoQ_{10} helps protect vitamin E in the body and gives it a hand by recycling it back to an active form after it's been oxidized in biochemical reactions. (We are big fans of the synergistic effects of nutrients.)

The other half of the vitamin E story concerns the four components known as the *tocotrienols.* Tocotrienols are turning out to be the real heavy lifters in the vitamin E family, at least when it comes to benefits for the heart. They have more potent antioxidant activity than tocopherols do.[34] They also increase the number of LDL receptors, which helps with LDL removal.[35] Tocotrienols provide significant lipid-lowering effects in experimental animals, and most prospective studies have demonstrated the same thing in humans.[36]

If you take vitamin E, we recommend that you always get it from a supplement labeled "mixed tocopherols" in order to avoid the problems that can occur with pure alpha-tocopherol supplementation. A vitamin E supplement that is 100 percent alpha-tocopherol is less effective and may even be problematic in high doses. Virtually all the studies showing negative results used the alpha-tocopherol form or, worse, the synthetic dl-alpha-tocopherol form. (The dl-alpha-tocopherol form should be left on the shelf to rot!)

If you add 100 to 200 IUs of mixed tocopherols and gamma vitamin E to a regimen that also includes vitamin C and CoQ$_{10}$, you should be fine! We also like the tocotrienols and especially delta tocotrienol as the research clearly demonstrates the remarkable benefits of these compounds.

OMEGA-3: THE ULTIMATE WELLNESS MOLECULE

If you've read this book sequentially, you're already familiar with omega-3 fatty acids from our extensive discussion of them in chapter 10, so here we'll highlight just a few of the many studies demonstrating the value of omega-3 fats for the heart. (We should also point out that there is equally compelling research documenting the positive effect of omega-3s on the brain as well,[37] but because this is a book on cholesterol and cardiovascular disease, we'll focus on the heart.)

More than thirty years ago, scientists began to notice very low rates of cardiovascular disease among Greenland Eskimos compared to age- and sex-matched Danish control subjects. Shortly afterward, they were able to link these low rates of heart disease to high consumption of omega-3s in the Greenland diet.[38] This discovery triggered an enormous amount of research on the role of fish oil in preventing heart disease. (As of this writing—January 2020—a National Library Medicine [pubmed.gov] search for "omega-3 cardiovascular benefit" produced 378 peer-review journal articles.)

One recent review of omega-3s and cardiovascular disease by Dariush Mozaffarian, M.D., of the Harvard School of Public Health, concluded that omega-3 consumption "lowers plasma triglycerides, resting heart rate, and blood pressure and might also improve myocardial filling and efficiency, lower inflammation, and improve vascular function."[39] Mozaffarian also noted that the benefits of omega-3s seem most consistent for coronary heart disease mortality and sudden cardiac death.

In case your eyes were beginning to glaze over from all the medical journal speak, let's sum it up in plain English: There is reliable and consistent research evidence demonstrating that omega-3 fats, mainly from fish, lower the death rate from heart disease and lower the risk of sudden cardiac death. This is hard-core evidence that fish oil saves lives.

One of the landmark clinical studies of omega-3 supplementation in a high-risk population was published in 1999 and was known as the GISSI-Prevenzione trial.[40] More than 11,000 patients who had suffered a heart attack within the past three months were randomly assigned to receive either 1 g a day of omega-3s, 300 mg of vitamin E, both, or neither, in addition to whatever standard therapy they were receiving. Vitamin E had no effect, but omega-3s were associated with a 20 percent reduction in mortality and a whopping 45 percent reduction in the risk of sudden death. These effects were apparent within a mere three months of therapy.[41]

International guidelines recommend 1 g of omega-3 fats daily for all people who've already had a heart attack or for patients with elevated triglycerides.[42] Experts believe these guidelines will soon be extended to patients with heart failure as well.[43]

It's worth mentioning that the overwhelming majority of research on omega-3s and heart disease was done using the two omega-3s that are found in fish, EPA and DHA. But other studies have also found that ALA—the omega-3 found in plant foods such as flax and flaxseed oil—has benefits for the heart as well. One review of the literature pointed out that both *in vitro* (test-tube) studies and animal studies have shown that ALA can prevent ventricular fibrillation, the chief mechanism of cardiac death, and that it might be even more efficient at preventing this than EPA and DHA are. The review also noted that ALA was effective at lowering platelet aggregation, which is an important step in thrombosis (a stroke or nonfatal heart attack).[44]

Even if you're already on a statin drug and have decided to remain on one, fish oil can still help you. One study found that among more than 3,600 people with a history of cardiovascular disease—many of whom were on antiplatelet drugs, antihypertensive agents, and nitrates—daily fish oil supplementation led to a sta-tistically significant 19 percent reduction in major coronary events compared to the control group.[45]

Omega-3 fats, particularly from healthy, wild fish, are your heart's best friend, whether you're recovering from a heart attack or hoping to prevent one. They lower triglycerides. And they lower blood pressure. And best of all, omega-3s are among the most anti-inflammatory compounds on the planet, meaning they have a beneficial effect on the root causes of heart disease.

We recommend that you take 2 to 3 g of fish oil daily. Since the publication of the first edition, recommendations by functional medicine doctors in the know tend to run closer to 3 to 4 g a day, and that's of combined EPA and DHA (see below for explanation). We also recommend that you eat cold water fish (such as wild salmon) as often as you can. We *both* recommend Vital Choice, an impeccable source of wild salmon from pristine Alaskan waters that is reasonably priced and shipped in dry ice directly to your door. Like many health professionals, we buy nearly all of our fish—and 100 percent of our salmon—from Vital Choice. You can find links to this terrific company on our websites.

When you supplement with fish oil, remember that the total amount of omega-3s is not what's important. Bargain-basement omega-3 supplements often tout on their labels how much omega-3 they contain. This number by itself is meaningless. You want to know specifically how much EPA and DHA are contained within each capsule. These are the gold nuggets in the prospector's tin—you don't care about the *total* amount of stones in that pan, you care about the *gold*. EPA and DHA are the gold. Try to get at least 2 g daily of combined EPA and DHA. (Jonny is a fan of even higher doses—3 to 4 g a day of combined EPA and DHA.

PANTETHINE: YOUR SECRET WEAPON

Pantethine is a metabolically active (and somewhat more expensive) form of vitamin B$_5$ (pantothenic acid). The blood tests of patients with dyslipidemia—a fancy way of saying that their blood levels of cholesterol are too high—significantly improve with pantethine supplementation. And although this can't be seen on a blood test, pantethine also reduces the oxidation of LDL.[46]

No fewer than twenty-eight clinical trials in humans have shown that pantethine produces significant positive changes in triglycerides, LDL cholesterol, and VLDL, along with increases in HDL cholesterol.[47] In all of these trials, virtually no adverse effects were noted. The mean dose of pantethine in these studies was 900 mg per day given as 300 mg three times daily. This appears to be the optimal dosage, and it is the one we recommend.

According to a review of the literature on pantethine published in *Progress in Cardiovascular Diseases*, Mark Houston, M.D., noted that in most studies, at the end of four months pantethine reduced total cholesterol by 15.1 percent, LDL by 20.1 percent, and triglycerides by 32.9 percent, with an increase in HDL of 8.4 percent.[48] Houston also noted that in studies of longer duration, there appeared to be continued improvement. (The only adverse reactions were mild gastrointestinal side effects in less than 4 percent of the subjects.) As previously stated, we recommend

900 mg of pantethine divided into three daily doses of 300 mg each.

GLUCOSAMINE SULFATE

If you're familiar with glucosamine sulfate, you might be surprised to find it listed here as a potential supplement for heart health. Actually, we were also surprised. For decades, glucosamine—together with a synergistic nutrient called chondrotrin sulfate—have been known as supplements for joint health.

Indeed, almost all the research on glucosamine—a natural component of cartilage—has been done on arthritis patients. And the results, though generally positive, have not always been conclusive. Sometimes it works for knee arthritis, but not for hip arthritis. (Why? Who knows?) Sometimes it works for people with *moderate-to-severe* arthritic pain, but not for *mild* pain. But overall, it's a very researched supplement that has generally helped people with pain related to joints, and those who use it swear by it.

(Full disclosure: One of us—Jonny—has severe arthritis of the shoulder and is a competitive tennis player. Jonny takes a daily dose of 1500 mg of glucosamine sulfate—together with 1250 mg of chondroitin—as part of his joint supplement routine, and has found it. together with CBD, fish oil, and a few other things, to be extremely helpful.)

So why is glucosamine making a surprise appearance in the heart supplement section of this book?

Well, one thing we know about glucosamine is that it's *anti-inflammatory*. Another thing we know is that glucosamine works even better when it's combined with fish oil, the combo providing a double whammy of anti-inflammatory power.[49]

Given its anti-inflammatory actions, it really shouldn't be all that remarkable that glucosamine might have a place in a supplement program designed to protect the heart. And in fact, that's exactly what a recent study in the *British Medical Journal* found.

Researchers led by Dr. Lu Qi at the Tulane University Obesity Research Center in New Orleans did a lifestyle survey involving more than 466,000 men and women, none of whom had been diagnosed with heart disease when survey polling began. They were tracked for an average of seven years. Those taking the supplement had a 15 percent lower risk for heart disease. Glucosamine was also associated with a significant drop in the experience of coronary heart disease, stroke, or death from heart-disease related issues.

Dr. Qi, commenting on his own findings, said, "I am a bit surprised but not very much, because previous studies from humans or animals have shown that glucosamine may have protective effects on inflammation, which is a risk factor for cardiovascular disease." Dr. Qi added. "In addition, glucosamine use may mimic effects of a low-carbohydrate diet, which has been also related to lower CVD risk."[50]

Now let's be clear about two things. One, this is an observational/association study. Association does not prove causality; it simply shows that two things are consistently found together, more so than they would be by chance. So while there's now evidence that taking glucosamine is related to a reduction in the risk for heart disease, we don't know for sure that one caused the other.

Two, the effect was small. Though it was statistically significant—unlikely to have been found by accident—it was not a huge effect. Glucosamine use was associated with a 15 percent lower risk of total CVD (cardiovascular disease) events, 22 percent lower risk of CVD death, 18 percent lower risk of coronary heart disease (slightly different from cardiovascular disease), and a 9 percent lower risk for stroke.[51]

Still. That's not nothing.

Glucosamine sulfate wouldn't be our first choice for a heart supplement. But it definitely is one you should consider adding to your heart supplement routine.

OMEGA-7

By now you've heard us talk about inflammation quite a bit. That's because there is no disease either of us can think of that doesn't involve inflammation, and that's especially true with heart disease. Therefore, anything that can be demonstrated to reduce systemic inflammation gets our attention.

Enter Omega-7.

Most people have never heard of omega-7, but it's proving to be incredibly important. The main omega-7 fat in the body is called palmitoleic acid, and it's been shown to work on the cycle of events we refer to as "diabetic physiology" (see chapter 9)—high blood sugar, elevated lipids (fats), excessive body fat, and, inevitably, insulin resistance. It's this cycle—nearly always triggered by too much sugar and starch—that we believe is the number one set of risk factors for heart disease. (You'll see why in Chapter 12.)

Omega-7 actually enhances insulin *sensitivity* (the exact opposite of the dreaded insulin *resistance*!).[52] Since insulin resistance and fat accumulation tend to go hand in hand, and since omega-7 helps fight insulin resistance, it's not entirely surprising that omega-7s also helps with breaking down fat and increasing the enzymes that are needed for fat burning in the first place.[53]

Fat cells produce inflammatory cytokines, as well as other bad actors. They release molecules called *adipokines* that can change the metabolic activity of tissues and ultimately produce higher levels of inflammation.[54] That's why reducing excess body fat is *always* a good idea if you're trying to prevent heart disease. Remember, heart disease is in large measure an inflammatory disease, and anything that reduces inflammation—like losing weight—is a net gain for your heart.

Which brings us to the remarkable study on omega-7 performed at the Cleveland Clinic.[55]

The first randomized control trial of omega-7 supplements in humans was done at the Cleveland Clinic Wellness Institute. Overweight or obese adults with evidence of inflammation—defined as CRP levels between 2 mg/L and 5 mg/L—were randomly assigned to two groups. One group got 220 mg of purified omega-7 supplementation, one group got a placebo. The "outcome" measure was CRP score (see page 198), which, you may remember stands for C-reactive protein and is a blood measure for systemic inflammation.

The average baseline C-reactive protein (CRP) level for all subjects in the study was 4.3 ml/DL, considered "high risk" for cardiovascular disease. But after only thirty days, there was a 44 percent reduction in CRP levels in the omega-7 group compared to the placebo group. Those who took the supplement wound up with an average CRP of 2.1, which, while not ideal, is well within the "average risk" range for inflammation-induced cardiovascular disease.

This study—having been done at one of the most prestigious medical centers in the world, and producing such a significant result—is why we think omega-7 may well have a place in the treatment and prevention of cardiometabolic disease. One company—Barlean's—makes a product with the exact dose used in the study, 210 mg. It's called Heart Remedy. (Full disclosure: Barlean's also makes a 440 mg dose of the same omega-7 in a product called Joint Relief. We see no reason not to take the higher dose, but either will provide high quality omega-7.)

OTHER SUPPLEMENTATION YOU SHOULD CONSIDER

Picking the "top" supplements for treating any health issue is always difficult. In trying to keep the list from being too overwhelming, you're always going to leave a few good things out. There's also the very real issue of compliance. Most people don't like to take a lot of pills, even if the pills in question are natural substances that will boost or protect their health. We consider the following supplements important, and we suggest that you read about what they do and consider using them in addition to the key supplements discussed above.

Vitamin C. Vitamin C is one of the most powerful antioxidants in the world, and because heart disease is initiated by oxidative damage (damage caused by free radicals), any help you can get in the antioxidant department is a good thing. And the evidence is not just theoretical: A large 2011 study published in the *American Heart Journal* found that the lower the

NATURAL CLOT BUSTERS: NATTOKINASE AND LUMBROKINASE

Hyperviscosity refers to sticky, or sludgy, blood. When blood thickens, it bogs down as it moves through the blood vessels, causing platelets to stick together and clump. Blood vessels become more rigid, less elastic, and frequently calcified. The danger lies in the tendency to form clots that can block vessels leading to vital organs.

Nattokinase is extracted from the traditional fermented soy food natto, believed by many researchers to contribute to the low incidence of coronary heart disease in Japan. It provides a unique, powerful, and safe way to eliminate clots, or reduce the tendency to form clots, and thus decrease the risk of heart attack and stroke.[64]

Lumbrokinase, developed in both Japan and China, comes from an extract of earthworm, a traditional source of healing in Asian medicine. These two separate products of dynamic Asian research share a powerful and common property of great interest to anyone who wants to protect their cardiovascular system: They are natural clot eaters.

Here's how it works: Your body naturally produces *fibrin*, a fibrous protein formed from fibrinogen. (A fibrinogen test is one of the blood tests we recommend—see appendix B— because it is a good marker of how much fibrin you're making.) Fibrin is both good and bad. Its clot-forming action is immediately activated when bleeding occurs, so that's a good thing. But excess fibrin activity can produce consistently thick blood, and that's a big problem.

To offset the danger—and to create thinner blood—the body produces another substance called *plasmin*, an enzyme whose job is to break down excess fibrin. A nice system of checks and balances. But if plasmin, the natural anticlotting agent, becomes overwhelmed and can't keep up with the job, there's trouble in River City. And that's where nattokinase and lumbrokinase come in. If blood clots in an already narrowed blood vessel, you're basically screwed. So if you can dissolve the clotted material, you can open arteries and improve blood flow. If you reduce the clot even just a tiny bit, you get a significant blood flow boost.

Nattokinase and lumbrokinase are natural blood thinners. They can literally turn your blood from the consistency of ketchup to the consistency of red wine! Best of all, they work pretty quickly, within minutes to hours.

If you take these supplements preventively, you may not form clots in the first place.

level of vitamin C in the blood, the higher the risk for heart failure.[56] Take 1,000 to 2,000 mg a day.

Worth knowing: Vitamin C is extremely safe, and side effects are rare because the body can't store the vitamin. (In some cases, doses exceeding 2,000 mg a day can lead to a little harmless stomach upset and diarrhea.) The bigger danger is the fact that vitamin C increases the amount of iron absorbed from foods. People with hemochromatosis, an inherited condition in which too much iron builds up in the bloodstream, should not take more than 100 mg of supplemental vitamin C.

Curcumin. This extract from the Indian spice turmeric has multiple benefits, not the least of which is that it's highly anti-inflammatory. Scientific research has demonstrated its anti-inflammatory, antioxidant, anti-thrombotic, and cardiovascular protective effects.[57] Curcumin also reduces oxidized LDL cholesterol.[58] In animal studies, it was shown to protect the lining of the artery walls from damage caused by homocysteine.[59] The synergistic relationship of curcumin with resveratrol is especially important.

Resveratrol. Resveratrol is the ingredient in red wine that's best known for its "anti-aging" activity. It helps protect the arteries by improving their elasticity, inhibits blood clots, and lowers both oxidized LDL and blood pressure.[60] Not a bad resume! It's both a strong antioxidant and a strong anti-inflammatory, inhibiting a number of inflammatory enzymes that can contribute to heart disease. It also inhibits the ability of certain molecules to stick to the arterial walls, where they can take up residence and contribute to inflammation.[61] The recommended daily dose is 30 to 200 mg of trans-resveratrol, the active compo-

nent of resveratrol. Read labels carefully to see what percentage of the capsule is actually the "trans" variety, because that's the only kind that counts.

Citrus Bergamot. Citrus bergamot is a fruit that's endemic to the Calabrian region in Southern Italy and if it lives up to its promise—which it seems to be doing—it may turn out to be one of the most important supplements for the prevention of metabolic syndrome (aka insulin resistance syndrome or pre-diabetes). Metabolic syndrome, you'll remember, is a collection of symptoms (high blood sugar, high triglycerides, high blood pressure, abdominal fat, etc.) that greatly increases the risk for heart disease.

Citrus bergamot lowers blood sugar. It lowers triglycerides. And it lowers blood pressure. Dr. Sinatra calls this, " a trifecta of cardiovascular health."

As with all of the other supplements, but especially with resveratrol, curcumin, and fish oil, you need to pay attention to the label and the amount of active ingredients. Look for bergamot products with a high percentage of polyphenols (at least 30 percent if not more). Citrus bergamot extract of 38 percent polyphenols has been demonstrated to suppress inflammation, inhibit plaque formation, and improve arterial responsiveness, thus contributing mightily to cardiovascular health.[62]

Berberine. Berberine is an active biological compound that can be extracted from a number of plants, notably shrubs. Although it has a long history of use in traditional Chinese medicine, it's now earning a reputation among modern day health practitioners in the west as an effective adjunct treatment for a number of cardiometabolic issues.

It is a powerful antioxidant and anti-inflammatory

that also decreases triglycerides and blood sugar. And some research shows it may increase insulin receptors (which would increase insulin sensitivity and reduce insulin resistance). It also increases nitrous oxide.

A meta-analysis of sixteen berberine studies done in 2018 showed significant improvements in conventional measures of cardiovascular risk, including, by the way, a reduction in triglycerides of 25 mg/dl. And another meta-analysis—this one looking at reductions in blood sugar—concluded that *"(b)ased on the existing evidence reviewed, berberine has beneficial effects on blood glucose control in the treatment of type 2 diabetic patients and exhibits efficacy comparable with that of conventional oral hypoglycaemics."* In other words, berberine's blood sugar lowering capacity was found to be comparable to several well-established pharmaceutical medicines.[63]

Cocoa flavanols. Plant chemicals in cocoa known as *flavanols* help the body synthesize a compound called nitric oxide, which is critical for healthy blood flow and healthy blood pressure. Nitric oxide also improves platelet function, meaning it makes your blood less sticky. It also makes the lining of the arteries less attractive for white blood cells to attach to and stick around. Researchers in Germany followed more than 19,000 people for a minimum of ten years and found that those who ate the most flavanol-rich dark chocolate had lower blood pressure and a 39 percent lower risk of having a heart attack or stroke compared to those who ate almost no chocolate.[65]

Astaxanthin. Dr. Sinatra first got acquainted with astaxanthin at a Japanese symposium on CoQ_{10} over a decade ago. Astaxanthin is what gives the orange-red color to salmon, shrimp, lobster, and crab to mention a few. It has more antioxidant power than vitamin C and even pycnogenol. He was so enthusiastic about what he heard that he started to incorporate astaxanthin into his Omega Vitalisea product at Healthy Directions.

Over the last few years, there have been more than 1,400 publications in the medical literature regarding the powerful antioxidant and anti-aging aspects of astaxanthin. These improvements have not only been seen in heart and brain function, but also in eye and skin health as well. Astaxanthin from algae is a unique potent carotenoid that is a terrific free-radical fighter supporting the brain, eye, heart, and skin. Both of us believe this powerful antioxidant should be incorporated in one's supplemental program on a daily basis. (One very good food source of astaxanthin is wild-caught salmon and krill!)

CONVINCING YOUR DOCTOR

If you show this chapter to your doctor, and he or she is still skeptical, we suggest you direct him or her to the superb review paper on nonpharmacological treatment for dyslipidemia written by Mark Houston, M.D., and published in *Progress in Cardiovascular Diseases*.[66] This paper has 421 citations and should go a long way toward reassuring him or her that there is plenty of research to support the use of these natural, non-toxic substances.

◀ WHAT YOU NEED TO KNOW

- Coenzyme Q_{10} (CoQ_{10}) is a kind of "energy fuel" for the heart. Statins deplete CoQ_{10}; supplementation is an absolute necessity if you're on a statin drug, and it is a very good idea even if you're not.
- L-carnitine supplementation after a heart attack increases survival rate and makes it less likely you'll suffer a second heart attack.
- Magnesium relaxes the artery walls, reduces blood pressure, and makes it easier for the heart to pump blood and for the blood to flow freely.
- Niacin will lower both triglycerides and the "bad" kind of LDL cholesterol. It also reduces a toxic substance called lipoprotein(a)–Lp(a) for short–and raises HDL. Don't use the time-release kind.
- Omega-3s–especially from fish–lower the death rate from heart disease. They also lower triglycerides, resting heart rate, and blood pressure. Omega-3s are highly anti-inflammatory.
- Other supplements worth considering include vitamin C, curcumin, resveratrol, citrus bergamot, berberine, and cocoa flavanols.

CHAPTER 12

THE SCIENCE OF HEALTHY LIVING: EAT, LAUGH, PLAY, LOVE

BOTH OF US, DURING OUR GRADUATE SCHOOL YEARS, trained in psychology. Jonny earned a master's in psychology from the New School for Social Research, and Steve trained for two years in gestalt therapy and then followed up with a six-year certification in bioenergetic psychotherapy. Perhaps that's why both of us, throughout our careers, have been keenly aware of the role that attitude, thought, feeling, emotion, and the subconscious play in our physical health. We have both seen the collapse of the old-fashioned way of thinking about "mind" and "body" as two separate areas of study. Today, every scientist worth his weight in Bunsen burners understands that "mind" and "body" are *not* two discrete entities, but two completely entwined and interrelated parts of a whole that operate together and are impossible to disentangle.

In fact there's an entire field of legitimate scientific study that actually studies how mind and body influence each other. It's called psychoneuroimmunology, or sometimes psychoneuroendocrinology, and it's been around since 1975.[1] It specifically studies how what we think about (psychoneuro) affects our immune system (immunology) or our hormones (endocrinology). The findings are profound and incontrovertible—what we think about affects virtually all of our physiology, including (if not especially) the cardiometabolic ones.[2]

Here's a perfect example: stress. Now, textbooks have been written detailing exactly how excessive levels of stress hormones–known as chronic stress–do long-term metabolic damage. And as fascinating as that story is, it will take us way too far afield to detail here. So we're going to ask you, for the purposes of this book, to accept our conclusion based on decades of study and a close reading of the research: Chronic stress is either a promoter, contributor, accompaniment, multiplier, or proximate cause of just about every disease on the planet.

It's also, by the way, a major instigator of inflammation. And weight gain (particularly around the middle). And elevated blood pressure.

The term "chronic stress" has become an all too familiar accompaniment to daily life. And here's what chronic stress does: It damages and weakens your heart (and your immune system). It weakens your resistance to bad stuff. It lowers your resilience.

And it can even bring on a heart attack.

Virtually every one of the recommended activities below lowers stress hormones. We can't overstate the importance of this. You can test to your heart's content, eat all the right foods, and even exercise regularly, but if you're not managing your stress hormones, you're draining your health bank account, and eventually, it will catch up with you.

And this is not just speculation. Dozens of studies have now shown that what you think about profoundly affects your physiology, your immune system, your blood pressure, your stress hormones, and everything that's affected by them. We can simply no longer treat "heart disease" like it's a solely physical phenomenon.

Opening your heart to your feelings and learning how to express them in a healthy way will do far more for your heart and your overall health than you might imagine. This final section offers some specific tech-

Everyone reading this book needs to know this: Diet, exercise, and/or nutritional supplements are important tools that help prevent and even heal heart disease. But they are only a part of the picture. The many hidden emotional and psychological risk factors that are hardly ever addressed by conventional medicine are equally important–and sometimes even more so. They include suppressed anger, rage, the loss of love (what Dr. Sinatra calls "heartbreak"), and the emotional isolation that results from lack of intimacy with other people.

niques you can use to accomplish this.

BREATHE DEEPLY

When people are subjected to chronic stress, they oftentimes become tense and rigid. They take shallow breaths. High chest breathing can, over the course of time, result in actual physical changes in the body, such as a more rigid upper body, including the chest and shoulders. Slow, rhythmic, deep abdominal breathing, however, is physiologically more suited to the body and has the added benefit of allowing a greater intake of oxygen.

Proper breathing has been the subject of many stress-management programs. It's the first place you start when you learn to meditate, and it's a principle focus of yoga. In Gestalt psychotherapy, deep breathing is used as a vehicle to loosen up the energy of the chest and to free emotions.

A more prolonged form of deep breathing is meditation, which has an impressive amount of research showing that it lowers blood pressure effectively. Cardiologist Herbert Benson, M.D., has been doing pioneering research on meditation and deep breathing for decades. An associate professor of medicine at Harvard Medical School and founder of the Benson-Henry Institute for Mind Body Medicine at Massachusetts General Hospital, he coined the term "the Relaxation Response" to refer to a physical state of deep rest that changes the physical and emotional responses to stress. And it's all based on deep breathing and calming the mind.

Benson was able to show time and again that the relaxation response decreases the heart rate, lowers blood pressure, slows the rate of breathing, and relaxes the muscles. It also increases levels of nitric oxide—a molecule that's important for circulation and improved blood flow. Tai chi, meditation, yoga, and mindfulness are all able to elicit the relaxation response.

According to the Benson-Henry Institute, between 60 and 90 percent of all doctor visits are for complaints related to, or affected by, stress. "Scores of diseases and conditions are either caused or made worse by stress," Benson has said. "These include anxiety, mild or moderate depression, anger, hostility, hot flashes of menopause, infertility, PMS, high blood pressure, and heart attacks. Every one can be caused by stress or exacerbated by it. And to the extent that that's the case, the relaxation response is helpful."[3]

HOW CRYING AND LAUGHING CAN HELP

Next to love, crying is perhaps the most healing activity for the heart. It frees the heart of muscular tension and rigidity. Sobbing enhances oxygen delivery. Man is the only primate able to weep for emotional reasons. Weeping is nature's way of releasing the pain of heartbreak and preventing death. Any expression of feeling will help to heal your heart. Despite what we're taught, it's not weak to show your feelings. In fact, it's far healthier than "stuffing" your feelings and seething silently.

Laughing is a way of experiencing strong feelings, just as crying is. (In fact, strenuous laughter often turns into tears.) When you laugh fully, breathing increases, freeing up the rigidity in the chest, diaphragm, and even deep down in the psoas muscles. As a spontaneous release of energy, laughter has the

HOW TO DO "THE RELAXATION RESPONSE"

Allow ten to twenty minutes to try this simple technique:

- Sit quietly in a comfortable position.
- Close your eyes.
- Deeply relax all your muscles beginning at your feet and progressing up to your face. Keep them relaxed.
- Breathe through your nose. Become aware of your breathing. As you breathe out, say the word "one" silently to yourself. For example, breathe in...out, ("one"), in...out ("one"), etc. Breathe easily and naturally.
- Continue for ten to twenty minutes.
- You may open your eyes to check the time, but don't use an alarm. When you finish, sit quietly for several minutes at first with your eyes closed and later with your eyes open. Don't stand for a few minutes.

"Don't worry about whether you are successful in achieving a deep level of relaxation. Maintain a passive attitude and permit relaxation to occur at its own pace. When distracting thoughts occur, try to ignore them by not dwelling upon them and return to repeating one."
    –From *The Relaxation Response* by Herbert Benson, M.D., used with permission

NOTE: Try not to do this within a couple hours of eating. According to Benson, the digestive process seems to interfere with eliciting the relaxation response.

potential to be extremely therapeutic.

Laughing Your Way to Health

Over the course of his lifetime, Norman Cousins, the legendary journalist and editor of the *Saturday Evening Post*, suffered from a number of serious medical conditions, including heart disease and ankylosing spondylitis, a disease characterized by chronic inflammation along the axial skeleton. At one point, doctors gave him little hope of surviving. He ignored their doomsaying and developed his own program for recovery that involved love, hope, faith, and, courtesy of the Marx Brothers films he loved to watch, an awful lot of laughter.

Although he eventually died of heart failure at age seventy-five, Cousins lived far longer than his doctors predicted, a full thirty-six years after first being diagnosed with heart disease. (Cousins also did research on the biochemistry of human emotions at the School of Medicine at the University of California, Los Angeles, and wrote two important books on emotion, healing, and illness–*Anatomy of an Illness* and *The Healing Heart*.)

SEX: THE ADVANTAGES OF INTIMACY

Have you ever wondered why some elderly people look much younger than their stated age while some younger people look so much older? This observation was studied by a Russian gerontologist who examined 15,000 individuals over the age of eighty in provinces of the former Soviet Union. He found several common denominators or markers for longevity. People who lived the longest reported working outdoors, high levels of physical activity, and a diet high in vegetables, fruits, and fresh whole grains. But several of the common denominators involved relationships, intimacy, and sexuality.

Many of these individuals continued to have an active sex life well into their eighties and nineties. And why not? Aging couples who are committed to one another's pleasure can adapt sexually to the aging process. On an emotional level, sexuality provides a sense of security, connectedness, and emotional intimacy. When sexuality is an expression of love, the energies of the partners can fuse in harmony like two tuning forks vibrating with the same frequency. Feelings of warmth, connectedness, and emotional intimacy can help open our hearts.

EXPRESSING EMOTIONS (ESPECIALLY FOR MEN!)

Showing and expressing feelings can be a huge challenge for some people, particularly men. But getting in touch with your feelings doesn't have to be embarrassing at all. You don't have to get up in front of some encounter group and spill your guts to strangers. All it may take is a pencil and paper.

A writing exercise developed by social psychologist James Pennebaker has been tested in dozens of studies in which subjects were assigned to write about either mundane activities, such as running errands, or personal traumas. The technique is pure simplicity. You write your deepest thoughts and emotions about any event, situation, person, or even trauma for about fifteen minutes on four consecutive nights. Pennebaker has found that people who do this simple, private exercise show improvements in immune system functioning, are less likely to visit doctors, get better grades in school, and miss fewer days of work.[4]

THE POWER OF TOUCH AND MASSAGE

Touch therapy or massage appears to be associated with a decreased heart rate, decreased blood pressure, and increased endorphin release, resulting in an increased sense of relaxation and heightened well-being. In humans, massage can be considered a tranquilizer with absolutely no side effects!

Massage activates the parasympathetic system and provides a nice, healing balance to the typical sympathetic overdrive experienced by type-A, coronary-prone individuals.

PLAY

Play is one of the most healing things you can do for your heart health and your emotional well-being. And most adults have no idea how to do it. Sure, we talk about "playing" tennis or golf, but sports are different—though enjoyable, they're not healing because they involve performance, competition, and the need to win! (Just ask Dr. Jonny how he feels after losing a tennis match!)

Play is totally different. True play is spontaneous and has no agenda, rules, or regulations, or even a desired outcome. When we play, we are totally free. That is, we do things solely for joy and pleasure. When we play, we become totally absorbed in what we are doing; we are taken out of our heads (and down into our bodies).

Time stops for us.

Think of how completely absorbed five- or six-year-olds become when they're painting a picture. Within minutes, nothing else matters to them but the colors, the feel of the brush on the paper, the way the paint drips and blobs and runs, the way the colors mix, and how closely they can match the picture with the image in their minds. Being carried away by their imaginations and getting their inspirations down on paper is, for a short time, the single most important thing in the world to them. Everything else falls away—worries, fears, wants, needs, hunger—and is replaced by a sense of total involvement, excitement, satisfaction, and gratification.

If you can play even partially this way, it can completely cut you free from stress and worry and help heal your mind and heart. Because of this nearly miraculous benefit of play, we encourage you to play like children. If, like most adults, you've forgotten how, observe children and see what they do.

Remember, play has no outcome, no goal. You need to play for play's sake alone, and, when you play, try to bring out the little child inside you. Once you connect with your inner child—believe us, we all have one—it will bring you to another level of healing.

HEARTMATH™

And speaking of another level of healing . . . Bringing the heart and brain into balance—also called coherence—is an effective way to reduce stress, improve overall health (including heart health), and foster well-being. HeartMath offers an easy-to-do technique to accomplish this.

Coherence—a term used in fields as diverse as quantum physics and social science—always implies a harmonious relationship between part of a system.[5] In the case of HeartMath, it refers to a harmonious relationship between the heart and the brain.

The Institute of HeartMath—a non-profit organization dedicated to researching the principle that the heart and the brain are deeply connected—is where much of the research on heart-brain coherence originated.[6] The Institute was founded on the premise that the heart has a natural intelligence of its own. Intuitively, we all understand this. Just consider how we speak about the heart—"I knew it in my heart!" is just one of countless examples. We seem to "know" that the heart has something to tell us, but HeartMath goes a bit further and puts that knowledge to practical use.

You see, according to the founders of HeartMath, the heart isn't just a detached organ whose job it is to beat regularly like a metronome, passively responding to signals from the central nervous system. It actually has its own responses to events—which is what the HeartMath folks mean when they refer to the heart's native "intelligence." The way the heart communicates those responses back out to the rest of the body is by varying its rhythms. (Those rhythms—known as heart rate variability or HRV—can actually be measured. You can see the results on an app called Inner Balance—more on that in a minute.) The variations in heart rhythm are the equivalent of a kind of Morse code for the rest of the body, and those varying rhythms of the heart actually impact your physiology, in a kind of endless feedback loop.

Remember when we talked earlier about psychoneuroimmunology, the study of how our thoughts affect the rest of our body? Well this is similar, only it's the study of how the heart's "thoughts"—expressed through variable rhythms—also affect the rest of our body!

According to Rollin McCraty, Ph.D., director of research at HeartMath Institute, the heart sends more information to the brain and the CNS than the other way around.[7] The brain is always interpreting these signals from the heart to create how we feel. And the quality of the informational signals sent from the heart to the brain have profound effects on brain function—mental clarity, emotional experience—as well as on physical health. The idea is that if you shift the rhythms of the heart—which you can do using the Inner Balance app as a biofeedback tool—you can quickly improve brain function, not to mention overall physical health.

The overall purpose of HeartMath technology is to bring the rhythms of the heart into balance with what's going on in your brain. Which goes a long way toward reducing stress and all the associated health problems that are aggravated or caused by it.

The Inner Balance app—available for both IOS and Android and downloadable wherever you get your apps—works with a little device* that clips onto your ear and lets you monitor your own heart rate variability in real time, so you can see instantly what it's doing and whether or not it's congruent with what you're "thinking" or focused on. If, for example, you focus on a word like appreciation or gratitude, but your heart rate variability is in the red zone, your heart and brain are not "thinking" the same thing. On the other hand, if you focus on appreciation or gratitude and your heart rate variability is in the green zone, you are in convergence. Congrats!

* The app is free but there is a charge for the device. Full disclosure: Jonny is a regular user of the Inner Balance app and personally thinks the cost is worth it.

When you are in convergence—when the heart and brain are on the same metaphorical page—good stuff happens. Remember that appreciation and gratitude are incompatible with anger and stress. (That's why people say to take a deep breath when you're angry! Deep breathing and anger aren't good bedmates!) One of the goals of a HeartMath practice is to be able to focus on things like gratitude, love, appreciation, service, peace, and joy—and to know that your heart will respond in kind, with all the health benefits that accrue with that. Since both of us fully subscribe to the notion that heart, brain, mind, spirit, and physical health are all interconnected, we included HeartMath as an option for accessing that interconnectedness—and using it to improve your overall health. At the very least, the app helps you get in touch with your own body and what it's doing—and that kind of mindfulness is always a positive thing.

FINAL WORDS

Foods can fuel your heart, supplements can support it, and exercise can strengthen it. But never neglect the "hidden" emotional and psychological risk factors that contribute to the development of heart disease as surely as smoking, a high-sugar diet, stress, high blood pressure, and lack of exercise do.

Building and maintaining strong emotional connections with other people is one of the best stress-management strategies on the planet. It's also one of the best ways to keep your heart healthy and your soul nourished. Next to exercise, it's the closest thing we have to a panacea. It also makes life a lot more rich, a lot more fun, and a lot more gratifying.

Enjoy the journey.

APPENDIX A

The ALLHAT Study: Not a Single Life Was Saved

The Antihypertensive and Lipid-Lowering Treatment to Prevent Heart Attack Trial (ALLHAT), conducted between 1994 and 2002, was the largest North American cholesterol study ever undertaken, and as of 2002, it was the largest study ever done using the statin drug pravastatin (brand name Pravachol). Ten thousand participants with high LDL cholesterol levels were divided into two groups. One group was treated with pravastatin, and the other group was simply given the standard advice on "lifestyle changes."

Twenty-eight percent of the pravastatin takers did lower their cholesterol by a small but statistically significant amount (compared to 11 percent who did so in the "lifestyle change" group). This allowed the pravastatin folks to trumpet a significant reduction in cholesterol and declare the trial a success.

Not so fast.

When the death rates from heart attack were examined, there was no difference between the two groups. The statin drug lowered cholesterol in 28 percent of the people taking it, but not a single life was saved. Pravastatin neither significantly reduced "all-cause" mortality (death from any reason whatsoever), nor reduced fatal or nonfatal coronary heart disease in the patients who took it.[1]

The ASCOT-LLA Trial: Not Exactly a Slam Dunk for Lipitor

The Anglo-Scandinavian Cardiac Outcomes Trial-Lipid Lowering Arm (ASCOT-LLA) was a multicenter randomized controlled trial in which more than ten thousand patients with high blood pressure and at least three other cardiovascular risk factors were assigned to one of two groups. Half were given atorvastatin (aka Lipitor), and half were given a placebo (an inactive substance in a pill form). Remember, too, that all patients in this study were hypertensive. Most were overweight (average BMI 28.6), 81 percent were male, and about a third were smokers. And importantly, because it makes this study pretty unique for its time, all the participants had either average or *lower* than average cholesterol—in contrast to the vast majority of statin studies that test their drug on folks with high cholesterol.[2]

First, the good news—at least as far as Lipitor's stockholders were concerned: After a mean follow-up time of 3.3 years, those taking Lipitor appeared to benefit. No doubt about it. Risk of heart disease dropped by 36 percent, and on the whole, fatal and nonfatal strokes, total cardiovascular events, and total coronary events were significantly lowered between 21 and 29 percent. Although the study was supposed to span five years, it was terminated early—ostensibly because the Lipitor group was outperforming the placebo group with such fanfare.

Of course, as we've pointed out, all these results may be because of the many other things statin drugs do besides lower cholesterol. And the folks in this study certainly had risk factors (e.g., being overweight and having high blood pressure), so any one of the positive effects of statin drugs—such as its antioxidant, blood-thinning, or anti-inflammatory qualities—could easily have made a difference. (This is particularly likely given that the participants didn't have any cholesterol-lowering needs to begin with!)

Nonetheless, with all those cardiovascular disease reductions, it sure *looks* like a slam dunk for Lipitor, doesn't it?

Not so fast. Here's where the story takes a turn for the ugly.

For one, the fine print: After three years, there was no statistical difference in the number of deaths between the two groups. (In fact, there were actually a few more deaths among the women taking Lipitor than among the women taking the placebo.) So approximately $100 million was spent, and not a single life was saved.

Secondly, a closer examination of the study's findings revealed some serious cracks in the "three cheers for Lipitor" story. Here's why. When ASCOT-LLA's findings were published in 2003 in the *Lancet*, its authors gave the drug an unsurprising thumbs up, stating that "The reductions in major cardiovascular events with atorvastatin are large, given the short follow-up time." (We say "unsurprising," because all fourteen of those authors served as consultants to—and received travel expenses, speaking fees, or research funding from—pharmaceutical companies

marketing cholesterol-lowering drugs. That fact alone doesn't make the results invalid, but it certainly plants a potential bias among the folks who ran the study.)

In response to the ASCOT-LLA paper, though, a number of other researchers—especially ones who *weren't* on any statin company's payroll—submitted commentary that was far less flattering. In one response published in the *Lancet*, Uffe Ravnskov pointed out that in the Lipitor group, there was a higher (albeit not quite statistically significant) rate of heart failure, diabetes, and kidney impairment compared to the placebo—and what's more, that the study's early termination made it hard to assess the possible effects of Lipitor on cancer rates.[3] Dirk Devroey and Leslie Vander Ginst likewise wrote that they "dispute the conclusions" of the ASCOT-LLA's authors, noting that the benefits of Lipitor weren't significant in patients aged sixty or younger, in those with diabetes, in those with left-ventricular hypertrophy, in those with previous vascular disease, and in those without renal dysfunction. Likewise—and we quote—"Among women, placebo even had nonsignificantly better results than atorvastatin."[4]

In another reply, physician Peter Trewby highlighted the low level of absolute benefit for Lipitor takers—stating "It is not the significance . . . of the reduction in relative risk that causes us concern, but whether the reduction in absolute risk with atorvastatin is sufficient for patients to take another drug for the rest of their lives from which they have under 1% chance per year of benefiting."[5]

Speaking of relative versus absolute risk, let's dive in to our third and final point: that "36% reduction in heart disease risk" wasn't actually all that impressive once we take off the reality-distorting "relative risk" goggles. Among the Lipitor group, 1.9 percent of the study subjects experienced fatal heart disease or a non-fatal heart attack, compared to 3 percent of the placebo group. That's an absolute difference of only *1.1 percent*—the number Trewby deftly cited.

So, slam dunk for Lipitor? More like an air ball.

The Heart Protection Study: Pretty Weak Protection

The Heart Protection Study (HPS) divided more than twenty thousand adults with either coronary artery disease or diabetes into two groups and gave one group 40 mg of the statin Zocor daily while the other group received a placebo.[6] It was claimed that "massive benefits" were obtained by lowering cholesterol with the statin drug, and indeed fewer people died in the Zocor group than in the placebo group.

But let's look at the absolute numbers. Those in the Zocor group had an 87.1 percent survival rate after five years, but those in the placebo group had an 85.4 percent survival rate, an absolute difference of 1.8 percent. Most important, the survival rates were independent of lowering cholesterol. In other words, lowering LDL levels made essentially no difference in the risk of death from heart disease. (This is not difficult to understand when you factor in the other things statins do besides lower cholesterol. If anything, it simply shows that statin drugs may be useful in certain populations, but if they are, it's independent of their ability to lower cholesterol. In fact, it increasingly looks like lowering cholesterol may be the least significant thing statins do.)

As Uffe Ravnskov, M.D., Ph.D., stated in a letter to the editor of the *British Medical Journal* regarding the Heart Protection Study results, "Tell a patient that his chance not to die in five years without statin treatment is 85.4 percent and that [statin] treatment can increase this to 87.1 percent. With these figures in hand I doubt that anyone should accept a treatment whose long-term effects are unknown."[7]

Japanese Lipid Intervention Trial: No Relationship between LDL and Dying

In this trial, more than forty-seven thousand patients received Zocor over the course of six years. There was quite a variety in their response to this treatment. Some folks saw dramatic lowering of their LDL levels, some saw a moderate fall in their levels, and some experienced essentially no reduction in their levels.

After five years, the researchers examined the death rate among the participants and cross-referenced these deaths with the patients' LDL levels. You'd think this would be the perfect study to demonstrate a correlation between lower LDL levels and a decreased risk for heart disease, right? Clearly, those whose LDL levels had dropped dramatically would have been far more likely to live, while those whose cholesterol levels had not dropped at all would have been far more likely to die, and those who had lowered their cholesterol only a modest amount would have fallen somewhere in between.

We're sure that's what the researchers expected to see.

But they didn't.

After five years there was exactly no correlation

between LDL levels and death rate in the three groups. In other words, whether your cholesterol had been lowered or not had no correlation to whether or not you died. Patients with the highest levels of LDL died at pretty much the exact same rate as patients with the lowest LDL levels (and as patients with LDL levels in between the highest and the lowest). Bottom line: Lowering LDL levels didn't give you even a drop of protection against dying.

LRC-CPPT: Escape Heart Disease So You Can Die from Something Else (And Some More Fuzzy Math, While We're At It)?

The Lipid Research Clinics Coronary Primary Prevention Trial (LRC-CPPT), published in 1984, is an interesting case—one that takes a little digging to see where we've been duped. In this study, researchers put 3,800 middle-aged men with very high cholesterol on either a cholestyramine resin (which lowers cholesterol by binding to bile acids) or a placebo, with both groups also following a moderate cholesterol-lowering diet.[8] After an average of 7.4 years, the cholestyramine drug group slashed their total and LDL cholesterol compared to the placebo—an 8.5 percent greater reduction in total cholesterol and 12.6 percent greater reduction in LDL, to be exact. More importantly, the cholestyramine group reduced their rate of death from heart disease by 24 percent and their rate of nonfatal heart attacks by 19 percent.

It wouldn't be an exaggeration to call this study groundbreaking: It was the first trial that actually showed people could cut their risk of dying from heart disease by lowering their cholesterol.

The problem? This rosy picture changes when we look at what happened with *total* mortality—or rather, what didn't happen. By the end of the study, there was no significant difference—nada, zilch, goose egg—in total deaths between the cholestyramine group versus the placebo group. Despite lowering their cholesterol and dying less from heart disease, the cholestyramine group just ended up dying *more* from other things—making their total mortality a wash.

Not exactly a reason to whip out the bubbly, right?

And that's not all. LRC-CPPT is another shining example of how *relative risk* can fool us into thinking a study's findings are more dramatic than they really are. When we put that "24 percent reduction in heart disease death" into absolute terms, the whole house of cards falls apart: The cholestyramine group's rate of heart disease death was 1.6 percent, while the placebo group had a microscopically higher rate of 2 percent—a difference of only 0.4 percent.

And the number of participants driving that difference? A mere eight men out of 3,800.

In other words, another study for the slush pile.

PROSPER: Some Benefits, but Only for Certain People

The Prospective Study of Pravastatin in the Elderly at Risk (PROSPER) was interesting for a number of reasons. In this study, older patients were divided into two groups. The first group consisted of patients with no history of heart disease (primary prevention group), and the second group consisted of patients with current or past cardiovascular disease (secondary prevention group). Half of each group received Pravachol (a statin drug), while the other half received a placebo.

There was some reduction in heart attacks or strokes, but only in the secondary prevention group (those who had current heart disease or a history of heart disease). There was, however, no reduction in heart attacks or strokes in the primary prevention group, the group that had no history of heart disease to begin with. This is pretty much in keeping with the findings of the vast majority of other studies.

But there were two other interesting findings, one of them quite troubling.

When pharmaceutical reps spin the data from the PROSPER study, they concentrate on the single fact that Pravachol reduced heart attacks and strokes (while downplaying the fact that it did so only in the group that already had heart disease). Okay, that's good; the prevention of a few heart attacks and strokes, even in a limited population, is always nice. But what about other measures of health, disease, and well-being besides heart attacks and strokes?

To answer this question, researchers decided to look at other measures of total health impact. They looked at "total deaths" and "total serious adverse events" and found that both were completely unchanged by Pravachol. Once again, a statin drug had a beneficial effect on heart attacks and strokes in the secondary prevention population but not in the primary prevention population, and once again, not a single life was saved overall.

The second finding was more troubling. Both groups receiving Pravachol had an increased risk of cancer. Amazingly, the investigators simply dismissed this statistically significant finding as "the play of chance."

The JUPITER Trial: "Flawed"

We saved this one for last, because it's the juiciest, most perfect example of utter cholesterol madness, media hype, behind-the-scenes manipulation, and intellectual dishonesty.

If you read the papers or watched the news in 2009, you probably heard about this study, though you may not have known what it was called. Its name—JUPITER—stands for the Justification for the Use of Statins in Primary Prevention: An Intervention Trial Evaluating Rosuvastatin. (Even the title of the study should give you pause; you don't do a study to justify the use of a drug you've already decided to use. What if the results of the study indicated the opposite? An objective scientific study wouldn't know the results in advance.)

Anyway, on to the study, about which there's much to dislike and critique—for example, everything.

The JUPITER trial looked at nearly 18,000 people whose cholesterol was perfectly normal or even on the low side. What these folks did have, however, were elevated levels of C-reactive protein (CRP). As we've said, CRP is a general measure of inflammation, and for the record, it's a measure we consider important. (You'll read more about CRP testing in appendix B.) Now it's abundantly clear that what the manufacturers of the drug were aiming for here was a demonstration that statin drugs help prevent deaths even in people with normal cholesterol!

So here's the party line on the JUPITER trial, the line that was robotically repeated in virtually every news outlet in America: The JUPITER trial was such a resounding success that they had to stop it early because it would be "unethical" to continue, given that the group being treated with the drug (Crestor) experienced half as many deaths, strokes, and heart attacks as the control (untreated) group.

The JUPITER trial was touted everywhere as proof that the cholesterol guidelines needed to be changed. Clearly, the drug manufacturers argued, people who met or exceeded the existing standards for cholesterol were demonstrably helped by lowering their "normal" cholesterol even further, virtually cutting their risk for all kinds of terrible things in half! Obviously, they argued to anyone who would listen, we need to make the recommended "normal" levels even lower! (Can you imagine the cheers that would erupt at stockholders' meetings if your product just expanded its market by roughly 11 million people?[9] Why that's almost as good as expanding an adult market by targeting children! Oh, that's right. Ever since 2011, that's exactly what the statin lobbyists were doing. Never mind.)*

Well that was then. This is now.

Nine respected authors, including a Harvard Medical School faculty member, teamed up to write a critical reappraisal of the JUPITER trial, a reappraisal that was published in 2010 in *Archives of Internal Medicine*, one of the most respected, and conservative, medical journals in the world.[10] "The trial was flawed," they wrote. "It was discontinued (according to pre-specified rules) after fewer than two years of follow-up, with no differences between the two groups on the most objective criteria." The authors also said, "The possibility that bias entered the trial

is particularly concerning because of the strong commercial interest in the study." They concluded that "[t]he results of the trial do not support the use of statin treatment for primary prevention of cardiovascular diseases."

So how did this study manage to garner headlines like this one: "Heart Attack Risk Lowered More Than 50 Percent by Taking Crestor!"?

Let's take a look.

The JUPITER trial took 17,800 people—men over sixty, women over fifty—and put them into two groups. One group received 20 mg of Crestor daily, while the other group received a placebo.

Now before we tell you the results, let's recall the distinction between relative versus absolute numbers, a distinction we talked about earlier.

The study went on for 1.9 years, and at the end of that time it was determined that the risk of having a heart attack in the placebo group was 1.8 percent, while the risk of having a heart attack in the Crestor group was 0.9 percent.

So, yes, there was a 50 percent reduction in risk! Relatively speaking. But let's do the math on the number that really matters, the absolute risk.

The placebo group had a 1.8 percent risk, and the Crestor group had a 0.9 percent risk, so the absolute, real reduction in risk was 1.8 minus 0.9, or 0.9 percent. In absolute numbers, this means that if you took a group of 100 untreated people, 1.8 of them would have a heart attack at some point over the course of almost two years. If you took that same group of 100 people and treated them all with Crestor for the same period, 0.9 of them would have a heart attack. Researchers calculate that this translates into 120

* When the results of JUPITER came out, the stock of AstraZeneca—the company that makes Crestor—shot up by double digits.

people needing treatment for 1.9 years in order to prevent one event. At a cost of well over a quarter of a million dollars for almost two years' worth of Crestor, that's an awful lot to spend to prevent one event. Especially when there's a significant chance of experiencing really bad side effects from the medicine that's costing you a fortune.

Commenting on the JUPITER study in the *New England Journal of Medicine* in November 2008, Mark A. Hlatky, M.D., wrote: "[A]bsolute differences in risk are more clinically important than relative reductions in risk in deciding whether to recommend drug ther-apy, since the absolute benefits of treatment must be large enough to justify the associated risks and costs." He added that "[l]ong-term safety is clearly important in considering committing low-risk subjects without clinical disease to twenty years or more of drug treatment."[11]

Did we mention that there was a significantly higher incidence of diabetes in the group treated with Crestor?[12] (In her studies on statin side effects, Stephanie Seneff also observed a highly significant correlation—p = 0.006—between mentions of diabetes and statin drug side effect reports.)

APPENDIX B

BEYOND CHOLESTEROL TESTING: WHAT TESTS SHOULD I GET?

We hope by now you're convinced that total cholesterol is a meaningless number and should be the basis for absolutely nothing in your treatment plan. The old division into "good" (HDL) cholesterol and "bad" (LDL) cholesterol is out of date and provides only marginally better information than a "total" cholesterol reading.

As we've said, both good and bad cholesterol have a number of different components (or subtypes) that behave quite differently, and the twenty-first-century version of a cholesterol test should always tell you exactly which subtypes you have and, most important, your total number of particles. Anything less than this up-to-date test—sometimes called the NMR particle test or the NMR Lipo-Profile panel—is not particularly useful and should never be the sole basis on which a treatment plan or a statin drug is recommended.

PARTICLE SIZE TEST (THE NMR LIPO-PROFILE TEST)

Although LDL cholesterol is known as the "bad" cholesterol, the fact is that it comes in several shapes and sizes, as does HDL cholesterol, the so-called "good" kind. These different subtypes of cholesterol behave very differently. Seen under a microscope, some LDL particles are big, fluffy, and much less likely to do any damage. Some are small, dense, "angry," and much more likely to become oxidized and inflamed, slipping through the cells that line the walls of the arteries (the endothelium) and beginning the inflammatory cascade that leads to heart disease.

Tests are now available that measure LDL particle size and total particle number, and that's the information you really want to have. If you have a pattern A cholesterol profile, most of your LDL cholesterol is the big, fluffy kind; but if you have a pattern B profile, most of your LDL cholesterol is composed of the small, dense, atherogenic particles that cause inflammation and ultimately plaque. (Pattern B is much more likely to be associated with insulin resistance and metabolic syndrome.)[1] (Fortunately, you can change the distribution from small to buoyant by following the dietary and supplement recommendations in this book.)

The LDL particle test is available through a number of labs. One of the best-known and most established particle tests is known as the NMR Lipo-Profile. Taking a statin drug, or any other medication, based solely on the standard cholesterol test is a really bad idea. Ask your doctor for one of the newer particle tests. If he objects, make sure he has a darn good reason. It's the only cholesterol test that matters.

C-REACTIVE PROTEIN (CRP)

CRP is a marker for inflammation that is directly associated with overall heart and cardiovascular health. In multiple studies, CRP has been identified as a potent predictor of future cardiovascular health—and, in our opinion, one that is far more reliable than elevated cholesterol levels. Biological characteristics that are associated with high CRP levels include infections, high blood sugar, excess weight, and hypercoagulability of blood (sticky blood).

Fortunately, there is a simple test that your doctor can conduct to find out how much CRP is in your blood. Just make sure the high-sensitivity test **(hs-CRP)** is used. This test doesn't take much time: Typically, blood is drawn from a vein located either on your forearm or on the inside of your elbow. The blood is then analyzed in several tests to determine the level of CRP present. (Dr. Sinatra's recommendation for an optimal CRP level is less than 0.8 mg/dL.)

FIBRINOGEN

Fibrinogen is a protein that determines the stickiness of your blood by enabling your platelets to stick together. You need adequate fibrinogen levels to stop bleeding when you've been injured, but you also want to balance your fibrinogen levels to support optimal blood circulation and prevent unnecessary clotting. (In women younger than forty-five, Dr. Sinatra has seen far more heart attacks caused by improper blood clotting than by anything else.) Normal levels

are between 200 and 400 mg/dL, and they may be elevated during any kind of inflammation.

Fibrinogen has been identified as an independent risk factor for cardiovascular disease and is associated with the traditional risk factors as well. In one study, fibrinogen levels were significantly higher among subjects with cardiovascular disease than among those without it.[2]

If you have a family history of heart concerns, you must check your serum fibrinogen level. Women who smoke, take oral contraceptives, or are post-menopausal usually have higher fibrinogen levels.

Worth noting: This test hasn't caught on with many doctors because there are no direct treatments for elevated levels. But supplements such as nattokinase, discussed in chapter 11 on supplements, can work well to "thin" the blood and prevent unwanted clotting. Adding omega-3 fatty acids to your diet may also help.

SERUM FERRITIN

Ever wonder why so many vitamin manufacturers offer multiple vitamins "without iron"? Here's why: Iron is one of those weird substances where if you don't have enough you can have some real problems (e.g., iron-deficiency anemia), but if you have too much, look out! Iron is highly susceptible to oxidation. (Imagine someone leaving a barbell from your gym outside in the rain for a couple of days. It's going to rust like crazy. That's oxidation.)

Iron levels in the body are cumulative (stored in the muscles and other tissues), and unless iron is lost through menstruation or by donating blood, over the years toxic levels can build up in the system. Although this danger always exists for men, it becomes a real risk for women after menopause. Both of us are adamant that no one but premenopausal women should ever take vitamins with iron, or supplemental iron of any kind, unless prescribed by a health practitioner.

Iron overload—technically called *hemochromatosis*—can actually contribute to heart disease. Researchers measure iron in the blood by measuring a form of it called *ferritin*. A 1992 study by Finnish researchers examined the role of iron in coronary artery disease. After studying 1,900 Finnish men between the ages of forty-two and sixty for five years, the researchers found that men with excessive levels of ferritin had an elevated risk of heart attack, and that every 1 percent increase in ferritin translated into a 4 percent increase in heart attack risk.[3]

Those with high levels of ferritin were more than twice as likely to have heart attacks than those with lower levels. The authors of this study concluded that ferritin levels may be an even stronger risk factor for heart disease than high blood pressure or diabetes is.[4] It's certainly a more important risk factor than high cholesterol.

If your ferritin levels are high, consider donating blood every so often, or ask your doctor to consider a therapeutic phlebotomy. (Dr. Sinatra's recommendation for an optimal serum ferritin level is less than 80 mg/L for women and less than 90 mg/L for men.)

Worth noting: One consideration regarding supplemental vitamin C is that it helps the body absorb iron better. If you have a problem with iron levels, keep your supplemental vitamin C to less than 100 mg a day.

LP(A)

Lp(a) is a type of cholesterol-carrying molecule that contains one LDL (low-density lipoprotein) molecule chemically bound to an attachment protein called *apolipoprotein(a)*. In a healthy body, Lp(a) isn't much of a problem. It circulates and carries out repair and restoration work on damaged blood vessels. The protein part of it promotes blood clotting. So far, so good.

The problem is, the more repair you need on your arteries, the more Lp(a) is utilized, and that's when things get ugly. Lp(a) concentrates at the site of damage, binds with a couple of amino acids within the wall of a damaged blood vessel, dumps its LDL cargo, and starts to promote the deposition of oxidized LDL into the wall, leading to more inflammation and ultimately to plaque.

Also, Lp(a) promotes the formation of blood clots on top of the newly formed plaque, which narrows the blood vessels further. If the clots are large enough, they can block an artery. (Most heart attacks are due to either a large clot developing in vessels with moderate-to-severe narrowing or a plaque rupture that blocks the artery.)

Elevated Lp(a) is a very serious risk factor. A very high percentage of heart attacks happen to people with high Lp(a) levels. Dr. Sinatra thinks Lp(a) is one of the most devastating risk factors for heart disease and one of the hardest to treat.

One reason doctors aren't running out to test for Lp(a) all the time is that there are no real pharmaceutical interventions that work to lower it. In addition, Lp(a) levels are largely genetically determined and not very modifiable by lifestyle choices.

However, your Lp(a) level can give you a good idea of your real risk for heart disease, and a high level may serve as a wake-up call to inspire you to work harder to improve your heart health using the strategies, foods, supplements, and lifestyle changes suggested in this book. That said, Dr. Sinatra feels that Lp(a) can be lowered with a combination of 1 to 2 g of fish oil, 500 to 2,500 mg of niacin (not the slow-release kind), and 20 mg of lumbrokinase.

Worth noting: Statin drugs can sometimes raise Lp(a) levels! This is mentioned on the warning labels of statin drug ads in the Canadian edition of the *New England Journal of Medicine*, but such labeling is not required by the Food and Drug Administration, so you won't see it in ads published in the United States.[5]

HOMOCYSTEINE

Homocysteine is an amino acid by-product that causes your body to lay down sticky platelets in blood vessels. Having some homocysteine is normal, but an excess might affect your cardiovascular health. Evidence shows that homocysteine contributes to atherosclerosis, reduces the flexibility of blood vessels, and helps make platelets stickier, thus slowing blood flow. Net result: There's a direct correlation between high homocysteine levels and an increased risk of heart disease and stroke.

Elevated homocysteine strongly predicts both a first and a recurring cardiovascular incident (including death).[6] Too much homocysteine adversely affects the function of the endothelium, the all-important lining of the artery walls. It also increases oxidative damage and promotes inflammation and thrombosis—a regular evil trifecta for heart disease.[7] One study looked at

more than 3,000 patients with chronic heart disease and found that a subsequent coronary event was 2.5 times more likely in patients with elevated levels of homocysteine. What's more, each 5 ↔mol/L of homocysteine predicted a 25 percent increase in risk![8]

Fortunately, there's an easy way to bring down homocysteine levels. All you have to do is give the body the three main nutrients it needs to metabolize homocysteine back into harmless compounds. The three nutrients are folic acid, vitamin B_{12}, and vitamin B_6. All it takes is about 400 to 800 mcg of folic acid, 400 to 1,000 mcg of B_{12}, and 5 to 20 mg of B_6. If you've had a heart attack or other cardiovascular event; if you have a family history of early heart disease; or if you have hypothyroidism, lupus, or kidney disease, consider asking your doctor to test your homocysteine levels. Finally, if you take drugs that tend to elevate homocysteine—theophylline (for asthma), methotrexate (for cancer or arthritis), or L-dopa (for Parkinson's)—you should be tested. (Dr. Sinatra's recommendation for an optimal homocysteine level is between 7 and 9 μmol/L.)

INTERLEUKIN-6

Interleukin-6 is important because it stimulates the liver to produce CRP. And we are learning that this inflammatory cytokine has a strong association with not only heart disease but also asthma. (Asthma is the result of airways swelling and constricting, so it makes sense that an inflammatory agent is behind the curtains here as well.) The Iowa 65+ Rural Health Study demonstrated that elevated levels of interleukin-6 and CRP were associated with an increased risk for both cardiovascular disease and general mortality in healthy older people.

Interleukin-6 may be an even better marker for inflammation than CRP is because these "precursor" levels rise earlier. If you're concerned about inflammation and its effect on your heart, ask your doctor to do an interleukin-6 test. (Dr. Sinatra's recommendation for an optimal interleukin-6 level is 0.0 to 12.0 pg/mL.)

CORONARY CALCIUM SCAN

Calcium is great—as long as it stays in the bones and teeth. One place you don't want it is in the coronary arteries.

Coronary calcification is one of the major risk factors that predicts coronary heart disease and future heart attacks.[9] The more calcium present, the greater the risk of suffering a heart attack. Men develop calcifications about ten to fifteen years earlier than women do. Calcification can be detected in the majority of asymptomatic men over fifty-five years of age and in women over sixty-five.

As far back as 1991, cardiologist Stephen Seely, M.D., published a paper in the *International Journal of Cardiology* titled "Is Calcium Excess in the Western Diet a Major Cause of Arterial Disease?" He pointed out that cholesterol only makes up 3 percent of arterial plaque while calcium makes up 50 percent![10]

The Florida cardiologist Arthur Agatston, M.D., is best known for his wildly popular South Beach diet, but what many people don't know is that he also developed a widely accepted test for coronary calcification known as the **Agatston test**. Individuals who score less than 10 on the Agatston test have minimal calcification; those with Agatston scores of 11 to 99 have moderate calcification; those with scores of 100 to 400 have increased calcification; and those with scores above 400 have extensive calcification.

It is well established that individuals with Agatston scores above 400 have an increased occurrence of coronary procedures (bypass, stent placement, and angioplasty) and events (myocardial infarction and cardiac death) within the two to five years following the test. Individuals with very high Agatston scores (over 1,000) have a 20 percent chance of suffering a heart attack or cardiac death within a year. Even among patients over the age of seventy who frequently have calcification, an Agatston score above 400 was associated with a higher risk of death.[11]

The American Heart Association and the American College of Cardiology provide guidelines for coronary calcification testing, available online, www.ahajournals.org/misc/sci-stmts_topindex.shtml. These guidelines currently suggest—and we agree—that screening for calcification is of value for an individual who is considered to be at intermediate ten-year risk, which means that he or she has a 10 to 20 percent likelihood of experiencing a cardiac event within the next ten years.[12]

CARDIAC AND GENETIC MARKERS

In the years since the original edition of this book was published, genetic testing has gone mainstream. From 23 and Me to the most advanced genetic testing[13] it's now possible for the average person to get all kinds of cardiometabolic genetic profiles that weren't available even a decade ago. And the price is coming down. Quest Labs now offers an advanced lipid panel called the Cardio IQ as well as an advanced inflammatory markers test, and more cardiac genetic tests are just around the corner.

If you really want to dig beneath the surface, here are some of the tests that are getting traction with doctors and that are worth discussing with your physician.

Measuring Oxidative Damage: F2-isoprostanes (F2-IsoPs)

As you read in chapter 5, inflammation and oxidation are the twin towers of cellular destruction. And heart disease is, in large measure, an inflammatory disease. (Remember, oxidation and inflammation are like inseparable twins and are always found together.) Some of the things that trigger the oxidation/inflammation cascade include poor diet, smoking, and sedentary lifestyle. F2-isoPs are the by-products of that damage, the evidence that the oxidation/inflammation cascade leaves behind.

F2-isoprostanes are compounds that are formed from oxidation, specifically from the oxidation of arachidonic acid (an important omega-6 fat). You can think of F2-IsoPs as "by-products" of the "rusting" (oxidation) process. And they can be measured. The F2-IsoPs contribute to heart disease by, among other things, constricting the arteries and contributing to platelet aggregation (blood clotting).

Elevated levels of F2-IsoPs more than double the risk for coronary artery disease (making it 2.6x more likely). They almost double the risk for death—people with high levels are 1.8x more likely to die from cardiovascular disease than those with low levels.[14]

Measuring Inflammation and the Vulnerability of Plaque: Myeloperoxidase (MPO)

Myeloperoxidase is an inflammatory enzyme that gets released in the *lumen*, the "inner tube" of the artery. It gets released when white blood cells start going crazy and mount a counterattack in response to fissures, erosions, or degradation of the fibrous cap that protects the plaque. Measuring MPO gives us a specific marker of vascular inflammation. It's also a measure of how vulnerable your plaque is (and remember that plaque only does real damage to your heart when it ruptures, which begins with damage to the fibrous cap). Elevated levels of MPO independently predict 2.0-2.4x increased risk of future cardiovascular events such as a heart attack or CVD-related death.[15] One of the best treatments for elevated MPO is high-dose fish oil.

Oxidized LDL (oxLDL)

Oxidized LDL (oxLDL) is associated with a 4.3x increased risk of cardiovascular events. By anyone's standards, that's a pretty serious increase in risk.

Oxidized LDL—as you read in chapter 5—is cholesterol that has been damaged by oxidation. You'll recall that this is what initiates the problem in the first place, as a damaged LDL particle lodges itself inside the wall of the artery and begins the process of atherosclerosis. Prior to being attacked by free radicals and oxidized, LDL is simply going about its business in the bloodstream and not causing much mischief. But once it's oxidized, that's another story.

This test measures damage to the protein attachment on the surface of the LDL molecule. That protein is called Apo-B, and any damage that's done to it is due to oxidation. Oxidized LDL (or oxidation of ApoB) is one of the events that initiates the process of macrophage recruitment, the formation of foam cells from the dead macrophages, and the whole cycle of vascular inflammation inside the artery wall. Elevated OxLDL levels are associated with a 4.3x increased risk of having a CHD event[16] and a 3.5x increased risk of developing metabolic syndrome (see chapter 9, The *Real* Cause of Heart Disease).[17]

The Plaq™ Test (LP-PLA2): Measures How Likely Plaque Is to Rupture

As we explained in chapter 4, a fibrous cap eventually forms around plaque, kind of like a scab forms on a wound. Stable plaque may never cause a problem, but the when it ruptures, look out. Plaque "disruption" (rupture) is one of the primary causes of heart attacks and sudden death[18] and is significantly associated with stroke.[19]

Lp-PLA2 is considered a specific marker for vascular inflammation and for the vulnerability of plaque to rupturing. When the artery walls become inflamed, the plaque itself makes this enzyme—Lp-PLA2. High levels may indicate a likelihood that the plaque is likely to rupture through the inside of the lining of the artery wall and get into the bloodstream, leading to a dangerous clot. The result could be heart attack or stroke.

The presence of Lp-PLA2 indicates arterial inflammation and is a recognized risk factor for heart disease. Lp-PLA2 is now included in four major guidelines, including the American Heart Association and the American College of Cardiology.

The 9p21 Test: Measures Susceptibility to Inflammation

Although technically not a gene, 9p21 is an important genetic marker that can give you an idea of how resistant or susceptible you are to inflammation.

Our friend, Dr. Mansoor Mohammed, clinical genomicist at the YouTrients personalized nutrition company in Canada, explains the 9p21 genetic marker by using the example of a Teflon pan as a stand-in for your arteries.

Imagine that you're got three different versions of a Teflon pan. One is the super-deluxe model that has a double coating of Teflon. The second is an ordinary but effective Teflon pan with a nice clean, unmarred surface. And the third is pretty scratched up and has a bunch of nicks and crevices.

The 9p21 genetic marker tells you what version of the Teflon pan you have. If you have the "double Teflon" version of the 9p21, you have "reduced sensitivity" to inflammatory agents (such as cigarette smoke and sugar). You may be able to handle some inflammatory substances a little better than most. If you have the ordinary Teflon version of the pan, you've got "average sensitivity" to inflammation, and if you've got the *scratched* version of the pan, you have *increased* sensitivity to things that cause inflammatory responses and a 2x increased risk of an early myocardial infarction (a heart attack).

In our opinion, everyone should consume as much anti-inflammatory foods and supplements as possible, regardless of genes. (Just because you're a fast swimmer doesn't mean you shouldn't avoid sharks!) But for those who have the "bad" version of this genetic marker, avoidance of things like smoke, overconsumption of vegetable oils, and sugar becomes even more critical.[20]

THE KIF-6 TEST: ARE YOU A GOOD CANDIDATE FOR A STATIN?

The KIF-6 test is controversial, but we're including it here because there's a good chance your doctor may actually recommend it, and there's some good research[21] to justify such a recommendation. (Full disclosure: There is also research to suggest that KIF-6 is not a very good predictor of cardiovascular risk.[22]) And so far, KIF-6 is not yet part of the recommendations of any major health organization (like the AMA), though insurance payers have been generally willing to pay for it. It's considered "an emerging cardiac marker."

Here's the story: There's a gene called KIF-6 that, like all genes, has different variants. One of those variants dramatically increases the risk for coronary heart disease, even independent of other factors like age, gender, smoking, and diabetes. And about 60 percent of patients have this variant.

The KIF-6 genetic test will basically tell you two things: one, which variant of the gene you have, and two, whether you are likely to benefit from statin therapy.

(Since not everyone benefits from statins, and since at some point it's likely that your doctor may talk to you about them, knowing your likelihood of your benefiting would be good info to have.)

If the KIF-6 test were a stock, our recommendation would be "wait and hold." There may well be some benefit to this test, but there's likely to be a lot of benefit for statin manufacturers as well. That doesn't mean it can't be good for the rest of us, but it is something to think about.

And consider any of the genetic tests discussed earlier, which your doctor may feel will give even more specific detail with which to design a treatment plan.

ABOUT THE AUTHORS

JONNY BOWDEN, PH.D, C.N.S., IS A BOARD-CERTIFIED NUTRITIONIST, the author of fifteen books including *The 150 Healthiest Foods on Earth*, *Living Low Carb*, and *The Great Cholesterol Myth*, and the creator of the best-selling weight loss program, *The Metabolic Factor*. Popularly known as "the Nutrition Myth Buster™", his no-nonsense approach to medical and nutritional misinformation has made him a popular guest on television (*Dr. Oz*, *The Doctors*, ABC-TV, MSNBC-TV, CNN, CBS-TV, CBN, Fox News, NBC-TV, and virtually every morning show in America). Dr. Bowden is a popular speaker at conferences all over the world and has spoken at such venues as Beijing University, The American Academy of Anti-Aging medicine, Paleo f(x), and Low Carb USA. He has written or contributed to articles in *The New York Times*, *Forbes*, *The Daily Beast*, *The Huffington Post*, *Vanity Fair Online*, *Men's Heath*, *Prevention*, *Forbes Online*, *O (The Oprah Magazine)*, *Vanity Fair Online*, and dozens of other print and online publications. He appears in the 2020 documentary, *The Big Fat Lie* (narrated by Dr. Mark Hyman), available on Amazon and streaming services.
www.jonnybowden.com / @jonnybowden / Dr. Jonny Bowden on Facebook

STEPHEN SINATRA, M.D., F.A.C.C., F.A.C.N., C.N.S., C.B.T., IS A BOARD-CERTIFIED CARDIOLOGIST and assistant clinical professor of medicine at the University of Connecticut School of Medicine. He is the author of many books, including *The Sinatra Solution: Metabolic Cardiology*, *Earthing: The Most Important Health Discovery Ever*, *Reverse Heart Disease Now*, and *Lower Your Blood Pressure in Eight Weeks*. Certified as a bioenergetic psychotherapist and nutrition and anti-aging specialist, Dr. Sinatra integrates psychological, nutraceutical, and electroceutical therapies in the matrix of healing. He is the founder of www.heartmdinstitute.com, an informational website dedicated to promoting public awareness of integrative medicine. He is a fellow in the American College of Cardiology and the American College of Nutrition. He is also the editor of a national newsletter titled *Heart, Health and Nutrition*. His websites include www.heartmdinstitute.com and www.drsinatra.com.

ACKNOWLEDGMENTS

MY DEAREST FRIENDS: Anja Christy, Sky London, Doug Monas, Susan Wood, Christopher Duncan, Peter Breger, Scott Ellis, Oliver Beaucamp, Chris Crabb, Jeannette Bessinger, Randy Graff, Mike Danielson, and Lauree Dash. You give my life meaning. Thank you.

My literary agent of over fifteen years, Coleen O'Shea, who has been a beacon of sanity and a great source of guidance.

The team at Fairwinds Press, especially my publisher, Jill Alexander, who saw the need for a new edition and greenlighted the project, and to my brilliant editor, Jenna Nelson Patton.

The writers who inspire me: William Goldman, Ed McBain, Nora Ephron, Robert Sapolsky. And the musicians who do the same: Allen Stone, Laura Nyro, Miles Davis, and John Coltrane.

Denise Minger, for her invaluable contributions to this book. We are enormously grateful for your insights, humor, wisdom, and intelligence.

Robert Crayhon whose influence and presence continues to be felt by all of us who studied with him.

My beloved family: Cadence, Jared, Logan, Jeffrey, Nancy, and Pace.

The island and the people of our "second home," St. Martin, FWI.

The wonderful doctors, researchers, scholars, and advocates who shared their work with me for this book, especially David Diamond, Ph.D., Robert DuBroff, M.D., and Jim Greenfield, M.D. and his team at Specialty Health in Nevada. And for all the giants—i.e., Uffe Ravnskov, M.D., Ph.D., Malcolm Kendrick, M.D., Anthony Colpo, and Michel de Lorgeril, M.D.,—on whose shoulders we stand.

And to my beloved Mischa—the great love of my life. Eleven years going on forever. I love you.

—Jonny

REFERENCES

WHY A NEW EDITION OF THIS BOOK WAS NEEDED

1. J. B. Meigs et al., "Impact of Insulin Resistance on Risk of Type 2 Diabetes and Cardiovascular Disease in People with Metabolic Syndrome," *Diabetes Care* 30, no.5 (2007): 1219-1225.

2. The National Institute of Diabetes and Digestive and Kidney Diseases Health Information Center, "Diabetes, Heart Disease, and Stroke," https://www.niddk.nih.gov/health-information/diabetes/overview/preventing-problems/heart-disease-stroke

3. D. Eddy et al, "Relationship of Insulin Resistance and Related Metabolic Variables to Coronary Artery Disease: A Mathematical Analysis," *Diabetes Care* 32, no. 2 (2009): 361-6.

WHY YOU SHOULD BE SKEPTICAL OF CHOLESTEROL AS AN INDICATOR OF HEART DISEASE

1. D. Mozaffarian et al., "Dietary fats, carbohydrate, and Progression of Coronary Atherosclerosis in Postmenopausal Women," *American Journal of Clinical Nutrition* 80, no. 5 (2004): 1175-84.

2. M. de Lorgeril et al. "Mediterranean Diet, Traditional Risk Factors, and the Rate of Cardiovascular Complications after Myocardial Infarction: Final Report of the Lyon Diet Heart Study," *Circulation* 99, no. 6 (1999): 779-85.

3. Channing Laboratory, "History," *The Nurses' Health Study*, www.channing.harvard.edu/nhs/?page_id=70.

4. Ibid.

5. M. de Lorgeril et al., "Mediterranean Alpha-Linolenic Acid-Rich Diet in Secondary Prevention of Coronary Heart Disease," *The Lancet*, no. 143 (1994): 1454-59.

6. J. Kastelein et al., "Simvastatin with or without Ezetimibe in Familial Hypercholesterolemia," *New England Journal of Medicine* 358, no. 14 (2008): 1431-43.

7. F. B. Hu et al., "Primary Prevention of Coronary Heart Disease in Women through Diet and Lifestyle," *New England Journal of Medicine* 343, no. 1 (2000): 16-12.

8. Ibid.

CHOLESTEROL IS HARMLESS!

1. University of Maryland, "Trans Fats 101," University of Maryland Medical Center, last modified November 3, 2010, www.umm.edu/features/transfats.htm.

2. G. V. Mann, "Coronary Heart Disease—'Doing the Wrong Things,'" *Nutrition Today* 20, no. 4 (1985): 12-14.

3. Ibid.

4. M. F. Oliver, "Consensus or Nonsensus Conferences on Coronary Heart Disease," *The Lancet* 325, no. 8437 (1985): 1087-89.

5. National Institutes of Health Consensus Development Conference Statement, December 10-12, 1984.

6. National Institutes of Health, "News from the Women's Health Initiative: Reducing Total Fat Intake May Have Small Effect on Risk of Breast Cancer, No Effect on Risk of Colorectal Cancer, Heart Disease, or Stroke," *NIH News*, last modified February 7, 2006, www.nih.gov/news/pr/feb2006/nhlbi-07.htm.

7. A. Ottoboni and F. Ottoboni, "Low-Fat Diet and Chronic Disease Prevention: The Women's Health Initiative and Its Reception," *Journal of American*

Physicians and Surgeons 12, no. 1 (2007): 10-13.

8. G. Kolata, "Low-Fat Diet Does Not Cut Health Risks, Study Finds," *New York Times*, February 8, 2006.

9. D. Lundell, *The Cure for Heart Disease* (Scottsdale: Publishing Intellect, 2012).

10. M. de Lorgeril, *A Near-Perfect Sexual Crime: Statins Against Cholesterol* (France: A4Set, 2011).

11. J. P. A. Ioannidis, "Why Most Published Research Findings Are False," *PLoS Medicine* 2(8): e124. https://doi.org/10.1371/journal.pmed.0020124; A. Berezow, "John Ioannidis Aims His Bazooka at Nutrition Science," *American Council on Science and Health* August 24, 2018; D. Robitzski, "Faulty Studies Mean Everything You Know About Nutrition Is Wrong," *Neoscope*, July 2, 2018.

12. National Cancer Institute, Division of Cancer Control & Population Sciences, "Usual Dietary Intakes: NHANES Food Frequency Questionnaire (FFQ)" https://epi.grants.cancer.gov/diet/usualintakes/ffq.html

13. Alan R Kristal et al., "Is It Time to Abandon the Food Frequency Questionnaire?" Cancer Epidemiology, Biomarkers and Prevention (AACR, December 2005) https://cebp.aacrjournals.org/content/14/12/2826

14. W. Walker, "The National Diet-Heart Study Final Report: American Heart Association Monograph. No. 19.," *Arch Intern Med* 123, no. 4 (1969): 473-474. doi:10.1001/archinte.1969.00300140119031

15. M. Gladwell: Revisionist History season 2, episode 10—"What Does a Son Owe His Father?"

16. V. Dhaka et al., "Trans Fats-Sources, Health Risks and Alternative Approach - A Review," *Journal of Food Science and Technology* 48, no. 5 (2011): 534-41. doi:10.1007/s13197-010-0225-8

17. Harvard School of Public Health. "Artificial Trans Fats Banned in U.S.," 2018: https://www.hsph.harvard.edu/news/hsph-in-the-news/us-bans-artificial-trans-fats

18. Perel, Esther, The State of Affairs: Rethinking Infidelity, (Harper Paperbacks: 2018)

THE REAL DEAL ON CHOLESTEROL

1. V. Marigliano, "Normal values in extreme old age," *Annals of the New York Academy of Sciences* 673 (1992): 23-28.

INFLAMMATION AND OXIDATION

1. D. Harman, "Aging: A Theory Based on Free Radical and Radiation Chemistry," Journal of Gerontology 11, no. 3 (1956): 298-300; D. Harman, "Free Radical Theory of Aging," in *Free Radicals and Aging*, eds. I. Emerit and B. Chance (Basel, Switzerland: Birkhäuser, 1992).

2. D. Lundell, *The Cure for Heart Disease* (Scottsdale: Publishing Intellect, 2012).

3. W. Cromwell et al., "LDL Particle Number and Risk of Future Cardiovascular Disease in the Framingham Offspring Study - Implications for LDL Management," *Journal of Clinical Lipidology* 1, no. 6 (2007): 583-92.

PART TWO

1. https://www.dhhs.nh.gov/dphs/nhp/documents/sugar.pdf

SUGAR: THE REAL DEMON IN THE DIET

1. M. Houston, M.D., M.S., director of the Hypertension Institute in Tennessee, May 2, 2012, telephone communication.

2. D. C. Goff et al., "Insulin Sensitivity and the Rise of Incident Hypertension," *Diabetes Care* 26, no. 3 (2003): 805-9.

3. "Too Much Insulin a Bad Thing for the Heart?" *Science Daily*, last modified April 19, 2010, www.sciencedaily.com/releases/2010/04/100419233109.htm.

4. V. Marigliano et al., "Normal Values in Extreme Old Age," *Annals of the New York Academy of Sciences* 673 (1992): 23-28.

5. J. O'Connell, *Sugar Nation: The Hidden Truth Behind America's Deadliest Habit and the Simple Way to Beat It*

(New York: Hyperion Books, 2011), 78.

6. Ibid.

7. G. Taubes, "Is Sugar Toxic?" *New York Times Magazine*, April 13, 2011.

8. "Findings and Recommendations on the Insulin Resistance Syndrome," American Association of Clinical Endocrinologists, Washington, D.C., August 25-26, 2002.

9. Ibid.

10. M. Miller, "What Is the Association Between the Triglyceride to High-density Lipoprotein Cholesterol Ratio and Insulin Resistance?" *Medscape Education*, www.medscape.org/viewarticle/588474; T. McLaughlin et al., "Use of Metabolic Markers to Identify Overweight Individuals Who Are Insulin Resistant," *Annals of Internal Medicine* 138, no. 10 (2003): 802-9.

11. "Type 2 Diabetes Reversed by Losing Fat from Pancreas," *Science Daily* December 1, 2015.

12. N. Avena et al., "Evidence for Sugar Addiction: Behavioral and Neurochemical Effects of Intermittent, Excessive Sugar Intake," *Neuroscience and Biobehavioral Reviews* 32, no. 1 (2008): 20-39.

13. A. Gearhardt et al., "The Addiction Potential of Hyperpalatable Foods," *Current Drug Abuse Reviews* 4 (2011): 140-45.

14. Taubes, "Is Sugar Toxic?"

15. G. V. Mann, *Coronary Heart Disease: The Dietary Sense and Nonsense* (London: Janus, 1993).

16. G. V. Mann et al., "Atherosclerosis in the Masai," *American Journal of Epidemiology* 95, no. 1 (1972): 26-37.

17. J. Yudkin, *Sweet and Dangerous* (New York: Wyden, 1972).

18. A. Keys, "Letter: Normal Plasma Cholesterol in a Man Who Eats 25 Eggs a Day," *New England Journal of Medicine* 325, no. 8 (1991): 584.

19. National Institutes of Health. "National Cholesterol Education Program," *National Heart, Lung, and Blood Institute*, last modified in October 2011, www.nhlbi.nih.gov/about/ncep.

20. World Health Organization, *Global Strategy on Diet, Physical Activity and Health* www.who.int/dietphysicalactivity/publications

21. J. Eilperin, "U.S. Sugar Industry Targets New Study," *Washington Post*, April 23, 2003, www.washingtonpost.com/ac2/wp-dyn/A17583-2003Apr22?language=printer.

22. "Historical Analysis Examines Sugar Industry Role in Heart Disease Research," For the Media, JAMA Network (9/12/16) https://media.jamanetwork.com/news-item/historical-analysis-examines-sugar-industry-role-in-heart-disease-research/

23. R. B. McGandy et al., "Dietary Fats, Carbohydrates and Atherosclerotic Vascular Disease," *New England Journal of Medicine*, 277(4), 186-192. doi:10.1056/nejm196707272770405

24. G. Taubes and C. Couzens, "Big Sugar's Sweet Little Lies," *Mother Jones* November/December 2012.

25. J. Casey, "The Hidden Ingredient That Can Sabotage Your Diet," *MedicineNet*, last modified January 3, 2005, www.medicinenet.com/script/main/art.asp?articlekey=56589.

26. C. Kearns et al., "Sugar Industry Sponsorship of Germ-Free Rodent Studies Linking Sucrose to Hyperlipidemia and Cancer: An Historical Analysis of Internal Documents," *PLoS Biology* November 2017.

27. C. Kearns and S. Glantz, "Sugar Industry Influence on the Scientific Agenda of the National Institute of Dental Research's 1971 National Caries Program: A Historical Analysis of Internal Documents," *PLoS Medicine* March 2015.

28. C. Kearns et al., "Sugar Industry and Coronary Heart Disease Research: A Historical Analysis of Internal Industry Documents," *JAMA Internal Medicine* 176, no. 11 (2016): 1680-1685.

29. Taubes, "Is Sugar Toxic?"

30. L. Tappy et al., "Metabolic Effects of Fructose and the Worldwide Increase in Obesity," *Physiological Reviews* 90, no. 1 (2010): 23–46; M. Dirlewanger et al., "Effects of Fructose on Hepatic Glucose Metabolism in Humans," *American Journal of Physiology, Endocrinology, and Metabolism* 279, no. 4 (2000): E907–11.

31. S. S. Elliott et al., "Fructose, Weight Gain, and the Insulin Resistance Syndrome," *American Journal of Clinical Nutrition* 76, no. 5 (2002): 911–22; K.A. Lê and L. Tappy, "Metabolic Effects of Fructose," *Current Opinion in Clinical Nutrition and Metabolic Care* 9, no. 4 (2006): 469–75; Y. Rayssiguier et al., "High Fructose Consumption Combined with Low Dietary Magnesium Intake May Increase the Incidence of the Metabolic Syndrome by Inducing Inflammation," *Magnesium Research Journal* 19, no. 4 (2006): 237–43.

32. K. Adeli and A. C. Rutledge, "Fructose and the Metabolic Syndrome: Pathophysiology and Molecular Mechanisms," *Nutrition Reviews* 65, no. 6 (2007): S13–S23; K.A. Lê and L. Tappy, "Metabolic Effects of Fructose."

33. "Fructose Metabolism by the Brain Increases Food Intake and Obesity, Study Suggests," *Science Daily*, www.sciencedaily.com/releases/2009/03/090325091811.htm.

THE TRUTH ABOUT FAT: IT'S NOT WHAT YOU THINK

1. F. B. Hu et al., "Meta-analysis of Prospective Cohort Studies Evaluating the Association of Saturated Fat with Cardiovascular Disease," *American Journal of Clinical Nutrition* 91, no. 3 (2010): 502–9.

2. R. S. Kuipers et al., "Saturated Fat, Carbohydrates, and Cardiovascular Disease," *Netherlands Journal of Medicine* 69, no. 9 (2011): 372–78.

3. R. Chowdhury et al., "Association of Dietary, Circulating, And Supplement Fatty Acids with Coronary Risk: A Systematic Review and Meta-Analysis," *Annals of Internal Medicine* 160, no. 6 (2014): 398–406.

4. R. de Souza et al., "Intake of Saturated and Trans Unsaturated Fatty Acids and Risk of All Cause Mortality, Cardiovascular Disease, and Type 2 Diabetes: Systematic Review and Meta-Analysis of Observational Studies," *BMJ* 351 (2015). doi: 10.1136/bmj.h3978

5. C. Ramsden et al., "Re-evaluation of the traditional diet-heart hypothesis: analysis of recovered data from Minnesota Coronary Experiment (1968-73)," *BMJ* 353(2016). doi:10.1136/bmj.i1246

6. "The effect of replacing saturated fat with mostly n-6 polyunsaturated fat on coronary heart disease: a meta-analysis of randomized controlled trials," Nutr. J 2017 May 19; 16(1): 30. https://www.ncbi.nlm.nih.gov/pubmed/28526025

7. F. de Meester and A. P. Simopoulos, eds., "A Balanced Omega-6/Omega-3 Fatty Acid Ratio, Cholesterol and Coronary Heart Disease," *World Review of Nutrition and Dietetics* 100 (2009): 1–21; T. Hamazaki, Y. Kirihara, and Y. Ogushi, "Blood Cholesterol as a Good Marker of Health in Japan," *World Review of Nutrition and Dietetics* 100 (2009): 63–70.

8. Japan Atherosclerosis Society, "Japan Atherosclerosis Society (JAS) Guidelines for Prevention of Atherosclerotic Cardiovascular Diseases," *Journal of Atherosclerosis and Thrombosis* 14, no. 2 (2007): 5–57; de Meester and Simopoulos, "A Balanced Omega-6/Omega-3 Fatty Acid Ratio, Cholesterol and Coronary Heart Disease."

9. T. Hamazaki, et al., "Blood Cholesterol as a Good Marker of Health in Japan," *World Review of Nutrition and Dietetics* 100 (2009): 63–70; de Meester and Simopoulos, "A Balanced Omega-6/Omega-3 Fatty Acid Ratio."

10. N. Panth et al., "Differential Effects of Medium- and

Long-Chain Saturated Fatty Acids on Blood Lipid Profile: A Systematic Review and Meta-Analysis," *The American Journal of Clinical Nutrition* 108, no. 4 (2018): 675-687.

11. F.B. Hu et al., "Dietary Saturated Fats and Their Food Sources in Relation to the Risk of Coronary Heart Disease in Women," *American Journal of Clinical Nutrition* 70, no. 6 (1999): 1001-08.

12. M-P. St-Onge et al., "Medium Chain Triglyceride Oil Consumption as Part of a Weight Loss Diet Does Not Lead to an Adverse Metabolic Profile When Compared to Olive Oil," *Journal of the American College of Nutrition* 27, no. 5 (2008): 547-52.

13. K-T. Khaw et al., "Randomised Trial of Coconut Oil, Olive Oil or Butter on Blood Lipids and Other Cardiovascular Risk Factors in Healthy Men and Women," *BMJ* 8, no. 3.

14. F. Rosqvist. "Potential Role of Milk Fat Globule Membrane in Modulating Plasma Lipoproteins, Gene Expression, and Cholesterol Metabolism in Humans: A Randomized Study," *American Journal of Clinical Nutrition* 102, no. 1 (2015): 20-30.

15. Rice, BH, "Dairy and Cardiovascular Disease: A Review of Recent Observational Research," Curr Nutr Rep 2014 Mar 15; 3: 130-180 eCollection 2014. https://www.ncbi.nlm.nih.gov/pubmed/24818071

16. D. M. Herrington, et al., "Dietary Fats, Carbohydrate, and Progression of Coronary Atherosclerosis in Postmenopausal Women," *American Journal of Clinical Nutrition* 80, no. 5 (2004): 1175-84.

17. Ibid.

18. R. H. Knopp and Barbara M. Retzlaff, "Saturated Fat Prevents Coronary Artery Disease? An American Paradox," *American Journal of Clinical Nutrition* 80, no. 5 (2004): 1102-3.

19. M. B. Katan et al., "Dietary Oils, Serum Lipoproteins, and Coronary Heart Disease," *American Journal of Clinical Nutrition* 61, no. 6 (1995): 1368S-73S.

20. S. Liu et al., "A Prospective Study of Dietary Glycemic Load, Carbohydrate Intake, and Risk of Coronary Heart Disease in U.S. Women," *American Journal of Clinical Nutrition* 71, no. 6 (2000): 1455-61.

21. M. U. Jakobsen et al., "Intake of Carbohydrates Compared with Intake of Saturated Fatty Acids and Risk of Myocardial Infarction: Importance of the Glycemic Index," *American Journal of Clinical Nutrition* 91, no. 6 (2010): 1764-68.

22. Ibid.

23. Ibid.

24. S.J. Nicholls et al., "Consumption of Saturated Fat Impairs the Anti-Inflammatory Properties of High-Density Lipoproteins and Endothelial Function," *Journal of the American College of Cardiology* 48, no. 4 (2006): 715-20.

25. R. S. Kuipers et al., "Saturated Fat, Carbohydrates, and Cardiovascular Disease," *Netherlands Journal of Medicine* 69, no. 9 (2011): 372-78.

26. Ibid; A. P. Simopoulos, "Overview of Evolutionary Aspects of w3 Fatty Acids in the Diet," *World Review of Nutrition and Dietetics* 83 (1998): 1-11.

27. R. O. Adolf et al., "Dietary Linoleic Acid Influences Desaturation and Acylation of Deuterium-labeled Linoleic and Linolenic Acids in Young Adult Males," *Biochimica et Biophysica Acta* 1213, no. 3 (1994): 277-88; Ghafoorunissa and M. Indu, "N-3 Fatty Acids in Indian Diets–Comparison of the Effects of Precursor (Alpha-linolenic Acid) vs. Product (Long Chain N-3 Polyunsaturated Fatty Acids)," *Nutrition Research* 12, nos. 4-5 (1992): 569-82.

28. A. P. Simopoulos, "Evolutionary Aspects of the Dietary Omega-6:Omega-3 Fatty Acid Ratio: Medical Implications," *World Review of Nutrition and Dietetics* 100 (2009): 1-21.

29. A. P. Simopoulos, "Overview of Evolutionary Aspects of w3 Fatty Acids in the Diet."

30. P. Reaven et al., "Effects of Oleate-rich and Linoleate-rich Diets on the Susceptibility of Low-density Lipoprotein to Oxidative Modification in Mildly Hypercholesterolemic Subjects," *Journal of Clinical Investigation* 91, no. 2 (1993): 668-76.

31. L. G. Cleland, "Linoleate Inhibits EPA Incorporation from Dietary Fish Oil Supplements in Human Subjects," *American Journal of Clinical Nutrition* 55, no. 2 (1992): 395-99.

32. W. E. M. Lands, "Diets Could Prevent Many Diseases," *Lipids* 38, no. 4 (2003): 317-21.

33. Ibid.

34. W. E. M. Lands, "A Critique of Paradoxes in Current Advice on Dietary Lipids," *Progress in Lipid Research* 47, no. 2 (2008): 77-106.

35. R. de Souza et al., "Intake of Saturated and Trans Unsaturated Fatty Acids and Risk of All Cause Mortality, Cardiovascular Disease, and Type 2 Diabetes: Systematic Review and Meta-Analysis of Observational Studies," *BMJ* 351 (2015); R. Chowdhury et al, "Association of Dietary, Circulating, and Supplement Fatty Acids with Coronary Risk: A Systematic Review and Meta-Analysis," *Annals of Internal Medicine* 2014. DOI:10.7326/M13-1788; A. Malhotra et al., "Saturated Fat Does Not Clog the Arteries: Coronary Heart Disease Is a Chronic Inflammatory Condition, The Risk of Which Can Be Effectively Reduced from Healthy Lifestyle Interventions," *British Journal of Sports Medicine* 51 (2017): 1111-1112; H. Nichols, "Artery-Clogging Saturated Fat Myth Debunked," *Medical News Today* 2017; P.W. Siri-Tarino et al., "Meta-Analysis of Prospective Cohort Studies Evaluating the Association of Saturated Fat with Cardiovascular Disease," *American Journal of Clinical Nutrition* 91, no. 3 (2010): 535-46.

THE STATIN DECEPTION

1. S. Subramanian et al., "High-Dose Atorvastatin Reduces Periodontal Inflammation,"*Journal of the American College of Cardiology* 62, no. 25 (2013): 2382-2391.

2. Y. Almog et al., "Statins, Inflammation, and Sepsis*: Hypothesis," *Chest* 124, no. 2 (2003): 740-743.

3. A. E. Dorr et al., "Colestipol Hydrochloride in Hypercholesterolemic Patients—Effect on Serum Cholesterol and Mortality," *Journal of Chronic Diseases* 31, no. 1 (1978): 5.

4. J. Stamler et al., "Effectiveness of Estrogens for the Long-Term Therapy of Middle-Aged Men with a History of Myocardial Infarction," *Coronary Heart Disease: Seventh Hahnemann Symposium*, eds. W. Likoff and J. Henry Moyer (New York: Grune & Stratton, 1963), 416.

45. D. Kuester, "Cholesterol-Reducing Drugs May Lessen Brain Function, Says ISU Researcher," *Iowa State University*, last modified February 23, 2009, www2.iastate.edu/~nscentral/news/2009/feb/shin.shtml.

6. Ibid.

7. M. Beck, "Can a Drug That Helps Hearts Be Harmful to the Brain?" *Wall Street Journal*, February 12, 2008.

8. D. Graveline, *Lipitor: Thief of Memory* (Duane Graveline, 2006), www.spacedoc.com/lipitor_thief_of_memory.html.

9. Martin, et al, "Statin therapy causes gut dysbiosis in mice through a PXR-dependent mechanism," Microbiome 2017; 5: 95. https://www.ncbi.nlm.nih.gov/pmc/articles/PMC5550934/

10. T. Khan et al., "Effect of Atorvastatin on the Gut Microbiota of High-Fat Diet-Induced Hypercholesterolemic Rats," *Scientific Reports* 8, no. 1 (2018): 662.

11. C. Iribarren et al., "Serum Total Cholesterol and Risk of Hospitalization and Death from Respiratory Disease," *International Journal of Epidemiology* 26, no. 6 (1997): 1191-1202; C. Iribarren et al., "Cohort Study of Serum Total Cholesterol and In-Hospital Incidence of Infectious

Diseases," *Epidemiology and Infection* 121, no. 2 (1998): 335-47; J.D. Neaton and D. N. Wentworth, "Low Serum Cholesterol and Risk of Death from AIDS," *AIDS* 11, no. 7 (1997): 929-30.

12. Harvard Women's Health Watch, "Statins and Women," June 2012: https://www.health.harvard.edu/heart-health/statins-and-women

13. J. Kantor, "Prevalence of Erectile Dysfunction and Active Depression: An Analytic Cross-Sectional Study of General Medical Patients," *American Journal of Epidemiology* 156, no. 11 (2002): 1035-42.

14. M. Kanat et al., "A Multi-Center, Open Label, Crossover Designed Prospective Study Evaluatiing the Effects of Lipid-lowering Treatment on Steroid Synthesis in Patients with Type 2 Diabetes (MODEST Study)," *Journal of Endocrinology Investigation* 32, no. 10 (2009): 852-56; R.D. Stanworth et al., "Statin Therapy is Associated with Lower Total but not Bioavailable or Free Testosterone in Men with Type 2 Diabetes," *Diabetes Care* 32, no. 4 (2009): 541-46; A. S. Dobbs et al., "Effects of High-Dose Simvastatin on Adrenal and Gonadal Steroidogenesis in Men with Hypercholesterolemia," *Metabolism* 49, no. 9 (2000): 1234-38; A. S. Dobs et al., "Effects of Simvastatin and Pravastatin on Gonadal Function in Male Hypercholesterolemic Patients," *Metabolism* 49, no. 1 (2000): 115-21; M. T. Hyyppä et al., "Does Simvastatin Affect Mood and Steroid Hormone Levels in Hypercholesterolemic Men? A Randomized Double-Blind Trial," *Psychoneuroendocrinology* 28, no. 2 (2003): 181-94.

15. B. Banaszewska et al., "Effects of Simvastatin and Oral Contraceptive Agent on Polycystic Ovary Syndrome: Prospective, Randomized, Crossover Trial," *Journal of Clinical Endocrinology & Metabolism* 92, no. 2 (2007): 456-61; T. Sathyapalan et al., "The Effect of Atorvastatin in Patients with Polycystic Ovary Syndrome: A Randomized Double-Blind Placebo-Controlled Study," *Journal of Clinical Endocrinology & Metabolism* 94, no. 1 (2009): 103-108.

16. C. Do et al., "Statins and Erectile Dysfunction: Results of a Case/Non-Case Study using the French Pharmacovigilance System Database," *Drug Safety* 32, no. 7 (2009): 591-97.

17. C. J. Malkin et al., "Low Serum Testosterone and Increased Mortality in Men with Coronary Heart Disease," *Heart* 96, no. 22 (2010): 1821-25.

18. S. Shrivastava et al., "Chronic Cholesterol Depletion Using Statin Impairs the Function and Dynamics of Human Serotonin (1A) Receptors," *Biochemistry* 49, no. 26 (2010): 5426-35; L.N. Johnson-Anuna et al., "Chronic Administration of Statins Alters Multiple Gene Expression Patterns in Mouse Cerebral Cortex," *Journal of Pharmacology and Experimental Therapeutics* 312, no. 2 (2005): 786-93. A. Linetti et al., "Cholesterol Reduction Impairs Exocytosis of Synaptic Vesicles," *Journal of Cell Science* 123, no. 4 (2010): 595-605.

19. T. B. Horwich et al., "Low Serum Total Cholesterol Is Associated with Marked Increase in Mortality in Advanced Heart Failure," *Journal of Cardiac Failure* 8, no. 4 (2002): 216-24.

20. S. Brescianini et al., "Low Total Cholesterol and Increased Risk of Dying: Are Low Levels Clinical Warning Signs in the Elderly? Results from the Italian Longitudinal Study on Aging," *Journal of the American Geriatrics Society* 51, no. 7 (2003): 991-96.

21. A. Alawi et al., "Effect of the Magnitude of Lipid Lowering on Risk of Elevated Liver Enzymes, Rhabdomyolysis, and Cancer," *Journal of the American College of Cardiology* 50, no. 5 (2007): 409-18.

22. M.R. Goldstein et al., "Primary Prevention of Cardiovascular Disease with Statins: Cautionary Notes," *QJM: An International Journal of Medicine* 102 no. 11 (2009): 817-820.

23. Corrao G, et al., Statins and the risk of diabetes, Diabetes Care 2014 Aug; 37(8): 2225-32. https://www.ncbi.nlm.nih.gov/pubmed/24969582

24. D. Preiss et al., "Risk of Incident Diabetes with Intensive-Dose Compared with Moderate-Dose Statin Therapy," *Journal of the American Medical Association* 305, no. 24 (2011): 2556-64.

25. J. Kreafle, "New Cholesterol Guidelines for Heart Health: What You Need to Know," *ABC News* November 12, 2018: https://abcnews.go.com/Health/cholesterol-guidelines-heart-health/story?id=59147980

26. M. Nakata et al., " Effects of Statins on the Adipocyte Maturation and Expression of Glucose Transporter 4 (SLC2A4): Implications in Glycaemic Control," *Diabetologia* 49, no. 8 (2006): 1881-92; M. Braulta et al., "Statin Treatment and New-Onset Diabetes: A Review of Proposed Mechanisms," *Metabolism* 63, no. 6 (2014): 735-745.

27. B. A. Golomb et al., "Physician Response to Patient Reports of Adverse Drug Effects," *Drug Safety* 30, no. 8 (2007): 669-75.

28. Ibid.

29. J. Stamler et al., "Is Relationship Between Serum Cholesterol and Risk of Premature Death from Coronary Heart Disease Continuous and Graded? Findings in 356,222 Primary Screenees of the Multiple Risk Factor Intervention Trial (MRFIT)," *JAMA* 256, no. 20 (1986): 2823-8.

30. David Diamond, Ph.D., "Demonization and Deception in Cholesterol Research." https://www.youtube.com/watch?v=yX1vBA9bLNk&t=3047s

31. T. Xuan-Mai et al., "Abstract 16619: Relationship Between Serum Cholesterol and Risk of Premature Death from Coronary Heart Disease in Male Veterans: is it Still Continuous and Graded?" *Circulation* 134 supp. 1 (2016).

32. H. S. Hecht and S. M. Harman, "Relation of Aggressiveness of Lipid-Lowering Treatment to Changes in Calcified Plaque Burden by Electron Beam Tomography," *American Journal of Cardiology* 92, no. 3 (2003): 334-36.

33. W. A. Flegel, "Inhibition of Endotoxin-Induced Activation of Human Monocytes by Human Lipoprotein," *Infection and Immunity* 57, no. 7 (1989): 2237-45; W.A. Flegel et al., "Prevention of Endotoxin-Induced Monokine Release by Human Low- and High-Density Lipoproteins and by Apolipoprotein A-I," *Infection and Immunity* 61, no. 12 (1993): 5140-46; H. Northoff et al., "The Role of Lipoproteins in Inactivation of Endotoxin by Serum," *Beitr Infusionsther* 30 (1992): 195-97.

34. Jacobs et al., "Report of the Conference on Low Blood Cholesterol."

35. Iribarren et al., "Serum Total Cholesterol and Risk of Hospitalization"; Iribarren et al., "Cohort Study of Serum Total Cholesterol."

36. Neaton and Wentworth, "Low Serum Cholesterol and Risk of Death from AIDS."

37. A. C. Looker et al., "Vitamin D Status: United States, 2001-2006," Centers for Disease Control and Prevention, NCHS Data Brief No. 59, March 2011, www.cdc.gov/nchs/data/databriefs/db59.htm.

38. W. Faloon, "Startling Findings About Vitamin D Levels in Life Extension Members," *Life Extension Magazine*, January 2010, www.lef.org/magazine/mag2010/jan2010_Startling-Findings-About-Vitamin-D-Levels-in-Life-Extension-Members_01.htm.

39. "Health Conditions," Vitamin D Council, last modified September 27, 2011, www.vitamindcouncil.org/health-conditions.

40. J. Abramson and J. M. Wright, "Are Lipid-Lowering Guidelines Evidence-Based?" *The Lancet* 369, no. 9557 (2007): 168-69.

41. Therapeutics Initiative, "Do Statins Have a Role in

Primary Prevention?" *Therapeutics Letter* #48, April-June 2003, www.ti.ubc.ca/newsletter/do-statins-have-role-primary-prevention.

42. M. Pignone et al., "Primary Prevention of CHD with Pharmacological Lipid-Lowering Therapy: A Meta-Analysis of Randomised Trials," *BMJ* 321, no. 7267 (2000): 983-86.

THE *REAL* CAUSE OF HEART DISEASE

1. A. Menke et al., "Prevalence of and Trends in Diabetes Among Adults in the United States, 1988-2012," *JAMA* 314, no. 10 (2015): 1021-29.

2. A. Boldt, "Starbucks' Pumpkin Spice Latte Nutrition Information," *Livestrong* Updated October 25, 2019: M.S. https://www.livestrong.com/article/274448-starbucks-pumpkin-spice-latte-nutrition-information

3. Starbucks, "Nutritional Information: Blueberry Muffin," https://www.starbucks.com/menu/food/bakery/bountiful-blueberry-muffin

4. M. Demasi et al., "The Cholesterol and Calorie Hypotheses are Both Dead – It Is Time to Focus on the Real Culprit: Insulin Resistance," *The Pharmaceutical Journal* July 14, 2017.

5. https://www.youtube.com/watch?v=UZoQiDaWnuE

6. A. Eenfeldt, "The Engineer Who Knows More Than Your Doctor," *Diet Doctor* June 13, 2016.

7. ibid.

8. Crofts, *Diabesity* 2015; 1 (4): 34-43

9. G. M. Fahy et al., "Reversal of Epigenetic Aging and Immunosenescent Trends in Humans," *Aging Cell* 18, no. 6 (2019): https://doi.org/10.1111/acel.13028.

10. N. Barzilai, Nir et al., "Metformin as a Tool to Target Aging," *Cell Metabolism* 23, no. 6 (2016): 1060-1065; W. Valencia et al., "Metformin and Ageing: Improving Ageing Outcomes Beyond Glycaemic Control,"
Diabetologia 60, no. 9 (2017): 1630-1638.

11. *Diabetes Epidemic and You* (Kraft, Trafford Publishing, 2008)

12. Meridian Valley Lab, "Kraft Prediabetes Profile," https://www.meridianvalleylab.com/services/kraft-prediabetes-profile

13. T. Hayashi et al., "Patterns of Insulin Concentration During the OGTT Predict the Risk of Type 2 Diabetes in Japanese Americans," *Diabetes Care* 36, no. 5 (2013): 1229-35.

14. J. DiNicolantonio et al, "Postprandial Insulin Assay as the Earliest Biomarker for Diagnosing Pre-Diabetes, Type 2 Diabetes and Increased Cardiovascular Risk," *Open Heart* 4, no. 2 (2017): doi:10.1136/openhrt-2017-000656

15. Ibid.

16. V. Ormazabal et al., "Association Between Insulin Resistance and the Development of Cardiovascular Disease," *Cardiovascular Diabetology* 17 (2018): https://cardiab.biomedcentral.com/articles/10.1186/s12933-018-0762-4

17. K.M. Flegal et al., "Excess Deaths Associated with Underweight, Overweight, and Obesity," *JAMA* 293, no. 15 (2005): 1861-7.

18. G. Howard et al., "Insulin Sensitivity and Atherosclerosis. The Insulin Resistance Atherosclerosis Study (IRAS) Investigators," *Circulation* 93, no. 10 (1996): 1809-17; A. Tenenbaum et al., "Insulin Resistance Is Associated with Increased Risk of Major Cardiovascular Events in Patients with Preexisting Coronary Artery Disease," *American Heart Journal* 153, no. 4: 559-65; K.B. Gast et al., "Insulin Resistance And Risk of Incident Cardiovascular Events in Adults Without Diabetes: Meta-Analysis," *PLoS One* 7, no. 12: doi: 10.1371/journal.pone.0052036; D. Eddy et al., "Relationship of Insulin Resistance and Related Metabolic Variables to Coronary Artery Disease: A

Mathematical Analysis," *Diabetes Care* 32, no. 2 (2009): 361-66; G. Reaven, "Insulin Resistance and Coronary Heart Disease in Nondiabetic Individuals," *Arteriosclerosis, Thrombosis, and Vascular Biology* 32, no. 8 (2012): 1754-59; D.J. Rader, "Effect of Insulin Resistance, Dyslipidemia, and Intra-Abdominal Adiposity on the Development of Cardiovascular Disease and Diabetes Mellitus," *American Journal of Medicine* 120, no. 3 supp. 1: S12-18; D.A. Savaino and J.A. Story, "Cardiovascular Disease and Fiber: Is Insulin Resistance the Missing Link?" *Nutrition Reviews* 58, no. 11 (2000): 356-58; C. Kong et al., "Insulin Resistance, Cardiovascular Risk Factors and Ultrasonically Measured Early Arterial Disease in Normotensive Type 2 Diabetic Subjects," *Diabetes/Metabolism research and Reviews* 16, no. 6 (2000): 448-53; H.N. Ginsberg, "Insulin Resistance and Cardiovascular Disease," *Journal of Clinical Investigation* 106, no. 4 (2000): 453-58; Z.T. Bloomgarden, "Insulin Resistance, Dyslipidemia, and Cardiovascular Disease," *Diabetes Care* 30, no. 8 (2007): 2164-70.

19. R.G. Garcia et al., "Hyperinsulinemia Is a Predictor of New Cardiovascular Events in Colombian Patients with a First Myocardial Infarction," *International Journal of Cardiology* 148, no. 1 (2011): 85-90.

20. K. Kotseva, "EUROASPIRE IV: A European Society of Cardiology Survey on the Lifestyle, Risk Factor and Therapeutic Management of Coronary Patients from 24 European Countries," *European Journal of Preventive Cardiology* 23, no. 6 (2016): 636-48; K. Kortseva, "Time Trends in Lifestyle, Cardiovascular Risk Factors, and Therapeutic Management in European Patients with Coronary Artery Disease. A comparison of Euroaspire IV and V surveys over 5 years in 21 countries.," NHLI Imperial College London, UK on behalf of the EuroAspire Investigators.

21. Healthline, "Type 2 Diabetes Statistics and Facts," https://www.healthline.com/health/type-2-diabetes/statistics#1; American Diabetes Association, "Statistics About Diabetes," https://www.diabetes.org/resources/statistics/statistics-about-diabetes

22. H.F. Bligh et al., "Plant-Rich Mixed Meals Based on Palaeolithic Diet Principles Have a Dramatic Impact on Incretin, Peptide YY and Satiety Response, but Show Little Effect on Glucose and Insulin Homeostasis: An Acute-Effects Randomised Study," *British Journal of Nutrition* 113, no. 4 (2015): 574-84.

23. G.B. Haber et al., "Depletion and Disruption of Dietary Fibre. Effects on Satiety, Plasma-Glucose, and Serum-Insulin," *Lancet* 2, no. 8040 (1977): 679-82. DOI: 10.1016/s0140-6736(77)90494-9; C. Desmarchelier et al., "Diet-induced Obesity in Ad Libitum-Fed Mice: Food Texture Overrides the Effect of Macronutrient Composition," *British Journal of Nutrition* 109, no. 8 (2013): 1518-27.

24. A.P. Simopoulos, "The importance of the ratio of omega-6/omega-3 essential fatty acids," *Biomedicine & Pharmacotherapy* 56, no. 8 (2002): 365-379.

25. The Blood Code: HOMA IR - Insulin Resistance Calculator: https://www.thebloodcode.com/homa-ir-calculator

26. LabCorp: https://www.labcorp.com/test-menu/31986/nmr-lipoprofile%C2%AE-with-insulin-resistance-markers-without-graph; https://www.labcorp.com/test-menu/26131/glyca; https://www.labcorp.com/assets/17167

27. M. Demasi et al., "The Cholesterol and Calorie Hypotheses Are Both Dead — It Is Time to Focus on the Real Culprit: Insulin Resistance," *Clinical Pharmacist* July 14, 2017: https://www.pharmaceutical-journal.com/opinion/insight/the-cholesterol-and-calorie-hypotheses-are-both-dead-it-is-time-to-focus-on-the-real-culprit-insulin-resistance/20203046.article?firstPass=false

BEYOND THE MEDITERRANEAN DIET: WHAT DO I EAT?

1. Faris, Stephan, "Eat Like an Italian," Time, (2/20/12). http://content.time.com/time/subscriber/article/0,33009,2106478-1,00.html

2. Sardinia Unlimited, "10 Sardinian Top Dishes," https://www.sardiniaunlimited.com/10-sardinian-top-dishes

3. Elizabeth David biography, Wikipedia. https://en.wikipedia.org/wiki/Elizabeth_David_bibliography

4. Su Cumbidu: https://www.sucumbidu.com/secondi-2

5. Lauren E O'Connor et al., "A Mediterranean-Style Eating Pattern with Lean, Unprocessed Red Meat Has Cardiometabolic Benefits for Adults Who Are Overweight or Obese in a Randomized, Crossover, Controlled Feeding Trial," The American Journal of Clinical Nutrition 108, no. 1, (2018): 33-40.

6. K. L. Stanhope et al., "Consumption of Fructose and High-Fructose Corn Syrup Increase Postprandial Triglycerides, LDL-Cholesterol, and Apolipoprotein-B in Young Men and Women," Journal of Clinical Endocrinology & Metabolism 96, no. 10 (2011): E1596-605; "Fructose Consumption Increases Risk Factors for Heart Disease: Study Suggests US Dietary Guideline for Upper Limit of Sugar Consumption Is Too High," Science Daily, July 28, 2011; K. L. Stanhope and P. J. Havel, "Endocrine and Metabolic Effects of Consuming Beverages Sweetened with Fructose, Glucose, Sucrose, or High-Fructose Corn Syrup," American Journal of Clinical Nutrition 88, no. 6 (2008): 1733S-37S.

7. S. Sieri et al., "Dietary Glycemic Load and Index and Risk of Coronary Heart Disease in a large Italian Cohort: The EPICOR Study," Archives of Internal Medicine 12, no. 170 (2010): 640-47.

8. "How High Carbohydrate Foods Can Raise Risk for Heart Problems," Science Daily, June 25, 2009, retrieved February 8, 2012, www.sciencedaily.com/releases/2009/06/090625133215.htm.

9. Tel Aviv University, "How High Carbohydrate Foods Can Raise Risk for Heart Problems," Science Daily, June 25, 2009, retrieved February 8, 2012, from www.sciencedaily.com/releases/2009/06/090625133215.htm

10. S. Liu et al., "Relation Between a Diet with a High Glycemic Load and Plasma Concentrations of High-Sensitivity C-Reactive Protein in Middle-Aged Women," American Journal of Clinical Nutrition 75, no. 3 (2002): 492-98.

11. Ibid.

12. C. Laino, "Trans Fats Up Heart Disease Risk," WebMD Health News, November 15, 2006, www.webmd.com/heart/news/20061115/heart-disease-risk-upped-by-trans-fats.

13. F. B. Hu et al., "Dietary Fat Intake and the Risk of Coronary Heart Disease in Women," New England Journal of Medicine 337, no. 21 (1997): 1491-99.143.

14. Institute of Medicine of the National Academies, Dietary Reference Intakes for Energy, Carbohydrate, Fiber, Fat, Fatty Acids, Cholesterol, Protein, and Amino Acids (Washington, D.C.: The National Academies Press, 2005), 504.

15. Harvard School of Public Health, "Eating Processed Meats, but Not Unprocessed Red Meats, May Raise Risk of Heart Disease and Diabetes," news release, May 17, 2010, www.hsph.harvard.edu/news/press-releases/2010-releases/processed-meats-unprocessed-heart-disease-diabetes.html.

16. Ibid.

17. J. Bowden, The 150 Healthiest Foods on Earth (Beverly, MA: Fair Winds Press, 2007).

18. L. Zhang et al., "Pterostilbene Protects Vascular Endothelial Cells Against Oxidized Low-Density Lipoprotein-Induced Apoptosis In Vitro and In Vivo," Apoptosis 17, no. 1 (2012): 25-36.

19. H. C. Ou et al., "Ellagic Acid Protects Endothelial

Cells from Oxidized Low-Density Lipoprotein-Induced Apoptosis by Modulating the PI3K/Akt/eNOS Pathway," Toxicology and Applied Pharmacology 248, no. 2 (2010): 134-43.

20. H. C. Hung et al., "Fruit and Vegetable Intake and Risk of Major Chronic Disease," Journal of the National Cancer Institute 96, no. 21 (2004): 1577-84.

21. Ibid.

22. F. J. He et al., "Increased Consumption of Fruit and Vegetables Is Related to a Reduced Risk of Coronary Heart Disease: Meta-Analysis of Cohort Studies," Journal of Human Hypertension 21, no. 9 (2007): 717-28.

23. F. J. He et al., "Fruit and Vegetable Consumption and Stroke: Meta-Analysis of Cohort Studies," The Lancet 367, no. 9507 (2006): 320-26.

24. H. C. Hung et al., "Fruit and Vegetable Intake and Risk of Major Chronic Disease," Journal of the National Cancer Institute 96, no. 21 (2004): 1577-84.

25. D. Mozaffarian et al., "Changes in Diet and Lifestyle and Long-Term Weight Gain in Men and Women," New England Journal of Medicine 364, no. 25 (2011): 2392-404.

26. M. Burros, "Eating Well; Pass the Nuts, Pass Up the Guilt," New York Times, January 15, 2003.

27. O. H. Franco et al., "The Polymeal: A More Natural, Safer, and Probably Tastier (than the Polypill) Strategy to Reduce Cardiovascular Disease by More Than 75%," BMJ 329, no. 7480 (2004): 1447.

28. D. M. Winham et al., "Pinto Bean Consumption Reduces Biomarkers for Heart Disease Risk," Journal of the American College of Nutrition 26, no. 3 (2007): 243-49.

29. E. K. Kabagambe et al., "Decreased Consumption of Dried Mature Beans Is Positively Associated with Urbanization and Nonfatal Acute Myocardial Infarction," Journal of Nutrition 135, no. 7 (2005): 1770-75.

30. Bazzano et al., "Legume Consumption and Risk of Coronary Heart Disease in U.S. Men and Women," Archives of Internal Medicine 161, no. 21 (2001): 2573-78.

31. A. Buitrago-Lopez et al., "Chocolate Consumption and Cardiometabolic Disorders: Systematic Review and Meta-Analysis," BMJ I 343 (2011): d4488.

32. S. Desch et al., "Effect of Cocoa Products on Blood Pressure: Systemic Review and Meta-Analysis," Abstract, American Journal of Hypertension 23, no. 1 (2010): 97-103.

33. B. Buijsse et al., "Cocoa Intake, Blood Pressure, and Cardiovascular Mortality," Archives of Internal Medicine 166, no. 4 (2006): 411-17.

34. M. Aviram et al., "Pomegranate Juice Consumption Reduces Oxidative Stress, Atherogenic Modifications to LDL, and Platelet Aggregation: Studies in Humans and in Atherosclerotic Apolipoprotein E-Deficient Mice," American Journal of Clinical Nutrition 71, no. 5 (2000): 1062-76; M. Aviram et al., "Pomegranate Juice Flavonoids Inhibit Low-Density Lipoprotein Oxidation and Cardiovascular Diseases: Studies in Atherosclerotic Mice and in Humans," Drugs Under Experimental and Clinical Research 28, no. 2-3 (2002): 49-62.

35. M. Aviram et al., "Pomegranate Juice Consumption for 3 Years by Patients with Carotid Artery Stenosis Reduces Common Carotid Intima-Media Thickness, Blood Pressure and LDL Oxidation," Clinical Nutrition 23, no. 3 (2004): 423-33.

36. L. J. Ignarro et al., "Pomegranate Juice Protects Nitric Oxide Against Oxidative Destruction and Enhances the Biological Actions of Nitric Oxide," Nitric Oxide 15, no. 2 (2006): 93-102.

37. D. K. Das et al., "Cardioprotection of Red Wine: Role of Polyphenolic Antioxidants," Drugs Under Experimental and Clinical Research 25, nos. 2-3 (1999): 115-20.

38. V. Ivanov at al., "Red Wine Antioxidants Bind to Human Lipoproteins and Protect them from Metal Ion-Dependent and Independent Oxidation," *Journal of Agriculture and Food Chemistry* 49, no. 9 (2001): 4442-49; M. Aviram and B. Fuhrman, "Wine Flavonoids Protect Against LDL Oxidation and Atherosclerosis," *Annals of the New York Academy of Sciences* 957 (2002): 146-61.

39. A. Lugasi et al., "Cardio-Protective Effect of Red Wine as Reflected in the Literature," Abstract, *Orvosi Hetilap* 138, no. 11 (1997): 673-78; T.S. Saleem and S.D. Basha, "Red Wine: A Drink to Your Heart," *Journal of Cardiovascular Disease Research* 1, no. 4 (2010): 171-76.

40. J. Sano, "Effects of Green Tea Intake on the Development of Coronary Artery Disease," *Circulation Journal* 68, no. 7 (2004): 665-70.

41. S. L. Duffy, "Short- and Long-Term Black Tea Consumption Reverses Endothelial Dysfunction in Patients with Coronary Artery Disease," *Circulation* 104 (2001): 151-56.

42. Medscape, "Black Tea Shown to Improve Blood Vessel Health," *Medscape News*, July 17, 2001, www.medscape.com/viewarticle/411324.

43. A. Trichopoulou et al., "Mediterranean Diet and Survival Among Patients with Coronary Heart Disease in Greece," *Archives of Internal Medicine* 165, no. 8 (2005): 929-35.

44. A. Ferrera et al., "Olive Oil and Reduced Need for Antihypertensive Medications," *Archives of Internal Medicine* 160, no. 6 (2000): 837-42.

45. "Olive Oil Contains Natural Anti-Inflammatory Agent," *Science Daily*, September 6, 2005, www.sciencedaily.com/releases/2005/09/050906075427.htm.

46. American Botanical Council, "Garlic," *Herbalgram*, http://cms.herbalgram.org/expandedE/Garlic.html.

HELP YOUR HEART WITH THESE SUPPLEMENTS

1. E. G. Campbell, "Doctors and Drug Companies–Scrutinizing Influential Relationships," *New England Journal of Medicine* 357 (2007): 1796-97; M. M. Chren, "Interactions Between Physicians and Drug Company Representatives," *American Journal of Medicine* 107, no. 2 (1999): 182-83.

2. Marchioli et al, "Early Protection Against Sudden Death by n-3 Polyunsaturated Fatty Acids After Myocardial Infarction: Time-Course Analysis of the Results of the Gruppo Italiano per lo Studio della Sopravvivenza nell'Infarto Miocardico (GISSI)-Prevenzione," *New England Journal of Medicine* 368 (2013): 1800-1808.

3. G. Kolata, "10 Findings That Contradict Medical Wisdom. Doctors, Take Note," *New York Times* July 1, 2019.

4. "NYHA Classification–The Stages of Heart Failure," Heart Failure Society of America, last modified December 5, 2011, www.abouthf.org/questions_stages.htm.

5. P. H. Langsjoen , S. Vadhanavikit, and K. Folkers, "Response of Patients in Classes III and IV of Cardiomyopathy to Therapy in a Blind and Crossover Trial with Coenzyme Q10," *Proceedings of the National Academy of Sciences of the United States of America* 82, no. 12 (1985): 4240-44.

6. P. H. Langsjoen et al., "A Six-Year Clinical Study of Therapy of Cardiomyopathy with Coenzyme Q10," *International Journal of Tissue Reactions* 12, no. 3 (1990): 169-71.

7. F. L. Rosenfeldt et al., "Coenzyme Q10 in the Treatment of Hypertension: A Meta-Analysis of the Clinical Trials," *Journal of Human Hypertension* 21, no. 4 (2007): 297-306.

8. S. Hendler, *PDR for Nutritional Supplements*, 2nd ed.

(Montvale, NJ: PDR Network, 2008), 152.

9. P. Davini et al., "Controlled Study on L-Carnitine Therapeutic Efficacy in Post-Infarction," *Drugs Under Experimental and Clinical Research* 18, no. 8 (1992): 355-65.

10. I. Rizos, "Three-Year Survival of Patients with Heart Failure Caused by Dilated Cardiomyopathy and L-Carnitine Administration," *American Heart Journal* 139, no. 2 (2000): S120-23.

11. L. Cacciatore et al., "The Therapeutic Effect of L-Carnitine in Patients with Exercise-Induced Stable Angina: A Controlled Study," *Drugs Under Experimental and Clinical Research* 17, no. 4 (1991): 225-35; G. Louis Bartels et al., "Effects of L-Propionylcarnitine on Ischemia-Induced Myocardial Dysfunction in Men with Angina Pectoris," *American Journal of Cardiology* 74, no. 2 (1994): 125-30.

12. L. A. Calò et al., "Antioxidant Effect of L-Carnitine and Its Short Chain Esters: Relevance for the Protection from Oxidative Stress Related Cardiovascular Damage," *International Journal of Cardiology* 107, no. 1 (2006): 54-60.

13. M. J. Bolland et al., "Effects of Calcium Supplements on Risk of Myocardial Infarction and Cardiovascular Events: Meta-Analysis," *BMJ* 341, no. c3691 (2010).

14. P. Raggi et al., "Progression of Coronary Artery Calcium and Risk of First Myocardial Infarction in Patients Receiving Cholesterol-Lowering Therapy," *Arteriosclerosis, Thrombosis, and Vascular Biology* 24, no. 7 (2004): 1272-77.

15. Ibid.

16. U. Hoffmann et al., "Use of New Imaging Techniques to Screen for Coronary Artery Disease," *Circulation* 108 (2003): e50-e53.

17. M. C. Houston and K. J. Harper, "Potassium, Magnesium, and Calcium: Their Role in Both the Cause and Treatment of Hypertension," *Journal of Clinical Hypertension* 10, no. 7 (2008): 3-11; L. Widman et al., "The Dose-Dependent Reduction in Blood Pressure Through Administration of Magnesium: A Double-Blind Placebo-Controlled Crossover Trial," *American Journal of Hypertension* 6, no. 1 (1993), 41-45.

18. P. Laurant and R. M. Touyz, "Physiological and Pathophysiological Role of Magnesium in the Cardiovascular System: Implications in Hypertension," *Journal of Hypertension* 18, no. 9 (2000): 1177-91.

19. R. Meerwaldt et al., "The Clinical Relevance of Assessing Advanced Glycation Endproducts Accumulation in Diabetes," *Cardiovascular Diabetology* 7, no. 29 (2008): 1-8; A. J. Smit, "Advanced Glycation Endproducts in Chronic Heart Failure," *Annals of the New York Academy of Sciences* 1126 (2008): 225-30; J. W. L. Hartog et al., "Advanced Glycation End-Products (AGEs) and Heart Failure: Pathophysiology and Clinical Implications," *European Journal of Heart Failure* 9, no. 12 (2007): 1146-55.

20. A. Sjögren et al., "Oral Administration of Magnesium Hydroxide to Subjects with Insulin-Dependent Diabetes Mellitus: Effects on Magnesium and Potassium Levels and on Insulin Requirements," *Magnesium* 7, no. 3 (1988): 117-22; L. M. de Lordes et al., "The Effect of Magnesium Supplementation in Increasing Doses on the Control of Type 2 Diabetes," *Diabetes Care* 21, no. 5 (1998): 682-86; G. Paolisso et al., "Dietary Magnesium Supplements Improve B-Cell Response to Glucose and Arginine in Elderly Non-Insulin Dependent Diabetic Subjects," *Acta Endocrinologica* 121, no. 1 (1989): 16-20.

21. F. Guerrero-Romero and M. Rodríguez-Morán, "Low Serum Magnesium Levels and Metabolic Syndrome," *Acta Diabetologica* 39, no. 4 (2002): 209-13.

22. "Magnesium, What Is It?" Office of Dietary Supplements, National Institutes of Health, http://ods.od.nih.gov/factsheets/magnesium-HealthProfessional.

23. S. Hendler, *PDR for Nutritional Supplements*, 2nd ed. (Montvale, NJ: PDR Network, 2008), 152.

24. E. S. Ford and A. H. Mokdad, "Dietary Magnesium Intake in a National Sample of U.S. Adults," *Journal of Nutrition* 133, no. 9 (2003): 2879-82.

25. R. Altschul et al., "Influence of Nicotinic Acid on Serum Cholesterol in Man," *Archives of Biochemistry and Biophysics* 54, no. 2 (1955): 558-59.

26. R. H. Knopp et al., "Contrasting Effects of Unmodified and Time-Release Forms of Niacin on Lipoproteins in Hyperlipidemic Subjects: Clues to Mechanism of Action of Niacin," *Metabolism* 34, no. 7 (1985): 642-50; J. M. McKenney et al., "A Comparison of the Efficacy and Toxic Effects of Sustained vs. Immediate-Release Niacin in Hypercholesterolemic Patients," *Journal of the American Medical Association* 271, no. 9 (1994): 672-77.

27. P. R. Kamstrup, "Genetically Elevated Lipoprotein(a) and Increased Risk of Myocardial Infarction," *Journal of the American Medical Association* 301, no. 22 (2009): 2331-39; M. Sandkamp et al., "Lipoprotein(a) Is an Independent Risk Factor for Myocardial Infarction at a Young Age," *Clinical Chemistry* 36, no. 1 (1990): 20-23; A. Gurakar et al., "Levels of Lipoprotein Lp(a) Decline with Neomycin and Niacin Treatment," *Atherosclerosis* 57, nos. 2-3 (1985): 293-301; L. A. Carlson et al., "Pronounced Lowering of Serum Levels of Lipoprotein Lp(a) in Hyperlipidaemic Subjects Treated with Nicotinic Acid," *Journal of Internal Medicine* 226, no. 4 (1989): 271-76.

28. J. Shepard et al., "Effects of Nicotinic Acid Therapy on Plasma High-Density Lipoprotein Subfraction Distribution and Composition and on Apolipoprotein A Metabolism," *Journal of Clinical Investigation* 63, no. 5 (1979): 858-67; G. Wahlberg et al., "Effects of Nicotinic Acid on Serum Cholesterol Concentrations of High Density Lipoprotein Subfractions HDL2 and HDL3 in Hyperlipoproteinaemia," *Journal of Internal Medicine* 228, no. 2 (1990): 151-57.

29. Shepard et al., "Effects of Nicotinic Acid Therapy"; Wahlberg et al., "Effects of Nicotinic Acid on Serum Cholesterol."

30. A. Gaby, *Nutritional Medicine* (Concord, NH: Fritz Perlberg Publishing, 2011).

31. A. Hoffer, "On Niacin Hepatitis," *Journal of Orthomolecular Medicine* 12 (1983): 90.

32. McKenney et al., "A Comparison of the Efficacy and Toxic Effects of Sustained Vs. Immediate-Release Niacin"; J.A. Etchason et al., "Niacin-Induced Hepatitis: A Potential Side Effect with Low-Dose Time-Release Niacin," Mayo Clinic Proceedings 66, no. 1 (1991): 23-28.

33. Gaby, Nutritional Medicine.

34. E. Serbinova et al., "Free Radical Recycling and Intramembrane Mobility in the Antioxidant Properties of Alpha-Tocopherol and Alpha-Tocotrienol," *Free Radical Biology & Medicine* 10, no. 5 (1991): 263-75.

35. R. A. Parker et al., "Tocotrienols Regulate Cholesterol Production in Mammalian Cells by Post-Transcriptional Suppression of 3-Hydroxy-3-Methylglutaryl-Coenzyme A reductase," *Journal of Biological Chemistry* 268 (1993): 11230-38; B.C. Pearce et al., "Hypocholesterolemic Activity of Synthetic and Natural Tocotrienols," *Journal of Medicinal Chemistry* 35, no. 20 (1992): 3595-606; B.C. Pearce et al., "Inhibitors of Cholesterol Biosynthesis. 2. Hypocholesterolemic and Antioxidant Activities of Benzopyran and Tetrahydronaphthalene Analogues of the tocotrienols," *Journal of Medicinal Chemistry* 37, no. 4 (1994): 526-41.

36. S. G. Yu et al., "Dose-Response Impact of Various Tocotrienols on Serum Lipid Parameters in Five-Week-Old Female Chickens," *Lipids* 41, no. 5 (2006): 453-61; M. Minhajuddin et al., "Hypolipidemic and Antioxidant Properties of Tocotrienol-Rich Fraction Isolated from

Rice Bran Oil in Experimentally Induced Hyperlipidemic Rats," *Food and Chemical Toxicology* 43, no. 5 (2005): 747-53; J. Iqbal et al., "Suppression of 7,12-Dimethyl-Benz[alpha]anthracene-Induced Carcinogenesis and Hypercholesterolaemia in Rats by Tocotrienol-Rich Fraction Isolated from Rice Bran Oil," *European Journal of Cancer Prevention* 12, no. 6 (2003): 447-53; A. A. Qureshi et al., "Novel Tocotrienols of Rice Bran Suppress Cholesterogenesis in Hereditary Hypercholesterolemic Swine," *Journal of Nutrition* 131, no. 2 (2001): 223-30; M. K. Teoh et al., "Protection by Tocotrienols against Hypercholesterolaemia and Atheroma," *Medical Journal of Malaysia* 49, no. 3 (1994): 255-62; A. A. Qureshi et al., "Dietary Tocotrienols Reduce Concentrations of Plasma Cholesterol, Apolipoprotein B, Thromboxane B2, and Platelet Factor 4 in Pigs with Inherited Hyperlipidemias," *American Journal of Clinical Nutrition* 53, no. 4 (1991): 1042S-46S; D. O'Byrne et al., "Studies of LDL Oxidation Following Alpha-, Gamma-, or Delta-Tocotrienyl Acetate Supplementation of Hypercholesterolemic Humans," *Free Radical Biology & Medicine* 29, no. 9 (2000): 834-45; A. A. Qureshi et al., "Lowering of Serum Cholesterol in Hypercholesterolemic Humans by Tocotrienols (Palm Vitee)," *American Journal of Clinical Nutrition* 53, no. 4 supplement (1991): 1021-26; Qureshi et al., "Response of Hypercholesterolemic Subjects to Administration of Tocotrienols," *Lipids* 30, no. 12 (1995): 1171-77; A. C. Tomeo et al., "Antioxidant Effects of Tocotrienols in Patients with Hyperlipidemia and Carotid Stenosis," *Lipids* 30, no. 12 (1995): 1179-83.

37. A. Stoll, *The Omega-3 Connection* (New York: Free Press, 2001).

38. J. Dyerberg et al., "Plasma Cholesterol Concentration in Caucasian Danes and Greenland West Coast Eskimos," *Danish Medical Bulletin* 24, no. 2 (1977): 52-55; H.O. Bang, et al., "The Composition of Food Consumed by Greenland Eskimos," *Acta Medica Scandinavica* 200, nos. 1-2 (1976): 69-73; H.O. Bang and J. Dyerberg, "Plasma Lipids and Lipoproteins in Greenlandic West Coast Eskimos," *Acta Medica Scandinavica* 192, nos. 1-2 (1972): 85-94; H.O. Bang et al., "Plasma Lipid and Lipoprotein Pattern in Greenlandic West Coast Eskimos," *The Lancet* 1, no. 7710 (1971): 1143-45; J. Dyerberg et al., "Fatty Acid Composition of the Plasma Lipids in Greenland Eskimos," *American Journal of Clinical Nutrition* 28, no. 9 (1975): 958-66.

39. D. Mozzafarian and J. H. Wu, "Omega-3 Fatty Acids and Cardiovascular Disease: Effects on Risk Factors, Molecular Pathways, and Clinical Events," *Journal of the American College of Cardiology* 58, no. 20 (2011): 2047-67.

40. GISSI-Prevenzione Investigators, "Dietary Supplementation with N-3 Polyunsaturated Fatty Acids and Vitamin E after Myocardial Infarction: Results of the GISSI-Prevenzione Trial," *The Lancet* 354, no. 9177 (1999): 447-55.

41. M. R. Cowie, "The Clinical Benefit of Omega-3 PUFA Ethyl Esters Supplementation in Patients with Heart Failure," *European Journal of Cardiovascular Medicine* 1, no. 2 (2010): 14-18.

42. "Clinical Guidelines, CG48," National Institute for Health and Clinical Excellence, last modified September 23, 2011, www.nice.org.uk/CG48.

43. Cowie, "The Clinical Benefit of Omega-3 PUFA Ethyl Esters."

44. D. Lanzmann-Petithory, "Alpha-Linolenic Acid and Cardiovascular Diseases," *Journal of Nutrition, Health & Aging* 5, no. 3 (2001): 179-83.

45. M. Yokoyama, "Effects of Eicosapentaenoic Acid (EPA) on Major Cardiovascular Events in Hypercholesterolemic Patients: The Japan EPA Lipid

Intervention Study (JELIS)" presentation, American Heart Association Scientific Sessions, Dallas, Texas, November 13-16, 2005; Medscape, "JELIS–Japan Eicosapentaenoic Acid (EPA) Lipid Intervention Study," Medscape Education, www.medscape.org/viewarticle/518574.

46. G. Bon et al., "Effects of Pantethine on In Vitro Peroxidation of Low-Density Lipoproteins," *Atherosclerosis* 57, no. 1 (1985): 99-106.

47. A. C. Junior et al., "Antigenotoxic and Antimutagenic Potential of an Annatto Pigment (Norbixin) Against Oxidative Stress," *Genetics and Molecular Research* 4, no. 1 (2005): 94-99; G. Kelly, "Pantethine: A Review of its Biochemistry and Therapeutic Applications," *Alternative Medicine Review* 2, no. 5 (1997): 365-77; F. Coronel et al., "Treatment of Hyperlipemia in Diabetic Patients on Dialysis with a Physiological Substance," *American Journal of Nephrology* 11, no. 1 (1991): 32-36; P. Binaghi et al., "Evaluation of the Hypocholesterolemic Activity of Pantethine in Perimenopausal Women," *Minerva Medica* 81 (1990): 475-79; Z. Lu, "A Double-Blind Clinical Trial: The Effects of Pantethine on Serum Lipids in Patients with Hyperlipidemia," *Chinese Journal of Cardiovascular Diseases* 17, no. 4 (1989): 221-23; M. Eto et al., "Lowering Effect of Pantethine on Plasma Beta-Thromboglobulin and Lipids in Diabetes Mellitus," *Artery* 15, no. 1 (1987): 1-12; D. Prisco et al., "Effect of Oral Treatment with Pantethine on Platelet and Plasma Phospholipids in Type II Hyperlipoproteinemia," *Angiology* 38, no. 3 (1987): 241-47; F. Bellani et al., "Treatment of Hyperlipidemias Complicated by Cardiovascular Disease in the Elderly: Results of an Open Short-Term Study with Pantethine," *Current Therapeutic Research* 40, no. 5 (1986): 912-16; S. Bertolini et al., "Lipoprotein Changes Induced by Pantethine in Hyperlipoproteinemic Patients: Adults and Children," *International Journal of Clinical Pharmacology and Therapeutics* 24, no. 11 (1986): 630-37; C. Donati et al., "Pantethine Improves the Lipid Abnormalities of Chronic Hemodialysis Patients: Results of a Multicenter Clinical Trial," *Clinical Nephrology* 25, no. 2 (1986): 70-74; L. Arsenio et al., "Effectiveness of Long-Term Treatment with Pantethine in Patients with Dyslipidemia," *Clinical Therapeutics* 8, no. 5 (1986): 537-45; S. Giannini et al., "Efeitos da Pantetina Sobrelipides Sangineos," *Arquivos Brasileiros de Cardiologia* 46, no. 4 (1986): 283-89; F. Bergesio et al., "Impiego della Pantetina nella Dislipidemia dell'Uremico Cronico in Trattamento Dialitico," *Journal of Clinical Medicine and Research* 66, nos. 11-12 (1985): 433-40; G. F. Gensini et al., "Changes in Fatty Acid Composition of the Single Platelet Phospholipids Induced by Pantethine Treatment," *International Journal of Clinical Pharmacology Research* 5, no. 5 (1985): 309-18; L. Cattin et al., "Treatment of Hypercholesterolemia with Pantethine and Fenofibrate: An Open Randomized Study on 43 Subjects," *Current Therapeutic Research* 38 (1985): 386-95; A. Postiglione et al., "Pantethine Versus Fenofibrate in the Treatment of Type II Hyperlipoproteinemia," *Monographs on Atherosclerosis* 13 (1985): 145-48; G. Seghieri et al., "Effetto della Terapia con Pantetina in Uremici Cronici Emodializzati con Iperlipoproteinemia di Tipo IV," *Journal of Clinical Medicine and Research* 66, nos. 5-6 (1985): 187-92; L. Arsenio et al., "Iperlipidemia Diabete ed Aterosclerosi: Efficacia del Trattamento con Pantetina," *Acta Biomed Ateneo Parmense* 55, no.1 (1984): 25-42; O. Bosello et al., "Changes in the Very Low Density Lipoprotein Distribution of Apolipoproteins C-III2, CIII1, C-III0, C-II, and Apolipoprotein E after Pantethine Administration," *Acta Therapeutica* 10 (1984): 421-30; P. Da Col et al., "Pantethine in the Treatment of Hypercholesterolemia: A Randomized Double-Blind Trial Versus Tiadenol,"

Current Therapeutic Research 36 (1984): 314-21; A. Gaddi et al., "Controlled Evaluation of Pantethine, a Natural Hypolipidemic Compound, in Patients with Different Forms of Hyperlipoproteinemia," *Atherosclerosis* 50, no. 1 (1984): 73-83; R. Miccoli et al., "Effects of Pantethine on Lipids and Apolipoproteins in Hypercholesterolemic Diabetic and Non-Diabetic Patients," *Current Therapeutic Research* 36 (1984): 545-49; M. Maioli et al., "Effect of Pantethine on the Subfractions of HDL in Dyslipidemic Patients," *Current Therapeutic Research* 35 (1984): 307-11; G. Ranieri et al., "Effect of Pantethine on Lipids and Lipoproteins in Man," *Acta Therapeutica* 10 (1984): 219-27; A. Murai et al., "The Effects of Pantethine on Lipid and Lipoprotein Abnormalities in Survivors of Cerebral Infarction," *Artery* 12, no. 4 (1983): 234-43; P. Avogaro et al., "Effect of Pantethine on Lipids, Lipoproteins and Apolipoproteins in Man," *Current Therapeutic Research* 33 (1983): 488-93; G. Maggi et al., "Pantethine: A Physiological Lipomodulating Agent in the Treatment of Hyperlipidemia," *Current Therapeutic Research* 32 (1982): 380-86; K. Hiramatsu et al., "Influence of Pantethine on Platelet Volume, Microviscosity, Lipid Composition and Functions in Diabetes Mellitus with Hyperlipidemia," *Tokai Journal of Experimental and Clinical Medicine* 6, no. 1 (1981): 49-57.

48. M. Houston et al., "Nonpharmocologic Treatment of Dyslipidemia," *Progress in Cardiovascular Disease* 52, no. 2 (2009): 61-94.

49. A. Mozes, "Glucosamine Joint Pain Supplement Could Help the Heart," *HealthDay* May 15, 2019.

50. Ibid.

51. H. Ma et al., "Association of Habitual Glucosamine Use with Risk of Cardiovascular Disease: Prospective Study in UK Biobank" *BMJ* 365(2019):l1628.

52. Z.H. Yang et al., "Chronic Administration of Palmitoleic Acid Reduces Insulin Resistance and Hepatic Lipid Accumulation in KK-Ay Mice with Genetic Type 2 Diabetes," *Lipids Health and Disease* 21, no. 10 (2011): 120.

53. A. Bolsoni-Lopes et al., "Palmitoleic Acid (N-7) Increases White Adipocyte Lipolysis and Lipase Content in a PPARÐ-Dependent Manner," *American Journal of Physiology, Endocrinology, and Metabolism* 305, no. 9 (2013): E1093-102.

54. Queiroz JC, Alonso-Vale MI, Curi R, et al. Control of adipogenesis by fatty acids. *Arquivos Brasileiros de Endocrinologia & Metabologia* 53, no. 5 (2009): 582-94.

55. A.M. Bernstein et al., "Purified Palmitoleic Acid for the Reduction of High-Sensitivity C-Reactive Protein and Serum Lipids: A Double-Blinded, Randomized, Placebo Controlled Study," *Journal of Clinical Lipidology* 8, no. 6 (2014): 612-7.

56. R. Pfister et al., "Plasma Vitamin C Predicts Incident Heart Failure in Men and Women in European Prospective Investigation into Cancer and Nutrition–Norfolk Prospective Study," *American Heart Journal* 162, no. 2 (2011): 246-53.

57. W. Wongcharoen and A. Phrommintikul, "The Protective Role of Curcumin in Cardiovascular Diseases," *International Journal of Cardiology* 133, no. 2 (2009): 145-51.

58. M. Houston, *What Your Doctor May Not Tell You About Heart Disease* (New York: Grand Central Life & Style, 2012).

59. G. Ramaswami, "Curcumin Blocks Homocysteine-Induced Endothelial Dysfunction in Porcine Coronary Arteries," *Journal of Vascular Surgery* 40, no. 6 (2004): 1216-22.

60. Houston, *What Your Doctor May Not Tell You.*

61. M. A. Carluccio et al., "Olive Oil and Red Wine Antioxidant Polyphenols Inhibit Endothelial Activation: Antiatherogenic Properties of Mediterranean Diet Phytochemicals," *Atherosclerosis, Thrombosis, and*

Vascular Biology 23, no. 4 (2003): 622-29.

62. W. Ross et al., "The Use of Bergamot-Derived Polyphenol Fraction in Cardiometabolic Risk Prevention and its Possible Mechanisms of Action," *Polyphenols in Human Health and Disease* 2 (2013): 1087-1105; V. Mollace et al., "Hypolipemic and Hypoglycaemic Activity of Bergamot Polyphenols: From Animal Models to Human Studies," *Fitoterapia* 82, no. 3 (2011): 309-16.

63. W. Chang et al., "Berberine as a Therapy for Type 2 Diabetes and Its Complications: From Mechanism of Action to Clinical Studies," *Biochemistry and Cell Biology* 93, no. 5 (2015): 479-86; J. Yin et al., "Efficacy of Berberine in Patients with Type 2 Diabetes Mellitus," *Metabolism* 7, no. 5 (2008): 712-17; L. Zheng et al., "Antioxidant and Anti-Inflammatory Activities of Berberine in the Treatment of Diabetes Mellitus," *Hindawi* 2014: https://doi.org/10.1155/2014/289264; T. Lou et al., "Berberine Inhibits Inflammatory Response and Ameliorates Insulin Resistance in Hepatocytes," *Inflammation* 34, no. 6 (2011): 659-67.

64. H. Sumi et al., "Enhancement of the Fibrinolytic Activity in Plasa by Oral Administration of Nattokinase," *Acta Haematologica* 84, no. 3 (1990): 139-43.

65. "Study Shows Chocolate Reduces Blood Pressure and Risk of Heart Disease," *European Society of Cardiology*, March 31, 2010, www.escardio.org/about/press/press-releases/pr-10/Pages/chocolate-reduces-blood-pressure.aspx.

66. M. Houston et al., "Nonpharmologic Treatment for Dyslipideia," *Progress in Cardiovascular Disease* 52, no. 2 (2009), 61-94.

THE SCIENCE OF HEALTHY LIVING: EAT, LAUGH, PLAY, LOVE.

1. R Ader and N Cohen. Behaviorally conditioned immunosuppression. *Psychosomatic Medicine*, Vol 37, Issue 4 333-340

"Robert Ader, Founder of Psychoneuroimmunology, Dies," University of Rochester Medical Center. December 12, 2011. Retrieved December 20, 2011.

2. M. Irwin and K. Vedhara, *Human Psychoneuroimmunology* (Oxford University Press, 2005); S. Segerstrom, *The Oxford handbook of psycho-neuroimmunology* (Oxford University Press, 2012).

3. J. Bowden, *The Most Effective Natural Cures on Earth* (Beverly, MA: Fair Winds Press, 2008).

4. J. W. Pennebaker, *Opening Up: The Healing Power of Expressing Emotions* (New York: Guilford Press, 1997); J. Frattaroli, "Experimental Disclosure and Its Moderators: A Meta-Analysis," *Psychological Bulletin* 132, no. 6 (2006): 823-65.

5. R. McCraty, "New Frontiers in Heart Rate Variability and Social Coherence Research: Techniques, Technologies, and Implications for Improving Group Dynamics and Outcomes," *Frontiers in Public Health* 5 (2017): doi: 10.3389/fpubh.2017.00267.

6. Ibid.

7. HeartMath, "The Science of HeartMath," https://www.heartmath.com/science

APPENDIX A

1. S. Jeffrey, "ALLHAT Lipid-Lowering Trial Shows No Benefit from Pravastatin," *Heartwire*, December 17, 2002, www.theheart.org/article/263333.do.

2. Sever, PS et al., "Reduction in cardiovascular events with atorvastatin in 2,532 patients with type 2 diabetes: Anglo-Scandinavian Cardiac Outcomes Trial--lipid-lowering arm (ASCOT-LLA)," Diabetes Care, 2005 May;28(5):1151-7. https://www.ncbi.nlm.nih.gov/pubmed/15855581

3. Uffe Ravnskov, "ASCOT-LLA: questions about the benefits of atorvastatin," The Lancet, Vol 361, issue 9373, P 1986, 6/7/03. https://www.thelancet.com/journals/lancet/article/PIIS0140-6736(03)13559-3/fulltext

4. Devroey, Dirk and Vander Ginst, Leslie, "ASCOT-LLA: questions about the benefits of atorvastatin," The Lancet, Vol 361, issue 9373, P 1985-86, 6/7/03 https://www.thelancet.com/journals/lancet/article/PIISO140-6736(03)13558-1/fulltext

5. Ibid.

6. Heart Protection Study Collaborative Drug, "MRC/BHF Heart Protection Study of Cholesterol Lowering with Simvastatin in 20,536 High-Risk Individuals: A Randomised Placebo-Controlled Trial," The Lancet 360, no. 9326 (2002): 7-22.

7. U. Ravnskov, "Statins as the New Aspirin," BMJ 324, no. 7340 (2002): 789.

8. "The Lipid Research Clinics Coronary Primary Prevention Trial Results. I. Reduction in Incidence of Coronary Heart Disease," JAMA 251, no. 3(1984): 351-64.

9. S. Boyles, "More May Benefit from Cholesterol Drugs," WebMD Health News, January 13, 2009, www.webmd.com/cholesterol-management/news/20090113/more-may-benefit-from-cholesterol-drugs.

10. M. de Lorgeril et al., "Cholesterol Lowering, Cardiovascular Diseases, and the Rousuvastatin-JUPITER Controversy: A Critical Reappraisal," Archives of Internal Medicine 170, no. 12 (2010): 1032-36.

11. M. A. Hlatky, "Expanding the Orbit of Primary Prevention—Moving Beyond JUPITER," New England Journal of Medicine 359 (2008): 2280-82.

12. Ibid.

APPENDIX B

1. J. Fan et al., "Small Dense LDL Cholesterol Is Associated with Metabolic Syndrome Traits Independently of Obesity and Inflammation," Nutrition & Metabolism 16, no. 7 (2019)

2. J. J. Stec et al., "Association of Fibrinogen with Cardiovascular Risk Factors and Cardiovascular Disease in the Framingham Offspring Population," Circulation 102, no. 14 (2000): 1634-38.

3. J. T. Salonen et al., "High Stored Iron Levels Are Associated with Excess Risk of Myocardial Infarction in Eastern Finnish Men," Circulation 86, no. 3 (1992): 803-11; L. K. Altman, "High Level of Iron Tied to Heart Risk," New York Times, September 8, 1992.

4. Salonen et al., "High Stored Iron Levels."

5. "Statins Can Damage Your Health," Vitamin C Foundation, www.vitamincfoundation.org/statinalert.

6. H. Refsum et al., "The Hordaland Homocysteine Study: A Community-Based Study of Homocysteine, Its Determinants, and Associations with Disease," Journal of Nutrition 136, no. 6 (2006): 1731S-40S; Homocystein Studies Collaboration, "Homocysteine and Risk of Ischemic Heart Disease and Stroke: A Meta-Analysis," Journal of the American Medical Association 288, no. 16 (2002): 2015-22; D.S. Wald et al., "Homocysteine and Cardiovascular Disease: Evidence on Casualty from a Meta-Analysis," BMJ 325, no. 7374 (2002): 1202.

7. D. S. Wald et al., "The Dose-Response Relation Between Serum Homocysteine and Cardiovascular Disease: Implications for Treatment and Screening," European Journal of Cardiovascular Prevention and Rehabilitation 11, no. 3 (2004): 250-53.

8. M. Haim et al., "Serum Homocysteine and Long-Term Risk of Myocardial Infarction and Sudden Death in Patients with Coronary Heart Disease," Cardiology 107, no. 1 (2007): 52-56.

9. M. Houston, What Your Doctor May Not Tell You About Heart Disease (New York: Grand Central Life & Style, 2012).

10. S. Seely, "Is Calcium Excess in Western Diet a Major Cause of Arterial Disease?" International Journal of Cardiology 33, no. 2 (1991): 191-98.

11. U. Hoffmann, T. J. Brady, and J. Muller, "Use of New Imaging Techniques to Screen for Coronary Artery

Disease," *Circulation* 108 (2003): e50-e53

12. Ibid.

13. M. Roest et al., "High levels of Urinary F2-Isoprostanes Predict Cardiovascular Mortality in Postmenopausal Women," *Journal of Clinical Lipidology* 2, no. 4 (2009): 298-303.

14. Ibid.

15. Y. Kataoka et al., "Myeloperoxidase Levels Predict Accelerated Progression of Coronary Atherosclerosis in Diabetic Patients: Insights from Intravascular Ultrasound," *Atherosclerosis* 232, no. 2 (2014): 377-83; R. Zhang et al., "Association Between Myeloperoxidase Levels and Risk of Coronary Artery Disease," *JAMA* 286, no. 17 (2001): 2136-42.

16. C. Meisinger et al., "Plasma oxidized low-density lipoprotein, a strong predictor for acute coronary heart disease events in apparently healthy, middle-aged men from the general population," *Circulation* 112, no.5 (2005): 651-57.

17. P. Holvoet et al., "Oxidized LDL and the Metabolic Syndrome," *Future Lipidology* 3, no.6 (2008): 637-49.

18. F. Erling et al., "Coronary Plaque Disruption," *Circulation* 92, no. 3 (1995): 657-671

19. A. Mauriello ete al., "A Pathobiologic Link Between Risk Factors Profile and Morphological Markers of Carotid Instability," *Atherosclerosis* 208, no. 2 (2010)): 572-80.

20. A. Pilbrow et al., "The Chromosome 9p21.3 Coronary Heart Disease Risk Allele Is Associated with Altered Gene Expression in Normal Heart and Vascular Tissues," *PLoS One* 7, no.6 (2012): e39574.

21. D. Allingham-Hawkins et al., "KIF6 p.Trp719Arg Testing to Assess Risk of Coronary Artery Disease and/or Statin Response," *PLoS Currents* 2 (2010): doi:10.1371/currents.RRN1191; D. Shiffman et al., "A Kinesin Family Member 6 Variant Is Associated with Coronary Heart Disease in the Women's Health Study," *Journal of the American College of Cardiology* 51, no. 4 (2008): 444-8; J. A. Hubacek et al., "Gene Variants at FTO, 9p21, and 2q36.3 are age-Independently Associated with Myocardial Infarction in Czech Men," *Clinica Chimica Acta* 454 (2016): 119-23.

22. R. Spector, "Stanford-led Study Disproves Link Between Genetic Variant, Risk of Coronary Artery Disease," *Stanford Medicine* October 7, 2010: https://med.stanford.edu/news/all-news/2010/10/stanford-led-study-disproves-link-between-genetic-variant-risk-of-coronary-artery-disease.html; B.J. Arsenault et al., "The 719Arg Variant of KIF6 and Cardiovascular Outcomes in Statin-Treated, Stable Coronary Patients of the Treating to New Targets and Incremental Decrease in End PointsThrough Aggressive Lipid-Lowering Prospective Studies," *Circulation: Cardiovascular Genetics* 5, no. 1 (2012): 51-57.

INDEX